MEDICAL RADIOLOGY

Diagnostic Imaging and Radiation Oncology

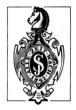

Current Topics in Clinical Radiobiology of Tumors

Contributors

K.K. Ang · M. Baumann · S.M. Bentzen · I. Brammer · W. Budach
E. Dikomey · Z. Fuks · M.R. Horsman · H. Johns · M.C. Joiner
H. Jung · S.A. Leibel · B. Marples · L.J. Peters · A. Taghian
H.D. Thames · K.R. Trott · G.D. Wilson · H.R. Withers

Edited by

Hans-Peter Beck-Bornholdt

Foreword by

Luther W. Brady and H.-P. Heilmann

With 61 Figures and 21 Tables

Springer-Verlag
Berlin Heidelberg New York
London Paris Tokyo
Hong Kong Barcelona
Budapest

Privat-Dozent Dr. rer. nat. Hans-Peter Beck-Bornholdt
Institut für Biophysik und Strahlenbiologie
Universität Hamburg
Martinistraße 52
20246 Hamburg
Germany

MEDICAL RADIOLOGY · Diagnostic Imaging and Radiation Oncology

Continuation of
Handbuch der medizinischen Radiologie
Encyclopedia of Medical Radiology

ISBN 3-540-56512-4 Springer-Verlag Berlin Heidelberg New York
ISBN 0-387-56512-4 Springer-Verlag New York Berlin Heidelberg

Library of Congress Cataloging-in-Publication Data
Current topics in clinical radiobiology of tumors/contributors, K.K. Ang... [et al.]; edited by Hans-Peter Beck-Bornholdt;
foreword by Luther W. Brady and H.-P. Heilmann. p. cm. Includes bibliographical references and index.
ISBN 0-387-56512-4. – ISBN 3-540-56512-4
1. Cancer – Radiotherapy. I. Ang, K.K. (K. Kian) II. Beck-Bornholdt, Hans-Peter, 1950– . [DNLM: 1. Radiobiology. 2.
Neoplasms – radiotherapy. 3. Radiotherapy – methods. QZ 269 C976 1993] RC271.R3C87 1993 616.99'40642 – dc20
DNLM/DLC 93-22941

© Springer-Verlag Berlin Heidelberg 1993
Printed in Germany

Typesetting: Thomson Press (I) Ltd., New Delhi
21/3130/SPS-5 4 3 2 1 0 – Printed on acid-free paper

Foreword

The impact of basic science radiobiological research is now being recognized of significant importance in clinical radiation oncology. Observations made in the laboratory using animals as well as tissue culture have led to a better biologic understanding of techniques for altered fractionation, techniques for measuring tumor cell proliferation, the possibilities and limitations of methods for evaluation of nonrandomized clinical studies in deriving time dose relationships for human tumors as well as a better understanding of repair kinetics in mammalian cells, fractionation sensitivity and the major impact of technologies to improve local/regional control with the subsequent impact on survival. These findings have led to changes in treatment schedules and have led to further close cooperation among the radiation oncologists and radiation biologists.

Well support research efforts in radiation biology have a major and significant impact on the clinical care of the cancer patient. Studies that originated in the laboratory are now finding their way into clinical practice resulting in better local and regional control and improved number of patients surviving without disease.

In 1993 surgery and radiation therapy remain the most effective treatment modalities in cancer management. More than 60% of all patients with malignant disease have radiation therapy as a part of their treatment regimen either for cure, palliation or as an adjunct to surgery and/or chemotherapy. There is no doubt but what molecular biologic research investigations may bring striking progress in cancer treatment in the future, the present is clearly directed toward the most effective implementation of technologies in surgery, radiation oncology, and medical oncology.

The volume by Hans-Peter Beck-Bornholdt is a timely forum setting forth the progress as well as the controversies in the contributions of radiation biology in cancer management. The book brings forth a significant focus on this important research subspecialty in cancer medicine.

Philadelphia/Hamburg, September 1993

L. W. BRADY
H.-P. HEILMANN

Preface

Extensive *controversial* discussions do not take place frequently at scientific meetings. Apart from sporadic debates in the correspondence sections of international journals, opportunities for lively disputes are rather rare. The aim of this book is to give a critical update on those subjects that at present are the main areas of controversy in the field of clinical radiobiology. It was not intended to write a comprehensive textbook on radiation biology. Since all authors completed their contributions within a few months, it was possible to reduce the delay between manuscript submission and publication to the length of time usually required for publication in journals.

The various chapters were carefully prepared by highly qualified specialists in the corresponding area of work. Chapter 1 gives a review of the clinical results obtained so far by applying accelerated fractionation. In direct relation to this contribution, Chapters 2 and 3 describe the possibilities and limitations of the methods for evaluation of nonrandomized clinical studies to derive time-dose relationships for human tumors and for the use of the BUdR technique for measurement of tumor proliferation. Chapter 4 gives an update of the current hyperfractionation studies. In this context, Chapter 5 reports on the most recent results obtained concerning the limitations of the linear-quadratic model at low doses per fraction and Chapter 6 provides a review of our knowledge on the dose dependence of repair kinetics in mammalian cells. The fractionation sensitivity of malignant melanomas is critically reviewed in Chapter 7. In Chapter 8 the predictive value of SF2 is discussed. This chapter is of special interest when considered along with Chapter 9, which describes the relevance of hypoxia in tumors. Chapter 10 discusses the impact of local tumor control on the outcome in human cancer and Chapter 11 describes the mechanisms of cell loss in irradiated tumors, an issue that has been overlooked for too long in radiobiology.

I hope that the work presented in this volume will provide valuable reading for the community of radiation oncologists, biologists and physicists.

Hamburg, August 1993   HANS-PETER BECK-BORNHOLDT

Acknowledgements. The editor wishes to thank DR. HANS-HERMANN DUBBEN, ANTJE PIECONKA, DR. ANNETTE RAABE, and HENNING WILLERS for their enthusiastic support in preparing this book.

Contents

1 Accelerated Fractionation

H.D. Thames, L.J. Peters, and K.K. Ang

1.1 Introduction

Other factors being equal, small tumors are easier to cure by radiotherapy than large ones, on account of there being fewer clonogens to sterilize. By analogy, if tumor clonogens proliferate appreciably during treatment, it is obvious that cure would be easier if the total number of clonogens to be sterilized were limited by shortening the overall treatment time. The way to accomplish this, i.e., shortening of the overall time by the strategy termed *accelerated fractionation*, is the subject of this chapter.

Accelerated fractionation is defined as a regimen of radiotherapy in which the duration of conventional treatment with daily fractions of 1.8-2 Gy, 5 days/week to total doses of ~ 70 Gy is reduced, without proportionate dose reduction and without

H.D. THAMES, PhD, Helen Buchanan and Stanley Joseph Seeger Research Professor, Department of Biomathematics, The University of Texas M.D. Anderson Cancer Center, 1515 Holcombe Blvd., Houston, TX 77030-4095, USA
L.J. PETERS, MD, Professor of Radiotherapy, Head, Division of Radiotherapy, John G. and Marie Stella Kenedy Chair, The University of Texas M.D. Anderson Cancer Center, 1515 Holcombe Blvd., Houston, TX 77030-4095, USA
K.K. ANG, MD, Professor of Radiotherapy, Department of Radiotherapy, The University of Texas M.D. Anderson Cancer Center, 1515 Holcombe Blvd., Houston, TX 77030-4095, USA

recourse to large dose fractions, by the delivery of two or more treatments on some or all of the treatment days. Thus it may be expected that acute reactions will be higher with accelerated fractionation, and the question is raised whether the increase in tumor control (relative to equally toxic conventional treatment) is high enough that a therapeutic gain will result. Moreover, the delivery of two or more doses per day entails the issue of recovery of normal tissues between doses, especially those whose response is delayed until after the end of treatment. In this chapter these issues are considered in the light of clinical experience to date.

1.2 Radiobiological Considerations

1.2.1 Normal Tissue

The overriding features of accelerated fractionation regimens are the *increased rate of dose delivery* and *reduced overall time*. The rate of dose delivery ("weekly dose rate") is an important determinant of the severity of acute reactions in epithelial and other tissues (such as bone marrow) organized into stem cell, maturation, and functional compartments (reviewed in THAMES et al. 1989). The level of injury in these tissues depends on the balance between the rate of cell killing by irradiation and the rate of regeneration of surviving stem cells, a balance that is a function primarily of the rate of dose accumulation. (The fraction size is also a factor in determining the severity of acute reactions, large fractions being more damaging per unit dose, but to a lesser extent than is the case for late reactions.) After the stem cell population is depleted to the point where it is unable to renew the functional layers of an epithelium, the acute reaction peaks and further depopulation produces no increase in severity of the reaction (MOULDER and FISCHER 1976). This means that the peak intensity of acute reactions is more influenced by the rate of dose accumulation than by the total dose, once a certain threshold of total dose has been reached. Conversely, the time taken to heal, as opposed to the peak intensity of the acute reactions, is dependent on total dose provided the weekly dose rate exceeds the regenerative ability of the surviving stem cells. This is because healing is a function of the absolute number of stem cells surviving the course of treatment, and the higher the total dose, the fewer stem cells will survive.

Since little, if any, regeneration occurs in late-reacting normal tissues over the time span of a course of radiotherapy, a reduction in overall treatment time would not be expected to affect the severity of late normal-tissue injury provided the size of dose per fraction is not increased. This is the case assuming that repair is complete between dose fractions, but since two or more of these are given each day when treatment is accelerated, there is the possibility of a reduction in late tolerance on this account. The time between doses is limited by logistic considerations to about 8 h for twice-daily treatment, and 6 h for thrice-daily treatment. The issue reduces to the kinetics of repair in late-reacting human tissue such as the cord, i.e., whether there is a detectable loss of tolerance with 6- or 8-h intervals relative to 24-h intervals, as has been reported for rat spinal cord (ANG et al. 1993).

Although most classical late radiation sequelae, e.g., spinal cord injury, show little or no dependence on overall time (provided full recovery occurs between dose fractions), overall time may be of significance for another class of late effects where total doses were less than or similar to conventional regimens, yet a higher incidence of late reactions was observed (PERACCHIA and SALTI 1981; SVOBODA 1984; VAN DEN BOGAERT et al. 1986). To explain these results, a distinction needs to be drawn between "true" late effects and "consequential" late reactions (PETERS et al. 1990). Many of the late effects seen in these studies can be attributed to severe and prolonged epithelial denudation rather than to direct radiation injury of the mesenchymal tissues normally associated with late reactions.

1.2.2 Tumors

The desired endpoint in tumors is sterilization of all cells capable of tumor regeneration, i.e., clonogens. Well differentiated carcinomas are more likely to retain the homeostatic characteristics of the epithelia from which they arise, and in these tumors a slightly unbalanced rate of cell production and loss in the unperturbed state could be upset by radiation-induced cell killing, leading to a controlled increase in net cell production by either an increased rate of proliferation or a reduced cell loss rate. In undifferentiated tumors this mechanism is less likely; rather, the most likely stimulus for stimulated repopulation is the increased availability, on account of radiation-induced cell killing, of nutrients and oxygen.

The importance of overall time with regard to acute normal-tissue reactions has long been recognized, but it has only recently been appreciated that the curability of many cancers (particularly squamous cell carcinomas) is also highly dependent on it. Evidence for accelerated regeneration of surviving tumor cells after initiation of treatment comes from three principal observations: (1) time-to-recurrence data for tumors that are not sterilized by radiation therapy, (2) a comparison of split-course and continuous treatment regimens, and (3) an analysis of tumor control doses as a function of time. In considering this evidence it is worthwhile to remember that the doubling time of tumor clonogens prior to treatment is likely to resemble the volume doubling time, e.g., for head and neck tumors a median value of about 60 days. This is so since the growth fraction should have reached a stable value in tumors large enough to be clinically manifest. Therefore, estimates that are considerably shorter than the volume doubling time would be indicative of significant acceleration in the net rate of production of tumor clonogens.

1. *Time to recurrence.* Recurrences of squamous cell carcinomas of the head and neck occur for the most part within 2 years of treatment, as exemplified by the time-to-recurrence data (from patients with squamous cell carcinomas of the pyriform sinus) in the report of EL BADAWI et al. (1982). The median time to recurrence was approximately 6 months, and 90% of all recurrences had occurred within 2 years. Since the recurrences were from a population of tumors where the majority was controlled, it follows that most recurrences must have arisen from one or a few surviving clonogenic cells. A clinically detectable recurrence from one surviving clonogen would require about 30 volume doublings, which is the same as saying that the mean doubling time of viable tumor cells must have been about 6 days.

2. *Split-course vs continuous treatments.* Split-course treatments generally give poorer results than continuous treatments if the dose is not higher in the split-course treatment. This was first reported for head and neck cancer by MILLION and ZIMMERMAN (1975); subsequently, BUDIHNA et al. (1980) calculated that the dose necessary to compensate for a

split in treatment was approximately 0.5 Gy per day. A recent report from OVERGAARD et al. (1988) established that a dose increment of 11–12 Gy was necessary to offset a treatment break of 3 weeks (i.e., 0.5–0.6 Gy/day) and achieve equal probability of tumor control of laryngeal cancers. Assuming that 2–3 Gy in 2-Gy fractions is necessary to reduce the surviving fractions of clonogenic cells by half, these data imply that four to six doublings must have occurred during the 3-week treatment split, yielding a clonogenic cell doubling time of 3.5–5.7 days.

3. *Tumor-control dose vs treatment time.* WITHERS et al. (1988) and MACIEJEWSKI et al. (1989) showed that after a variable lag period each additional day of treatment requires approximately 0.6 Gy for the same level of tumor control, and interpreted this to mean that surviving tumor clonogens regenerate during fractionated radiotherapy sufficiently rapidly as to require 0.6 Gy/day to compensate. This value for the dose equivalent of regeneration during therapy is similar to that obtained from analysis of the split-course data. The duration of the lag period has been questioned (BENTZEN and THAMES 1991).

In summary, evidence such as the above can be interpreted to indicate that after initiation of radiotherapy, surviving clonogens in squamous cell carcinomas of the head and neck are able to regenerate with doubling times on the order of 3–6 days).

It would be useful to confirm these findings with rodent tumors. However, since there is currently no known method to measure directly the proliferation kinetics of surviving clonogenic cells during treatment, it is difficult to substantiate these estimates in experimental systems. JUNG et al. (1990) found that the R1H rhabdomyosarcoma repopulated after single doses at rates no different from those observed in unirradiated tumors with the same number of clonogens. MILAS et al. (1991), on the other hand, showed that the clonogen doubling time in the murine mammary carcinoma MCA-4 was shorter in tumors that had been preexposed to a single high dose. BECK-BORNHOLDT et al. (1991) showed that repopulation during fractionated treatment of the R1H tumor was slower than in controls; after 3 weeks of treatment the repopulation rate increased somewhat, but was still slower than in controls.

KUMMERMEHR and TROTT (1982) made an extensive study of the relationship between various pretreatment kinetic parameters and the regenerative response during treatment in a variety of experimental tumors. Some of the experimental tumors showed accelerated regeneration during treatment

and others did not. Moreover, no single kinetic parameter consistently predicted the behavior of a tumor during treatment. The most useful, however, was the pretreatment potential doubling time (T_{pot}).

T_{pot} can be determined from a measure of the labeling index and the length of the S phase of the cell cycle. This type of study is now possible in humans using flow cytometric analyses of tumor cells labeled in vivo with bromodeoxyuridine (BUdR) which is tagged with a fluorescent monoclonal antibody. Preliminary data reported by BEGG et al. (1991) showed that in a series of 85 head and neck cancers, of which 60 had sufficient follow-up, the mean value of T_{pot} was 4.7 days, with a CV of 69% and a range of 1.4–17 days. TERRY et al. (1992) reported the distributions of kinetic parameters from 44 patients with head and neck cancer and 45 patients with large bowel (predominantly rectal) cancer. Median T_{pot} values were about 4 days for both sites; the quartiles were also strikingly similar (3 and 6 days), as were the ranges (1–31 days). RICH et al. (1993) have shown that for advanced rectal adenocarcinomas the extent of residual tumor after preoperative radiotherapy plus 5-fluorouracil is positively correlated with T_{pot}. Moreover, the complete responses were seen in patients with the longest T_{pot}s.

1.3 Accelerated Fractionation: Rationale and Strategies

A reduction in overall treatment time reduces the time available for regeneration of tumor clonogens during treatment, and therefore increases the probability of tumor control for a given total dose, if the rate of tumor clonogen regeneration does not increase in response to cell depletion, as occurs in normal tissues. With this caveat, a therapeutic gain should be realized from accelerated fractionation, since overall treatment time has little influence on the probability of late normal-tissue injury (provided the size of dose per fraction is not increased and the interval between dose fractions is sufficient for complete repair to take place).

Three basic strategies for accelerated fractionation (PETERS et al. 1988) have been tested and/or are being used at the present time (Fig. 1.1). Type A consists of an intensive short course of treatment in which the overall duration of treatment is markedly reduced with a corresponding substantial decrease in the total dose. Types B and C represent techniques where the duration of treatment is more modestly reduced but the total dose is kept in the same range

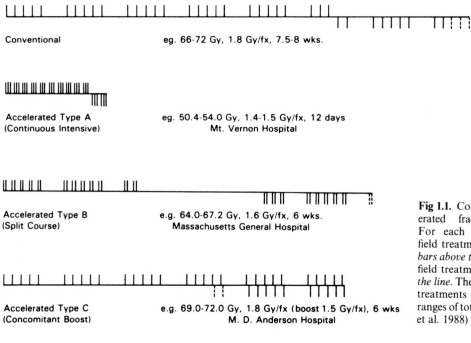

Conventional   eg. 66-72 Gy, 1.8 Gy/fx, 7.5-8 wks.

Accelerated Type A   eg. 50.4-54.0 Gy, 1.4-1.5 Gy/fx, 12 days
(Continuous Intensive)   Mt. Vernon Hospital

Accelerated Type B   e.g. 64.0-67.2 Gy, 1.6 Gy/fx, 6 wks.
(Split Course)   Massachusetts General Hospital

Accelerated Type C   e.g. 69.0-72.0 Gy, 1.8 Gy/fx (boost 1.5 Gy/fx), 6 wks
(Concomitant Boost)   M. D. Anderson Hospital

Fig 1.1. Conventional and accelerated fractionation schedules. For each schedule, the large-field treatment is denoted by the *bars above the line*, and the boost-field treatment by the *bars below the line*. The *dotted bars* represent treatments omitted in the lower ranges of total dose. (From PETERS et al. 1988)

as for a conventional treatment. This is accomplished by using either a split-course or concomitant boost technique. These techniques are conveniently distinguished on the basis of the strategy adopted to circumvent intolerable acute reactions: for type A a reduction in total dose; for type B a break in treatment; for type C a reduction in volume of mucosa exposed to accelerated treatment.

In order to compare the relative merits of schedules A–C it is necessary to establish a measure of therapeutic gain. One approach is to consider the difference between (1) the tumor dose for a specified level of local control and (2) the isoeffect dose for the dose-limiting normal tissue. Figure 1.2 depicts an isoeffect model of the zone of therapeutic gain in the treatment of head and neck cancers for these accelerated fractionation schedules, and is to be interpreted as follows.

The isoeffect curve for acute and consequential late reactions is based on maximum tolerated doses (MTD) for accelerated fractionation regimens reported by SAUNDERS et al. (1988a, b) 54 Gy in 36 fractions delivered in 12 days), LAMB et al. (1990) (59.4 Gy in 33 fractions delivered in 24 days), and ANG et al. (1990) (72 Gy in 42 fractions delivered in 40 days), and the report of ANDREWS (1965) that there was no mucositis in a series of 43 patients treated to

doses of up to 100 Gy in 43–44 fractions over 100 days. The curve for generic late (primary chronic) effects is based on abundant clinical experience that 70–72 Gy in 1.8- to 2-Gy fractions represents the

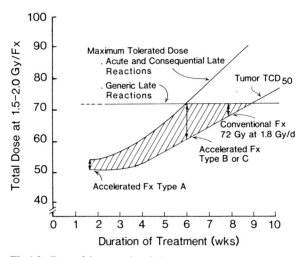

Fig 1.2. Zone of therapeutic gain in squamous cell carcinomas of the head neck for different accelerated fractionation schedules. Type A is 54 Gy in 36 fractions over 12 days (SAUNDERS et al. 1988b) and type B is 72 Gy in 42 fractions over 40 days (PETERS et al. 1988). Type C is 67.2 Gy in 42 fractions over 42 days (WANG et al. 1985). For explanation, see text (From PETERS et al. 1990)

limit of tolerance for late sequelae of head and neck radiotherapy. The time factor is negligible for primary chronic effects, providing sufficient time is allowed between fractions for complete recovery, and this is reflected by the flat late-isoeffect curve.

The isoeffect curve for tumors (assumed 50% control rate) is based on the composite for all head and neck sites generated by WITHERS et al. (1988) from a literature review. The shaded area represents the zone of therapeutic gain; the vertical separation between the isoeffect for dose-limiting normal-tissue reactions and for tumor control is a measure of the therapeutic gain for a given treatment. With a type A accelerated fractionation shedule, the therapeutic gain is limited by the tolerance of acutely reacting normal tissues. Conversely, with conventional fractionation it is limited by the tolerance of late-reacting normal tissues. The maximum gain is predicted with a type B or C accelerated fractionation schedule in which the treatment time is adjusted such that both acute and late reactions are simultaneously dose limiting; in other words, when the maximum dose that can be tolerated by late-responding tissues is given in the shortest time that permits its tolerance by acutely responding tissues.

This conclusion is unaffected in principle by the exact position of the tumor TCD_{50} curve. The only requirements are that the upward slope of this curve (representing regeneration of tumor clonogens) is less steep than the slope of the isoeffect curve for acute reactions, and that accelerated regeneration in the tumor clonogens does not begin significantly earlier during treatment than in the stem cells of the mucous membranes.

The possibility that the rate of regeneration may depend on the rate of dose delivery has been mentioned in the foregoing. The above conclusions would perhaps be modified if the rate of tumor-clonogen regeneration depended on the daily dose rate, in particular if it was higher after higher daily doses. In this event there would be different TCD_{50} curves for schedules A–C, and the differences in therapeutic gain would be difficult to evaluate. In general, however, this could only detract from the merit of schemes with an initial high rate of dose delivery.

A final point is that the therapeutic gain from accelerated fractionation depends on the overall duration of treatment being reduced to take advantage of the lack of overall time dependence on the tolerance of classically late-responding normal tissues. Some authors have characterized as accelerated fractionation regimens in which *segments* of treatment have been given on an accelerated basis, but in which the overall duration of the complete course of treatment is not reduced because of the insertion of rest intervals between the accelerated segments. This strategy offers no prospects of improved tumor control through reducing tumor cell regeneration during treatment, and is therefore termed *quasi-accelerated fractionation*.

1.4 Clinical Results

The clinical data will be reviewed according to the strategy employed. Results are summarized in Table 1.1.

1.4.1 Type A Continuous Short Intensive Courses

The pioneering study was that of NORIN and ONYANGO (1977), who showed that in the treatment of Burkitt's lymphoma thrice-daily treatment with fractional doses of 1–1.25 Gy yielded greatly improved response rates compared with once-daily fractionation to similar total doses.

Ultra-accelerated schedules in which total doses of around 50–55 Gy have been delivered in elapsed times of 2 weeks or less have been reported for three series of head and neck and one series of lung cancer patients. All three head and neck trials produced high tumor clearance rates but at the expense of severe acute reactions, usually requiring hospitalization. In addition, significant late toxicity was encountered. In two studies (PERACCHIA and SALTI 1981; SVOBODA 1984) most of the late effects can be interpreted as consequential in nature, but in the third study (DISCHE and SAUNDERS 1989) unexpected radiation myelopathy was also encountered at total doses well below those tolerated with conventional fractionation. Assuming no dosimetric error is uncovered, these results could be interpreted as evidence of the cumulative effect of incomplete repair in the spinal cord, even with 6-h interfraction intervals when three fractions per day were given on 12 consecutive days. However, this would require that repair in the human cord be slower than that measured in the rat cord (ANG et al. 1993; GUTTENBERGER et al. 1993). The study of SVOBODA (1984) on inoperable breast cancer with ultra-accelerated treatment was also characterized by increased late effects as a function of total dose and fraction size.

Treatment regimens of approximately 4 week's duration have been used in three studies, one head

Table 1.1. Clinical studies using accelerated fractionation

Tumor site	No. of patients	Dose/FX (cGy)	FX/Day (Interval in h)	Total dose (cGy)	Overall time (wk)	Tumor response	Complications	Authors
Type A: Continuous short intensive schedules								
Burkitt's lymphoma	34	100–125	3 (?)	2500–3100	~2 wk	CR: ~74% (better than once-daily treatment)	None	Norin and Onyango 1977
Head and neck	99	140–150	3 (6)	5040–5400	12 days	2-yr control: 51%	Severe mucositis, generally 2 wk hospitalization for nutritional support; myelopathy: 4	Dische and Saunders 1989
Various sites	59	170–230	3 (≥ 3)	5000–5500	10–14 days	CR at 3 mo: 86%; 3-yr survival: 44%	Peak mucositis 5–10 days posttreatment (occasional hospitalization); severe late complications (necrosis stenosis): 19%	Svoboda 1984
Various sites	22	200	3 (4)	4800–5400	9–11 days	CR at 8 mo: 68%	Confluent mucositis: 100%; mucosal necrosis: 55%; treatment-related deaths: 13	Peracchia and Salti 1981
Various sites	48	180	3 (≥ 4) 3 days/wk	5940	3.5 wk	CR at 2 mo: 56%; 2-yr DFS: 32%	Severe mucositis; patients with oral cavity lesions required hospitalization	Gray 1986
Breast Inoperable	39	140–300	3 (> 3)	4000–4750	5–14 days	CR: 56%; 3-yr TC: 27%	Skin thickening and fibrosis if > 4500 cGy and > 160 cGy/fx. Leathering and necrosis if > 4500 cGy and > 300 cGy/fx.	Svoboda 1984
Inflammatory	42	127–135	2 (≥ 3)	5100–5400 + boost 6600	4 wk	CR at 1–3 yr. 77%; 2-yr survival: 27%	Pneumonitis: 10%; severe fibrosis: 7%	Barker et al. 1980
Lung (NSCLC)	17	180–200	2 (~ 3)		< 4 wk	CR: 40%	Acute-chronic esophagitis: 100%; severe complication: 24%	Von Rottkay 1986
Lung (NSCLC)	75	140–150	3 (6)	5040–5400	12 days	2-yr survival 40%	Troublesome dysphagia from day 21–28	Dische and Saunders 1989
Brain: isolated melanoma	20	300–375	2 ≤ 6	3000–3750	1 wk	MST: 41 wk	Acute edema: 10%; late atrophy: 2	Choi et al. 1985a, b
metastases	23	190–240	2 (≥ 6)	3750–4800	2 wk	MST: 27 wk	Acute edema: 8%; late atrophy: 1	

Type B: Split-course accelerated fractionation schedules

			2 (≥4)					
Head and neck:								
Various sites	321	160	2 (≥4)	6720–7200	~6.5 wk	3-yr locoregional control: 6.8% (historical control: 46%)	Severe mucositis; late effects comparable to CF	Wang et al. 1985
Brain:								
malignant glioma (randomized)	295	200 / 200	3 (4) / 1	6000 ± misonidazole / 6000	4 wk / 6 wk	MST: no difference	No difference in brain necrosis	Horiot et al. 1988
Type C: Concomitant boost								
Head and neck:								
Various sites	53	180–200 +120–150 (boost)	1–2 (3–6)	7000–7400	6 wk	2-yr locoregional control: 65%	Severe mucositis: 35%; moderate late effects: 11% XRT only	Knee et al. 1985
Oropharynx (T2–3)	79	180 +150 (boost)	1–2 (4–6)	6900–7200	6 wk (including 10–12 days boost given b.i.d)	2-yr locoregional control: 68%	Severe mucositis (>6 wks after treatment): 9%; NG tube: 18%; late effects: 7%; 1 carotid rupture (after salvage surg.), 2 transient bone exposures, 1 mucosal ulceration	Ang et al. 1990
Quasi-accelerated								
Head and neck:								
Various sites (randomized)	149 / 159	160 / 170–200	3 (≥3) / 1	6720–7200 / 7000–7500	6–7 (4-wk rest) / 7–8	3-yr locoregional control: 35% 3-yr survival: 31% (for both arms)	Severe mucositis—4 patients did not complete treatment; late effects: 20% vs 11% (ulceration, trismus, dysphagia)	van den Boogaert et al. 1986
Prostate stage B and C	91	200	3 (4)	6000	6 (1 break of 3–4 wk or 2 breaks of 17 days)	Not stated	Severe complications (incontinence, stenosis, etc.): 19%	Vanuytsel et al. 1986

CR, *complete response;* DFS, *disease-free survival;* MST *median survival time*

and neck (GRAY 1986), one inflammatory breast (BARKER et al. 1980), and one lung (VON ROTTKAY 1986). In the inflammatory breast study, local tumor control rates were significantly improved over prior experience with the protracted Baclesse technique, without any undue acute toxicity. In the lung study, however, there is an indication that accelerated fractionation consisting of 1.8–2 Gy, twice daily to a total dose of 66 Gy in 4 weeks or less exceeds the tolerance of the esophagus: all patients developed severe acute esophagitis with secondary severe complications occurring in one-quarter of the patients.

Finally, schedules of this type have been used in the treatment of isolated brain metastases of malignant melanoma (CHOI et al. 1985a, b). The patients received either twice daily fractions of 3–3.75 Gy to total doses of 30–37.5 Gy in 1 week or 1.9–2.4 Gy per fraction to total doses of 37.5–48 Gy in 2 weeks. The median survival time of the patients treated in 1 week was significantly improved although whether this was due to the time factor, the size of dose per fraction, both, or other unknown factors, is unclear. With both regimens the incidence of acute edema and late brain atrophy was small, with the caveat that survival times were short so that the actuarial incidence of late injury may be higher.

1.4.2 Type B Split-Course Accelerated Fractionation Schedules

WANG et al. (1985) have reported improved local-regional control rates in a variety of head and neck sites with accelerated split-course treatment. The comparisons are to historical controls treated with relatively modest conventional doses. The regimen Wang characterizes as b.i.d.–b.i.d. consists of 1.6-Gy fractional doses given twice daily with a minimum 4-h interfraction interval to total doses of 64–67.2 Gy in 6–7 weeks in a split course (Fig. 1.1). An overall improvement in 3-year local-regional control from 46–68% was reported in a series of 321 patients. Although poorly documented in either series, late morbidity was said to be comparable to historical controls, while acute reactions were more severe, as expected. The EORTC conducted a randomized trial with accelerated split-course radiotherapy for the treatment of malignant gliomas (HORIOT et al. 1988, 1989). In both arms of the trial, a tumor dose of 60 Gy in 30 fractions was delivered in either 6 weeks with conventional fractionation, or 4 weeks using an accelerated split-course regimen. No difference in median survival time or in the incidence of late brain necrosis was observed.

1.4.3 Type C Concomitant Boost

Results of the concomitant boost schedule developed at UTMDACC (Fig. 1.1) were recently reported by ANG et al. (1990) in a series of 130 patients, most of whom had moderately advanced oropharyngeal primaries. The study was designed to test the optimum scheduling of the concomitant boost, either at the beginning, the end, or evenly distributed throughout the basic course of treatment. The best results were obtained when the concomitant boost was given during the *last* 2–2.5 weeks of the basic treatment course, and in this subset of patients 2-year local-regional control was 71%. By contrast, the 2-year control rate was 47% ($P = 0.043$) in patients in whom the boost was given either *throughout the basic course* or during the *first* 2–2.5 weeks. Severe acute reactions were increased compared with conventional fractionation, but no increase in late treatment complications was observed.

Quasi-accelerated fractionation was defined above as a regimen in which segments of accelerated fractionation have been interrupted by treatment breaks so that no reduction in overall treatment time was achieved (Table 1.1). There have been two trials, the first being a prospectively randomized trial in head and neck cancer in which a quasi-accelerated regimen consisting of 1.6 Gy three times daily in a split course delivering 67.2–72 Gy over 6–7 weeks was compared with standard fractionation (VAN DEN BOGAERT 1986). Local-regional control rates and 3-year survival figures were identical in both arms of the study. However, there was an increased incidence of late effects with the quasi-accelerated regimen. This may be attributable to the short minimum interfraction interval of 3 h specified in this protocol. The second study involved prostate cancer, where fractional doses of 2 Gy given three times daily with a 4-h interfraction interval were given to a total dose of 60 Gy in 6 weeks with one or two treatment interruptions (VANUYSTEL et al. 1986). This regimen produced an unexpected high incidence of severe late complications, again possibly attributable to incomplete repair between dose fractions.

1.5 Conclusions

1. Accelerated fractionation produces more severe acute reactions than does conventional treatment. In the case of type A regimens, acute normal-tissue reactions (and their sequelae) are major limitation to total dose.

2. Ultra-accelerated treatment with daily doses of 4.8 Gy or more have been associated with increased treatment-related deaths, sometimes with massive tumor hemorrhage.

3. The results of accelerated regimens of type B or C appear overall to be superior to those of type A. Prospective randomized studies comparing these strategies against best conventional fractionation are underway.

4. Accelerated fractionation regimens may be associated with unexpected late normal-tissue sequelae, of both a consequential and a generic nature. The risk of the latter is related to the size of dose per fraction, number of fractions delivered per day, and interfraction interval. The larger the dose per fraction, the greater the number of fractions per day, and the shorter the interfraction interval, the greater is the cumulative effect of incomplete repair in reducing the tolerance of late-responding normal tissues.

Acknowledgements. This investigation was supported in part by grants CA06294, CA29026, and CA16627 awarded by the National Cancer Institute, Department of Health and Human Services, USA.

References

Andrews JR (1965) Dose-time relationships in cancer radiotherapy: a clinical radiobiology study of extremes of dose and time. AJR 93: 56–74

Ang KK, Peters LJ, Weber RS, Maor MH, Morrison WH, Wendt CD, Brown BW (1990) Concomitant boost radiotherapy schedules in the treatment of carcinoma of the oropharynx and nasopharynx. Int J Radiat Oncol Biol Phys 19: 1339–1345

Ang KK, Jiang GL, Guttenberger R, Thames HD, Stephens LC, Smith CD, Feng Y (1992) The impact of spinal cord repair kinetics on the practice of altered fractionation schedules. Radiother Oncol 25: 287–294

Barker JL, Montague ED, Peters LJ (1980) Clinical experience with irradiation of inflammatory carcinoma of the breast with and without elective chemotherapy. Cancer 45: 625–629

Beck-Bornholdt H-P, Omniczynski M, Theis E, Vogler H, Würschmidt F (1991) Influence of treatment time on the response of rat rhabdomyosarcoma R1H to fractionated irradiation. Acta Oncol 30: 57–63

Begg AC, Hofland I, van Glabekke M, Bartelink H, Horiot J-C (1992) Predictive value of potential doubling time for radiotherapy of head and neck tumor patients: results from the EORTC cooperative trial 22581. Semin Radiat Oncol 2: 22–25

Bentzen SM, Thames HD (1991) Clinical evidence for tumor clonogen regeneration: interpretations of the data. Radiother Oncol 22: 161–166

Budihna M, Skrk J, Smid L, Furlan L (1980) Tumor cell repopulation in the rest interval of split-course radiation treatment. Strahlentherapie 156: 402–408

Choi KN, Withers HR, Rotman M (1985a) Intracranial metastases from melanomas: clinical features and treatment by accelerated fractionation. Cancer 56: 1–9

Choi KN, Withers HR, Rotman M (1985b) Metastatic melanoma in brain: rapid treatment or large dose fractions. Cancer 56: 10–15

Dische S, Saunders MI (1989) Continuous hyperfractionated, accelerated radiotherapy (CHART): an interim report upon late morbidity. Radiother Oncol 16: 65–72

El Badawi SA, Goepfert H, Hercon J, Fletcher GH, Oswald MJ (1982) Squamous cell carcinoma of the pyriform sinus. Laryngoscope 92: 357–364

Gray AJ (1986) Treatment of advanced head and neck cancer with accelerated fractionation. Int J Radiat Oncol Biol Phys 12: 9–12

Guttenberger R, Thames HD, Ang KK (1992) Is the experiences with CHART compatible with experimental data? A new model of repair kinetics and computer simulations. Radiother Oncol 25: 280–286

Horiot J, van den Bogaert W, Ang KK et al. (1988) European Organization for Research on Treatment of Cancer trials using radiotherapy with multiple fractions per day. A 1978–1987 survey. Front Radiat Ther Oncol 22: 149–161

Horiot JC, Le Fur R, Nguygen T (1989) Hyperfractionation versus conventional fractionation in curative radiotherapy of oropharynx carcinoma: updated results of a randomized EORTC trial. In: Abstracts of the Proceedings of the 17th International Congress of Radiology, Paris, p 231 (# 1067)

Jung H, Krueger H-J, Brammer I, Zywietz F, Beck-Bornholdt H-P (1990) Cell population kinetics of the rhabdomyosarcoma R1H of the rat after single doses of X-rays. Int J Radiat Biol 57: 567–589

Knee R, Fields RS, Peters LJ (1985) Concomitant boost radiotherapy for advanced squamous cell carcinoma of the head and neck. Radiother Oncol 4: 1–7

Kummermehr J, Trott K-R (1982) Rate of repopulation in a slow and fast growing mouse tumor. In: Karcher KH, Kogelnik HD, Reinartz G (eds) Progress in radio-oncology II. Raven, New York, pp 299–308

Lamb D, Spry N, Gray A, Johnson A, Alexander S, Dally M (1990) Accelerated fractionation radiotherapy for advanced head and neck cancer. Radiother Oncol 18: 107–116

Maciejewski B, Withers HR, Taylor JMG, Hliniak A (1989) Dose fractionation and regeneration in radiotherapy for cancer of the oral cavity and oropharynx: tumor dose-response and repopulation. Int J Radiat Oncol Biol Phys 16: 831–843

Milas L, Yamada S, Hunter N, Guttenberger R, Thames H (1991) Changes in TCD_{50} as measure of clonogen doubling time in irradiated and unirradiated tumors. Int J Radiat Oncol Biol Phys 21: 1195–1202

Million RR, Zimmerman RC (1975) Evaluation of University of Florida split-course technique for various head and neck squamous cell carcinomas. Cancer 35: 1533–1536

Moulder JE, Fischer JJ (1976) Radiation reaction of rat skin: the role of the number of fractions and the overall treatment time. Cancer 37: 2762–2767

Norin T, Onyango J (1977) Radiotherapy in Burkitt's lymphoma: conventional or superfractionated regime—early results. Int J Radiat Oncol Biol Phys 2: 399–406

Overgaard J, Hjelm-Hansen M, Johansen LV, Andersen AP (1988) Comparison of conventional and split-course radiotherapy as primary treatment in carcinoma of the larynx. Acta Oncol 27: 147–152

Peracchia G, Salti C (1981) Radiotherapy with thrice-a-day fractionation in a short overall time. Clinical experiences. Int J Radiat Oncol Biol Phys 7: 99–104

Peters LJ, Ang KK, Thames HD (1988) Accelerated fraction-ation in the radiation treatment of head and neck cancer: a critical comparison of different strategies. Acta Oncol 27: 185–194

Peters LJ, Brock WA, Travis EL (1990) Radiation biology at clinically revelant fractions. In: Devita V, Hellman S, Rosenberg SA (eds) Important advances in oncology 1990. J.B. Lippincott, Philadelphia, pp 65–83

Rich TA, Terry NHA, Meistrich ML et al. (1993) Tumor-cell kinetics of human rectal cancer: relationship between po-tential doubling times, response to irradiation and chemo-therapy, and patterns of failure. Int J Radiat Oncol Biol Phys (to be publ.)

Saunders M, Dische S, Fowler J et al. (1988a) Radiotherapy with three fractions per day for twelve consecutive days for tumors of the thorax, head and neck. Front Radiat Ther Oncol 22: 99–104

Saunders MI, Dische S, Fowler JF et al. (1988b) Radiotherapy employing three fractions on each of twelve consecutive days. Acta Oncol 27: 163–167

Svoboda V (1984) Accelerated fractionation: the Portsmouth experience 1972–1984. In: Proceedings of Varian's Fourth European Clinic Users Meeting, Malta, May 25–26, Zug, Switzerland, Varian, pp 70–75

Terry NHA, Meistrich ML, White RA, Rich TA, Peters LJ (1992) Cell kinetic measurements as predictors of response of human tumors to radiotherapy and chemotherapy. Cancer Bull 44: 124–129

Thames HD, Peters LJ, Ang KK (1989) Time-dose considera-tions for normal-tissue tolerance. Front Radiat Ther Oncol 23: 113–130

Van den Bogaert W, van der Schueren E, Horiot J et al. (1986) Early results of the EORTC randomized clinical trial on multiple fractions per day (MFD) and misonidazole in advanced head and neck cancer. Int J Radiat Oncol Biol Phys 12: 587–591

Vanuytsel L, Ang K, Vandenbussche L, Vereecken R, van der Schueren E (1986) Radiotherapy in multiple frac-tions per day for prostatic carcinoma: late complications. Int J Radiat Oncol Biol Phys 12: 1589–1595

von Rottkay P (1986) Remission and acute toxicity during accelerated fractionated irradiation of non-small cell bron-chial carcinoma. Strahlentherapie 162: 300–307

Wang CC, Blitzer PH, Suit H (1985) Twice-a-day radiation therapy for cancer of the head and neck. Cancer 55: 2100–2104

Withers HR, Taylor JMG, Maciejewski B (1988) The hazard of accelerated tumor clonogen repopulation during radio-therapy. Acta Oncol 27: 131–146

2 Time-Dose Relationships for Human Tumors: Estimation from Nonrandomized Studies

S.M. BENTZEN

CONTENTS

2.1 Introduction

Tumor cells proliferate before, during, and, unfortunately, in some cases after radiotherapy. With our

S.M. BENTZEN, PhD, Danish Cancer Society, Department of Experimental Clinical Oncology, Nørrebrogade 44, DK-8000 Aarhus C, Denmark

current radiobiological knowledge, we would expect this fact to result in a reduced probability of local tumor control if the same dose-fractionation schedule were to be applied in a longer overall time. However, independent of any mechanistic considerations at the cellular level, it is a problem for clinical science to decide to what extent an alteration of the treatment time alters the tumor control probability. At first sight this should be a simple task, but a multiple of methodological problems hamper the interpretation of the clinical studies published so far, and the magnitude of the time factor remains controversial at the time of writing. The aim of this chapter is to identify a number of these problems and to review critically our current knowledge of the time factor for human tumors.

2.2 Some Historical Notes on the Tumor Time Factor

Since the early days of radiotherapy it has been known that fractionated and protracted treatment had less biological effect than the same total dose given as a single irradiation. Yet, it is only within the last 25 years that the effects of fractionation and time have been clearly separated. Although through the years, "optimal" fractionation schedules have sometimes been proposed on the basis of normal-tissue considerations, cf. the concept of "treating to tolerance," the present discussion will concentrate on the tumor time factor.

2.2.1 The Strandqvist Plot

It was STRANDQVIST (1944) who pioneered the quantitative description of the "time factor" for human tumors and normal tissues. Strandqvist plotted data for local control and skin complications as a function of the logarithm of the total dose and the logarithm of the time since start of treatment and estimated a line separating (most of) the recurrences from (most of) the skin complications. He tested this relationship for several other data sets and concluded that the total dose, D, was related to the overall treatment time, T, by

$$D = k \cdot T^{0.22} \qquad (2.1)$$

where k is a constant to be determined from a fit to clinical data.

COHEN (1949) elaborated on Strandqvist's idea, but while he accepted the exponent of 0.22 for tumors, he estimated an exponent of 0.33 for skin complications. Although this observation was an artifact arising from inconsistent choices of how to represent single-dose data in the Strandqvist plot, the alleged difference in recovery exponents had a significant impact on the later derivation of the nominal standard dose (NSD) formula. An important detail is that Cohen interpreted T as being numerically equal to the number of fractions given.

2.2.2 The Ellis NSD Concept

In 1969 Frank ELLIS published a paper with the title "Dose, time and fractionation: a clinical hypothesis." Ellis was inspired by Strandqvist's and Cohen's studies and by experimental data reported by FOWLER et al. (1963) showing that, at least for a range of overall treatment times, the number of dose fractions was more important than time in itself. Ellis proposed that for normal tissue tolerance, the total dose, D, was related to number of fractions, N, and overall treatment time, T, by:

$$D = \text{NSD} \cdot N^{0.24} \cdot T^{0.11}, \qquad (2.2)$$

where NSD is a constant. Originally, the N exponent was 0.22 but Orton changed this to 0.24 to allow for treatment schedules employing five rather than six fractions per week. BENTZEN and OVERGAARD (1992) have given a more detailed discussion of the NSD formula and the severe criticism to which it has been subjected. What is of interest here, is that a tumor NSD was proposed as well. For tumor control after radiotherapy, Ellis suggested that the overall treatment time was of no importance. His argument was that the time factor in normal tissues resulted from the homeostatic control. He continued: "Malignant cells are not susceptible to homeostatic control as are normal cells. … We know that some tumours are hormone sensitive to some extent. In-so-far as they are sensitive to hormones they are not behaving like malignant cells." In other words, malignant cells have no time factor by definition! Furthermore, Ellis assumed that the N exponent was the same

for normal tissues and tumors, because both depended on the integrity of the connective tissue. Thus he proposed the relationship.

$$D = \text{NSD} \cdot N^{0.24} \qquad (2.3)$$

for tumor isoeffective dose.

2.2.3 The Strandqvist-Ellis Formulae and the Tumor Time Factor

The Strandqvist-Ellis formulae had a profound influence on radiotherapy practice in many institutions throughout the world in the 1970s and early 1980s, and played a major role in the attempts to calculate equivalent prescribed doses in treatment schedules involving a change in overall treatment time (BENTZEN and THAMES 1991). Support for this assertion is provided by the analysis by HENDRY and ROBERTS (1991) of the dose prescriptions for six surrogate cases in the Royal College of Radiologists' fractionation survey among 172 British radiotherapists. This analysis showed that the dose prescriptions were in good agreement with the NSD formula.

Taking the derivative of the Strandqvist formula with respect to time yields a dose of 0.44 Gy to compensate for an extra day in a schedule treating with 2 Gy per day (or per fraction in Cohen's interpretation of the Strandqvist formula). The NSD formula for tumors (Eq. 2.3) does not explicitly correct for treatment time. However, for a schedule applying one 2-Gy fraction per day 5 days per week, the total dose should be increased by 0.48 Gy per extra fraction, that is approximately 0.48 Gy per extra day (BENTZEN and THAMES 1991). It is a further illustration of the influence of the Strandqvist-Ellis formulae that these estimates are in rough agreement with the rule of thumb used in the Danish head and neck protocols in the 1970s, that a protraction of 1 week (5 treatment days) should be compensated by an extra 2-Gy fraction.

2.2.4 Cohen's Cell Population Kinetics Model

The cell population kinetics model of COHEN (1971) was based on the target cell hypothesis, i.e., that radiation reactions in human tissues depend on the depletion of some critical cell population below a certain threshold value. Cell survival was described by the two-component model or, in later studies by Cohen, by the linear-quadratic model. Cellular renewal was a key feature of the Cohen model. This was characterized by the growth rate of the target cell population and the number of available cell cycles in the tissue, as a growth-limiting factor. Apart from these two parameters the model included three parameters for the cellular dose-survival curve, the value of the critical threshold for cell depletion, and a field size correction for both tumors and normal tissues. The model parameters for specific tissues were to be estimated from clinical dose-response data using computer programs to obtain best-fitting values.

Cohen's model incorporated many sound biological concepts, but the fundamental difficulty was that few clinical data sets were available with a sufficient variability in treatment characteristics to allow reliable estimation of its many parameters.

Cohen's model became one of the arguments for split-course radiotherapy, that is fractionation schedules including a typically 2- to 4-week treatment-free break. The rationale for this type of schedule was that proliferation during the treatment pause would improve normal-tissue tolerance and thereby allow the tumor dose to be escalated (HJELM-HANSEN 1980). At the Department of Oncology in Aarhus, a 3-week split was introduced in the treatment of head and neck tumors and the total dose was raised by 10–12 Gy. Cohen's model predicted that tumor control would improve and that the incidence of early and late normal-tissue complications would decrease. When tried in the clinic, it turned out that tumor proliferation during the pause completely offset the gain in tumor control expected from the higher dose, and that late sequelae increased drastically (Fig. 2.1).

2.3 Quantitation of the Time Factor

Of the different ways to quantify the time factor, two predominate in the literature: the change in local control for a 1-week difference in treatment time and the dose required to compensate an extension of overall time by 1 day. The two measures are complementary and it is not possible to give a general preference for one of them. Unfortunately, conversion from one to the other is not straightforward as it involves knowledge of the steepness of the dose-response curve.

2.3.1 Loss of Local Control per Week

Provided that the biological doses and all other relevant characteristics, excepting treatment time,

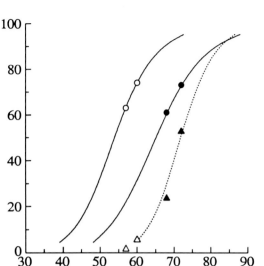

Fig. 2.1. The influence of overall treatment time on the dose-response relationship for local control of squamous cell carcinoma of the larynx (*circles*) and late edema (*triangles*). *Open symbols* show data for continuous-course radiotherapy (nominal duration 6 weeks); *closed symbols* show data for split-course radiotherapy (nominal duration 10 weeks). The 4-week protraction of treatment shifts the dose-response curve for local control towards higher doses, whereas the data for late edema fit onto a single dose-response curve independent of treatment time. (Modified from OVERGAARD et al. 1988)

are identical in two groups of patients, the observed difference in local control in percentage points for a given difference in treatment time is a simple way to quantify the time factor. This measure is often converted to the loss of local control per week, %/wk. The %/wk has the advantage of being easy to interpret. However, it also has some less attractive properties. First of all, the loss of local control depends on the position on the dose-response curve: if a 2-week protraction brings down the local control rate from 50% to 20% then a further 2-week protraction will yield a reduction of less than 30%! Another limitation of this measure, from the therapist's point of view, is that an observed %/wk gives no hint about the appropriate therapeutic countermeasure. An illustration of this is the reanalysis by LINDSTROM and FOWLER (1991) of tumor control data for T3 and T4 squamous cell carcinoma of the larynx (MACIEJEWSKI et al. 1983). The reanalysis showed a 62% [sic!] reduction in tumor control per week of prolonged treatment time. Lindstrom and Fowler suggested that this large value was influenced by patient selection. Nevertheless, the fitted model indicated that 1 extra week of treatment time could be balanced by raising the dose from 60 to 61 Gy, because of an extreme steepness of the dose-response curves in this study. A recovered dose per week of only 1.0 Gy would suggest that the split-course regimen employed in Aarhus from 1978 to 1979, in which in a 3-week break was typically accompanied by a 10–12 Gy increase in total dose, would yield an improved tumor control. This is in contrast with clinical observations (see Sect. 2.2.4).

2.3.2 Dose Recovered per Day

Assume that two groups of patients have the same local control rate despite different total treatment times and total doses. It is then possible to estimate the dose needed to compensate for the prolonged treatment time. Normally, this is converted to the dose needed to compensate for 1 extra day of treatment time, D_p. Tumor cells are assumed to grow exponentially, that is the natural logarithm of the number of cells, $\ln(N_0)$, increases linearly with time. Also, $\ln(N_0)$ decreases linearly with dose when a constant dose per fraction is employed. As a consequence, D_p is independent of the position on the dose-response curve.

In practice, an identical local control rate in two treatment groups would indeed be a lucky coincidence. There are basically two ways to get around this problem. One is to assume a certain steepness of the dose-response curve and to convert the doses resulting in the observed control rates into doses resulting in a common level of tumor control, most often 50%. If nonstandard fraction sizes are used, the nominal total doses are converted to equivalent doses with 2 Gy per fraction. The difficulty is that the result is critically dependent on the assumed values of the parameters, and that little is known about optimal values of these in most clinical series. The alternative to this approach is to apply mathematical modeling (see Sect. 2.3.4).

2.3.3 Clonogenic Doubling Time

A third measure, the tumor clonogen doubling time, T_{clon}, has also been used by some authors. One way to estimate this quantity has been to convert an observed recovery of dose into an equivalent number of doublings, assuming that a 2-Gy fraction halves the number of surviving clonogens. This latter as-

sumption cannot hold up for clinical data as this would mean that one 2-Gy fraction would change the local control rate from 36% to 60%. Therefore, the clonogen doubling time estimated in this way is not a biologically realistic quantity. Once again, the alternative to this approach is mathematical modeling.

2.3.4 Modeling Approaches

In this type of approach, it is necessary to assume a relationship between tumor control probability, TCP, and the tumor and treatment characteristics. There are two strategies, a "general" and a "mechanistic." The former refers to multivariate regression using standard models like the logistic or the Cox proportional hazards model. To some extent these methods may accommodate mechanistic elements, for example the terms "dose" and "dose × dose per fraction" may be included as explanatory variables to represent the isoeffective-dose concept of the linear-quadratic model. When the model parameters have been estimated, quantities like loss of local control per week and D_p are easily calculated. Such methods are often thought of as being assumption-free, which of course they are not. What is true, is that the investigator often tries a variety of different terms and combinations of these to arrive at a best-fitting model. This is in contrast to the mechanistic models, where a priori ideas about the biologically relevant mechanisms, and the way these affect the outcome, are built into the model. Each method has its pros and cons. The present author tends to favor the mechanistic models because of the insights provided by these, both in cases where they hold up and in cases where they fail to fit the data.

The starting point for most mechanistic models will be the Poisson formula for tumor control with cell killing described by the linear-quadratic model. For a total dose, D, given in dose per fraction, d, and overall treatment time, T, the TCP is

$$\text{TCP} = \exp[-N_0 \cdot \exp(-\alpha \cdot D - \beta \cdot D \cdot d + \lambda \cdot t)], \tag{2.4}$$

where N_0 is the number of tumor clonogens, α and β are the parameters of the linear-quadratic model, and λ is the growth constant for the assumed exponential growth of the tumor cells during treatment. The parameters, N_0, α, β, and λ are estimated from a direct fit to the clinical data. Other tumor characteristics, most importantly tumor volume, can easily be incorporated in the model.

While λ in itself is a quantitative measure of the tumor time factor (see Sect. 2.3.3), a more attractive measure is D_p:

$$D_p = \frac{\lambda}{\alpha + \beta \cdot d} = \lambda/\alpha_{\text{eff}}. \qquad (2.5)$$

Being the ratio of two parameters, D_p is a much more robust parameter, that is, its value can be more reliably established, when estimated from noisy data (TAYLOR and KIM 1989).

The clonogen doubling time, T_{clon}, is easily calculated from λ:

$$T_{\text{clon}} = \frac{\ln(2)}{\lambda}. \qquad (2.6)$$

In practice, values of T_{clon} estimated from clinical data are misleadingly high, thus giving a false impression of the deleterious effects of protracted treatment.

2.3.5 A Practical Example

It is illuminating to compare these three ways of quantifying the time factor by reference to a concrete clinical study. The analysis of the oropharynx material from Aarhus (BENTZEN et al. 1991) yielded the following estimates: a 7% loss of local control per week, a dose needed to compensate for protracted treatment time of 0.68 Gy/day, and an apparent clonogen doubling time of $T_{\text{clon}} = 21$ days. Several properties of these three measures should be noticed:

1. $D_p = 0.68$ Gy/day may seem a surprisingly high value. The reason why this translates into a relatively modest %/wk is the shallow dose-response curve seen in most human tumors.

2. Although $T_{\text{clon}} = 21$ days is the best fitting value, this gives only a vague, or even misleading, impression of the deleterious effect of a, say, 1-week protraction of treatment time. This is amplified by the popular rule of thumb that one 2-Gy fraction halves the number of surviving clonogens (see Sect. 2.3.3). Thus a 1-week protraction should be more than compensated by just one extra 2-Gy fraction. This is not correct, as shown by the estimate of D_p.

3. A 7% loss of local control per week may seem modest. However, about one in four or five patients actually gets a more than 10-day protraction of treatment for various reasons (see Sect. 2.4.2). This is equivalent to a 10% loss of local control in a potentially curable disease.

The reason for the high value of T_{clon} is probably inter- and/or intratumor heterogeneity. In a recent re-

analysis of the Aarhus oropharynx material (BENTZEN 1992a), variability in radiosensitivity was taken explicitly into consideration in a fit to the data of a model of the type in Eq. 2.4. The variability in radiosensitivity was derived from in vitro data with an empirical correction to allow for possible differences between in vitro and clinical radiosensitivities. Doing so, a $\tilde{T}_{\text{clon}}$ of only 3.2 days was obtained, whereas D_p only changed marginally to 0.75–0.77 Gy/day. $\tilde{T}_{\text{clon}}$ may be interpreted as the clonogen doubling time that would result if stratification according to intrinsic radiosensitivity was possible. In the absence of such stratification the best estimate of the apparent clonogenic doubling time is still the 21 days.

2.4 Sources of Variation in Overall Treatment Time

Overall treatment time may vary for a number of reasons. It is important to distinguish between variations in treatment time springing from a change of treatment policy and variations due to individual factors.

2.4.1 Treatment Policy

Different schools of radiotherapists have developed different "standard" fractionation schedules. This causes a *between-institutions* variability in dose-time schedules. The origin and scientific basis for these schedules, and also how experiences in different institutions have interacted over the years, are often unclear.

Radical changes of treatment policy have been implemented in some institutions and thereby caused a *within-institution* variation in the dose-time schedules. The two main modifications of overall treatment time have been the introduction of split-course regimens and multiple-fractions-per-day schedules.

2.4.2 Individual Factors

In practice, many radiotherapy patients are treated in an overall time that is longer than planned. In the study by LINDBERG et al. (1988), 70% of the patients with head and neck cancer had unplanned treatment interruptions of 1 day or more. Forty-nine percent of the patients had more than 5 days of unplanned interruptions, and 25% had more than 10 days. BENTZEN (1992b) defined the ideal treatment time for an individual patient as the time that would result from giving the actual number of fractions with the planned number of fractions per week and with allowance for the planned pause in patients receiving split-course radiotherapy. A comparison of the actual and the ideal treatment time in the Aarhus oropharynx series (BENTZEN et al. 1991) showed that 29% had a more than 5-day difference and 19% a more than 10-day difference, in good agreement with Lindberg et al.'s experience.

Individual patients may have a prolonged treatment time for a number of reasons. FYLES et al. (1992) have provided an interesting listing of the causes and the median duration of treatment interruptions in individual patients (Table 2.1). A total of 1314 unplanned treatment interruptions were distributed among 830 patients. The most frequent causes of interruptions were unrelated to stage of disease and patient prognosis, but the median duration of these interruptions was short, 1–2 days. By far the longest treatment interruptions were due to "failed attempts at intracavitary insertion" (median 18 days) and "disease complications" (median 14 days), which are directly associated with a poor prognosis.

Protracted treatment is quite simply more common in the unfavorable prognostic cases. In the University of Florida study on the effect of overall treatment time on local control in patients with adenocarcinoma of the prostate (AMDUR et al. 1990), the dose aim was 65 Gy for stage B1 patients and 65 to 70 Gy for patients with stage B2-C disease.

There was some individualization of treatment, but a major variability in treatment time came from the introduction of a 14- to 16- day treatment-free interval. Between 1967 and 1974 this split-course radiotherapy was the general policy. Nevertheless, with increasing stage of disease there was a highly statistically significant increase in the proportion of patients treated in more than 8 weeks, the cutoff point chosen by the authors in their analysis (Fig. 2.2). Stratification according to stage was performed in the authors' analysis, but it seems likely that poor prognosis was associated with an increased probability of prolonged treatment even within a specific stage. Another example is from PAJAK et al. (1991), who reported on 44 patients with an "unacceptably prolonged" treatment time in the RTOG randomized head and neck trials conducted since 1978. The median prolongation was 16 days, with a range from 11 to 88 (!) days. The 3-year locoregional control in this group was 13% compared with 27% for other patients. These patients constituted the majority of a group of 53 patients who had "major deviations from the protocol." Table 2.2 shows that the frequencies of four negative prognostic signs were all higher among the 53 patients than they were among the other patients. Even when this skewed distribution is not statistically significant, it may cause a significant bias in the comparison of the prognosis in the two groups.

There are at least two other important caveats in the analysis of data with individual variation in overall treatment time. First, these series will often

Table 2.1. Causes of treatment interruptions in 830 patients with carcinoma of the uterine cervix (FYLES et al. 1992) and the possible association with prognosis

Cause of interruption	Number of interruptions	Median duration (days)	Relation to prognosis
Holidays	488	1	None
Interval ERT–IRT	369	2	None (?)
Machine breakdown/ service	203	1	None
Failed IRT attempt	97	18	Related to "perforations, adhesions resulting from therapy and/or insufficient tumor regression"
Intercurrent illness	69	5	May be related to large tumor burden/poor performance status
RT complications	57	6	Possibly related to large treatment volume, i.e., locally advanced disease
			Locally advanced disease/poor performance status may lead to reduced tolerance
Disease complications	31	14	Related to locally advanced disease

ERT, external beam radiotherapy; IRT, intracavitary radiotherapy

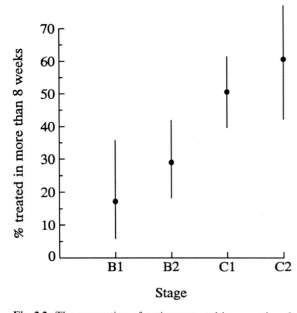

Fig. 2.2. The proportion of patients treated in more than 8 weeks versus clinical stage in a total of 211 patients with adenocarcinoma of the prostate as derived from the study by AMDUR et al. (1990). *Error bars* show the 95% confidence limits on the proportion. There is a statistically highly significant trend towards more frequent treatment protractions with increasing stage (Spearman's rank correlation significantly different from zero, $P < 10^{-5}$)

Table 2.2. Frequency of negative prognostic factors in patients with and without major deviations (MD) from protocol in the RTOG randomized head and neck trials since 1978 (from PAJAK et al. 1991)

	MD group $n = 53$	Other patients $n = 373$
T4	43%	38%
N3	47%	34%
Karnofsky score < 90	55%	44%
Base of tongue/oral cavity/nasopharynx	62%	45%

comprise a large proportion of patients treated with identical or only marginally different treatment schedules. Thus the estimate of the time factor may be very sensitive to a few patients with atypical schedules. An example is provided by HOEKSTRA et al. (1990), who noted that "the results [of their analysis of the time factor] were strongly dependent on the in- or exclusion of two patients with a small number of fractions...." The other problem is that some institutions have used individualized treatment schedules, where the therapist decides on a treatment schedule from a judgment of the chance for local control. This

means that long treatment times, and high total doses, will be found preferentially in the poor prognostic cases. A special situation is when the tumor response is evaluated during treatment and the poor responders are treated to higher total doses in longer overall times. Although the increased dose should counteract the treatment time extension, this is not necessarily sufficient to compensate for the poorer prognosis in this group of patients. With this treatment policy, there will often be no, or even a reverse, dose-response relationship and a strongly negative effect of treatment protraction (BATAINI et al. 1989).

2.5 Retrospective Studies: Overviews

The term "overview" refers to a retrospective analysis in which the results of several independent studies are pooled. There are two basic rationales for doing this. The first is to obtain greater variability in the total dose and treatment time than is normally found within a single institution. The second is that a larger number of patients should give the analysis a higher statistical power. The predominant problem in doing an overview is that heterogeneity in patient materials and radiotherapy practice—other than that related to dose-time schedule—may affect the conclusion. Clearly, heterogeneity may overshadow the effect being looked for, but the opposite might happen as well: dissimilarities between institutions/series could mimic an effect. An example of this is given in Sect. 2.5.2.1.

2.5.1 Head and Neck: the Withers Study

WITHERS et al. (1988) made a very comprehensive and well-analyzed overview of 59 data sets comprising 4668 patients with head and neck tumors of various stages and tumor sites. The idea was to plot corresponding values of the dose required to control 50% of the tumors, TCD_{50}, and the overall treatment time. To convert from the nominal total dose and dose per fraction to the TCD_{50} in 2-Gy fractions, the authors employed the linear-quadratic model with an α/β of 25 Gy and assumed the steepness of the dose-response curve to be characterized by a D_a of 5 Gy. The authors obtained a biphasic dose-time relationship, nicknamed the "dog leg," and they concluded that after a lag period of 4 ± 1 weeks, the increase in TCD_{50} with increasing overall time could be described by a straight line with a slope of 0.6 Gy/day.

2.5.1.1 Critique

WITHERS et al. (1988) mention several caveats in their own overview. The analysis pooled data for several anatomical sites within the head and neck, for tumors of various clinical stages (T1–T4 and N0–N3), and for both hyperbaric oxygen trials and kilovoltage x-ray treatments. Obviously, many differences existed in treatment technique and in the practice of reporting the treatment results. Series with very high or very low control rates were excluded from the analysis in order to minimize the potential error from extrapolating the actual doses to the TCD_{50}. However, it was not stated in the paper which series were excluded, thus making it impossible to judge whether these exclusions might have introduced a bias in the analysis. Also, the authors were aware of the possible influence of choosing different values for D_p and α/β. However, they thought any reasonable values for these parameters would not affect the conclusions as only modest extrapolations were involved.

BENTZEN and THAMES (1991) critically examined the interpretation of the "dog leg." They basically put forward two lines of criticism. One questions the existence of a 4-week lag before the onset of accelerated regeneration, as was suggested by Withers

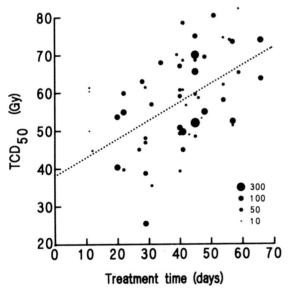

Fig. 2.3. TCD_{50} as a function of overall treatment time for squamous cell carcinoma of the head and neck. The figure is a replot of data from the review by WITHERS et al. (1988), but assuming a less steep clinical dose-response relationship than these authors did. The area of each data point is proportional to the number of patients in the corresponding data set. (From BENTZEN and THAMES 1991)

et al. If this lag period is real, any shortening of treatment time below 4 weeks, like the intensive CHART (continuous, hyperfractionated, accelerated radiotherapy) schedule completing treatment in only 12 days (DISCHE and SAUNDERS 1989), would not be worthwhile. The other criticism is that the dose-time relationship may reflect, or at least be influenced by, the historical acceptance of the NSD formula.

As for the lag period, this turns out to be dependent on details of the statistical analysis and the radiobiological parameters used in this. The choice of $\alpha/\beta = 25$ Gy is not so critical, as most studies applied dose per fraction close to 2 Gy, and therefore any α/β above 10 Gy would leave the dose-time plot essentially unchanged. The more objectionable part is the choice of D_a. Withers et al. applied a value of 5 Gy but stated that a lower value, e.g., 3.5 Gy, would be more relevant to clonogenic cell survival. The point, however, is that it is not the cellular D_0 that should be used, but rather the D_a derived from the steepness of the clinical dose-control relationship. Clinical D_a values are much higher: with a single exception, published values are all above 8 Gy, with the median of nine values being 14 Gy (BENTZEN and THAMES 1991). Bentzen and Thames replotted the data using a D_a of 18 Gy and at the same time plotted the data points as circles with an area proportional to the number of patients in the data set (Fig. 2.3). The conclusion was that the 4-week lag before the steep part of the dose-time relationship disappeared in the revised plot. But what D_a is the more realistic? HENDRY (1992) submitted all the data from the Withers' survey for a direct analysis and found support for a high value of D_a (29 Gy). Using this value would make the scatter of the data even greater and would further weaken the impression of a lag period.

The real trouble in deciding whether there is a lag period is that there are so few studies employing overall treatment times below 4 weeks. BENTZEN and THAMES (1992) estimated the TCD_{50} from the 12-day CHART schedule and found this to be consistent with a linear back-extrapolation of the dose-time relationship seen at times longer than 4 weeks. SLEVIN et al. (1992) have shown that also the 3-week schedule employed in Manchester is consistent with a linear back-extrapolation. Thus at the time of writing there is some indication that the lag period, if any, is likely to be shorter than 3 weeks and may be even shorter than the 12 days employed in CHART.

The other line of criticism is concerned with the historical choices of treatment practice that have almost certainly been influenced by the NSD formula.

BENTZEN and THAMES (1991) made the observation that if the prescribed doses were plotted in the time-dose plot without any conversion at all, the slope of the line was 0.48 Gy/day. This is exactly what the NSD formula would yield (see Sect. 2.2.3). Also, this is not statistically significantly different from the slope obtained when analizing the TCD_{50}-versus-time plot. In other words, it cannot be ruled out that the "dog-leg," at least partly, reflects the practice of dose prescriptions. Indeed, most of the data sets used for constructing the "dog-leg" originate from clinical experiences in the 1970s, when the NSD formula was at its peak popularity. The agreement with the NSD prediction does not disprove that 0.48 Gy is the correct estimate of the dose needed to compensate for 1 extra day of treatment time. The problem is that we cannot be sure, if this value simply arises because of a circular argument.

2.5.2 Bladder

MACIEJEWSKI and MAJEWSKI (1991) made an overview of 20 studies comprising a total of 2337 patients with transitional cell carcinoma of the bladder. The method of analysis was identical to that of WITHERS et al. (1988). The authors chose $D_a = 5$ Gy and an $\alpha/\beta = 15$ Gy for the bladder carcinomas. Also these authors concluded that there was no significant change in TCD_{50} with increasing overall time during the first 4–5 weeks after treatment. After this lag time, TCD_{50} increased with time at a rate of 0.36 Gy/day.

2.5.2.1 Critique

Most of the critique of the overview by Withers et al. also applies to the above-mentioned bladder tumor overview. There are, however, a few other concerns with the interpretation of the bladder study. KLEINEIDAM and DUBBEN (1992) have listed some of these:

1. Long overall treatment times were more frequently used for T3 tumors than for T1–T2 tumors.
2. Two data points appear to be erroneously plotted at too short times, whereby the slope of the dose-time relationship would be overestimated.
3. The difference in time of assessment of local control makes pooling of the sudies questionable.
4. Some of the data points in the overview represent very few patients.

Concerning point 1, the locally advanced tumors tended to be treated in longer overall times. Ten studies were exclusively concerned with T3 tumors. Six of these employed overall treatment times of more than 40 days. Of the other ten studies, four comprised T1–T2 tumors, four comprised T2 tumors, and two reported on T2–T3 tumors. Only one of these studies treated in more than 40 days. The proportion of studies treating in more than 40 days was significantly higher in reports on T3 tumors alone than in studies comprising tumors of lower T categories ($P = 0.003$). Regarding point 2, the original paper from which these two point are extracted agrees with the plot; thus this criticism is probably of no consequence for the conclusions drawn from the overview. Points 3 and 4 are indeed relevant, but it is not obvious that they would produce an artifactual dose-time relationship. The most serious concern is the correlation between tumor stage and treatment time. MARKS (1992) tried to overcome this problem by plotting the results for T3 tumors only. There was still a tendency towards increasing TCD_{50} values with increasing overall time. However, Marks pointed out that four of five studies treating in more than 45 days were from American centers where the physicians have a preference for cystectomy and therefore patients treated with definitive radiotherapy would be expected to be more locally advanced even within a specific clinical stage.

In addition to this, there are unclear criteria for inclusion of data points in the overview. The data from EDSMYR et al. (1985) are potentially very important in the analysis as these are the only data involving treatment times exceeding 50 days. But Edsmyr et al. actually report treatment results in two franctionation schedules: 84 Gy hyperfractionated (3 × 1.0 Gy per day) and 64 Gy in 2-Gy fractions. Both schedules were completed in about 60 days and local tumor clearances at 6 months is reported for T2 and T3 tumors separately. Maciejewski and Majewski only included data from the hyperfractionated arm (with an estimated TCD_{50} around 78 Gy) and not the results from the conventional arm (with an estimated TCD_{50} around 64–66 Gy).

In view of these problems, the importance of treatment time in bladder cancer remains controversial (see also Sect. 2.6.4).

2.6 Retrospective Single-Institution Studies

Single-institution studies (including multicenter studies employing a protocolar treatment schedule) are characterized by within-series variation in treatment time arising from changes in treatment policy or from individual causes.

2.6.1 Squamous Cell Carcinoma of the Head and Neck

Most reports on the tumor time factor have been concerned with squamous cell carcinoma of the head and neck. FOWLER and LINDSTROM (1992) reviewed the literature and estimated the maximum loss of local control per week, %/wk, from 12 studies. These, plus a few studies omitted from Fowler and Lindstrom's review, are summarized in Table 2.3. The range of estimates is wide, from a few percent to 62%, but all came out with a positive loss of control for prolonged treatments. Here, of course, there is a sort of publication bias: in a number of studies no significant effect of treatment time was demonstrated (a recent example is TAYLOR et al. 1991) and these are not included in the table.

Fowler and Lindstrom acknowledge that it is difficult or impossible to rule out the possibility that the estimates are confounded by factors unrelated to treatment time (cf. Sect. 2.4.2).

Even if we attribute the whole effect estimated in Table 2.3 to the treatment protraction, these estimates are not necessarily representative for the gain in local control after a 1-week shortening of treatment. The reason is that the %/wk depends on the control rate, that is on the position on the dose-response curve (see Sect. 2.3.1). For example, in the study by OVERGAARD et al. (1988), the local control probability in the continuous-course schedule de-livering 60 Gy in 2-Gy fractions was $74\% \pm 4\%$. This study yielded a loss of local control per week of 12%. However, the estimated control rate after a 1-week shortening of the treatment is 82%. This is not just a technicality but causes a drastic increase in the number of patients needed in a randomized trial of accelerated fractionation (see Sect. 2.8.2).

2.6.2 Squamous Cell Carcinoma of the Uterine Cervix

A significant does-time relationship was demonstrated in a large series of 830 patients treated with combined external beam and intracavitary radiotherapy for carcinoma of the uterine cervix FIGO stages I–IV from the Princess Margaret Hospital (FYLES et al. 1992). The actuarial probability of pelvic control at 5 years decreased by 1.1% for each day of treatment protraction in the interval 40–60 days. As total dose was not a statistically significant factor for local control, the dose recovered per day could not be estimated. Although the reasons for treatment prolongation were partly related to poor prognosis, the authors repeated their analysis without these cases and found that this "did not appreciably alter the time effect."

Split-course radiotherapy was introduced as a general treatment policy for locally advanced cervix cancer, FIGO stages IIb–IVa, in Aarhus from 1978 to 1984. These patients were compared with patients treated between 1974 and 1978 by continuous-course radiotherapy. A more comprehensive analysis is still in progress, but a preliminary analysis showed that

Table 2.3. Estimated loss of local control from a 1-week protraction of radiotherapy

Site	Observed	%/wk	Reference
Larynx[a]	Model	62	LINDSTROM and FOWLER (1991)[b]
Larynx	15%–25%/1 wk	15–25	TAYLOR et al. (1990)
Various	35%/2 wk	21	AMDUR et al. (1989)
Larynx	50%/20 d	20	MACIEJEWSKI et al. (1983)
Oropharynx	16%–34%/11 d	20	WANG (1988)
Tonsil	20%/10 d	14	BATAINI et al. (1989)
Tongue	13%–20%/10 d	9–14	MENDENHALL et al. (1989)
Larynx	45%/4 wk	12	OVERGAARD et al. (1988)
Various	14%/14 + d	12	PAJAK et al. (1991)
Larynx	13%–45%/1 wk	12	BUDIHNA et al. (1980)
Larynx	17%/10 d	12	BARTON et al. (1992)
Various	17%/12 wk	9	PARSONS et al. (1980)
Oropharynx[a]	Model	7	BENTZEN et al. (1991)
Neck nodes[a]	Model	3	BATAINI et al. (1988)
Supraglottic	4%/10 d	3	HOEKSTRA et al. (1990)

[a] The table is adapted from FOWLER and LINDSTROM (1992) except for these studies
[b] LINDSTROM and FOWLER (1991) is a reanalysis of data from MACIEJEWSKI et al. (1983)

split-course radiotherapy diminished the therapeutic ratio between local control and late complications (PEDERSEN et al. 1992).

2.6.3 Adenocarcinoma of the Prostate

Two large studies have looked for an effect of overall treatment time in localized prostate cancer. Both concluded that there is no significant reduction in the local control rate with increasing overall time, at least up to 10 weeks or more. LAI et al. (1991) analyzed 780 patients from the RTOG 75-06 and 77-06 protocols. Patients were stratified according to stage (TNM stages T1b, T2, and T3–T4) and treatment time with cutoff points $T \leq 7$, $7 < T \leq 9$, and $T > 9$ weeks. Actuarial analyses, with survival, disease-free survival, and locoregional control as the endpoints, revealed no significant relationship between treatment time and outcome of radiotherapy. In another study, LAI et al. (1990) analyzed the outcome of radiotherapy in a series of 542 patients from the Mallinckrodt Institute of Radiology. Four time strata ($T \leq 8$, $T \leq 9$, $T \leq 10$, and $T > 10$ weeks) were compared. There were no significant differences in actuarial survival or tumor control.

A third study from the University of Florida (AMDUR et al. 1990) reached the opposite conclusion from a series of 167 patients, namely that prolonged overall treatment time did reduce the local control rate. The two studies by Lai and colleagues are larger and have longer follow-up than the University of Florida study, and FOWLER (1991) has suggested that the result of the latter may be regarded as a statistical fluctuation. As discussed above (see Sect. 2.4.2), another likely explanation is that patient selection played a role in the Amdur et al. study.

Overall, there is quite strong evidence that treatment time is of no significant importance for local control in radiotherapy of adenocarcinoma of the prostate.

2.6.4 Other Tumors

There are a few other tumor types where a time factor has been sought.

2.6.4.1 Breast Cancer

Although no firm conclusions can be drawn, the experience with protracted treatment (the Baclesse technique) suggests that the time factor is less im-portant for adenocarcinoma of the breast than with squamous cell carcinoma of the head and neck (THAMES et al. 1990).

2.6.4.2 Bladder Cancer

HOLSTI and MÄNTYLÄ (1988) have published data from a series of 61 patients treated with definitive radiotherapy for bladder cancer. Of these, 28 were treated by continuous-course radiotherapy, and 33 by split-course radiotherapy with 2- to 3-week split. The average tumor dose was 3.3 Gy higher in the split-course group. No difference was seen in response rates, local control, or survival. This indicates a modest time factor but the number of patients is rather small, giving the study a low statistical power. This contrasts with the Gliwice experience, where 77 patients were treated with doses ranging from 50 to 75 Gy in overall treatment times of 35–75 days (MACIEJEWSKI and MAJEWSKI 1991). Thirty-six of these patients received split-course radiotherapy, but a variety of dose-time combinations were employed and it is not clear from the report what criteria were used for prescribing the treatment for an individual patient. A D_p of 0.36 Gy/day was estimated, which is less than for squamous cell carcinoma of the head and neck.

2.6.4.3 Malignant Melanoma

There was no demonstrable effect of overall treatment time (at least for $T < 10$ weeks) in 229 cutaneous and lymph node metastases treated by radiotherapy with variable doses, doses per fraction, and overall treatment time (BENTZEN et al. 1989b).

2.7 Nonrandomized Studies Involving a Change in Treatment Policy

Some of the problems concerned with patient selection are less pronounced when a change of treatment policy is the cause of variation in overall time. Examples of this are the use of split-course and multiple-fraction-per-day (accelerated) schedules where treatment time has been deliberately altered. Still, this type of study uses historical controls, which will not necessarily provide a valid estimate of the time effect. Variations over time in treatment technique, in local extension of disease at presentation, or even in the natural history of the disease may

Table 2.4. Expected gain from a 1-week shortening of radiotherapy based on experience from split-course studies

Site	Reference	Stage	Local control with conventional RT	Expected gain from a 1-week shortening of RT
Larynx	Overgaard et al. (1988)	All	74%	+ 8%
Larynx	Parsons et al. (1980)	T1–T2	79%	+ 4%
		T3	60%	+ 6%
		T4	32%	+ 9%
Oropharynx	Bentzen et al. (1991)	T3	63%	+ 7%

[a] Multivariate modeling in which a number of clinical characteristics must be specified to calculate the local control probability. The current value is for a male patient with a poorly differentiated T3 tumor and the median values of tumor size and hemoglobin concentration (Bentzen et al. 1991)

affect the prognosis. A special problem is stage migration, a phenomenon seen when more sensitive methods are included in the staging procedure. This will move prognostically poor patients from one stage into a higher stage, say, from stage I to stage III. The point is that such patients will have relatively good prognoses compared with other stage III patients, which may lead to improved results in both stages (Feinstein et al. 1985). Stage migration and all of the above changes in prognosis with time would tend to improve results in more recently treated patients. Thus a bias towards a (more) negative effect of protracted treatment may be introduced if patients treated by split-course radiotherapy are compared to more recent controls or if patients receiving accelerated fractionation are compared to controls from previous years.

Notwithstanding these caveats, studies involving a change of treatment policy are probably the most reliable source for estimating the time factor from clinical data at the time of writing. There are a few such studies in squamous cell carcinoma of the head and neck.

2.7.1 Split-Course Radiotherapy

Split-course schedules were initially devised to spare patients with a poor performance status (Sambrook 1962) but gained popularity in many centers in the 1960s and 1970s as a general schedule for radiotherapy. As the early toxicity is low, the compliance with split-course schedules is generally good.

Table 2.4 displays the estimated gain from a 1-week shortening of treatment as derived from the experience with split-course radiotherapy in head and neck cancer. The estimates fall within a relatively narrow range around 7% and are all in the low end of the spectrum seen in other single-institution studies (Table 2.3).

2.7.2 Multiple Fractions per Day

One problem is that treatments with multiple fractions per day are associated with an increased early toxicity relative to that of the standard treatment. This means that the standard treatment may still be used as a cross-over regimen for patients in a poor general condition, which again could mimic a benefit from shortening the treatment. The other problem is that many multiple-fractions-per-day schedules also involve the use of lower-than-standard doses per fraction with a simultaneous increase in the biological effective dose to the tumor, thus making an isolation of the time effect somewhat speculative. The only simple inference from such a study is an upper limit on the eventual gain from shorter treatment. As an example, Parsons et al. (1992) have updated the results of the moderately accelerated, hyperfractionated schedule tried at the University of Florida (Table 2.5). This schedule employed two

Table 2.5. Twice-a-day versus conventional radiotherapy (from Parsons et al. 1992)

Site	Stage	Observed change in local control[a]
Oropharynx	T2	7
	T3	2
	T4	17
Supraglottic larynx	T2	11
	T3	23
Vocal cord	T2	18
	T3	14

[a] The twice-a-day schedule was shorter by 1.5 weeks but at the same time the biological effective dose was increased by some 5%–10%

fractions of 1.2 Gy per day to a total dose of 74.4 Gy (PARSONS et al. 1988). This total dose is about 10%–15% higher than the dose used in the conventional schedule given to the historical controls. Assuming an $\alpha/\beta = 10$ Gy this corresponds to an increase in the biological effective tumor dose of at least 5%–10%. A range of gains from 2% to 23% were observed, but the only statistically significant improvement in local control was seen in the T2 vocal cord tumors. *Under the (unrealistic) assumption that all the gain may be attributed to the shorter overall time,* a 1-week shortening would be expected to yield a 14% improvement in tumor control. But obviously the 5%–10% increase in biological dose cannot be neglected and even if a quite shallow clinical dose-response curve is assumed, the increased biological dose would account for 5–10 percentage points of the improvement.

2.8 Randomized Trials of Accelerated Radiotherapy

2.8.1 Why Do We Need Randomized Trials?

A decrease in the probability of local control of head and neck squamous cell carcinoma with increasing overall treatment time has been consistently demonstrated in a large number of studies using various methods of analysis. From a clinical point of view, two important questions remain: Does the observed decrease in tumor control with increasing overall time imply that a clinically significant gain in control can be obtained by treatment acceleration? And exactly what is the price in terms of early and late treatment-related morbidity? There are so many loose ends in the retrospective studies analyzed so far, that further progress in this field requires well-conducted randomized trials. It is beyond the scope of the present chapter to discuss the treatment-related morbidity after acceleration of treatment. Two recent papers addressing this problem are BENTZEN and THAMES (1991) and HENDRY (1992). Concerning a possible gain in tumor control probability, a clinical trial is only ethical if on the one hand there is a reasonable expectation that the experimental therapy might be beneficial for the patient, but on the other hand it is not obvious that the conventional treatment is inferior. In this author's view, this is exactly where we are now regarding treatment acceleration.

2.8.2 Dimensioning a Trial

To calculate the number of patients needed in a two-arm randomized clinical trial, three quantities must be specified: the minimal clinically relevant differences between the two treatment arms, the significance level of the test α, and the power of the statistical test $1-\beta$. The choice of α is almost uniformly accepted to be 5%. The power of the test is the probability of dectecting a real existing difference of the specified magnitude between the two arms. Small clinical trials have a low power, or loosely speaking they bear a high risk of a false-negative outcome. Typically, the power is chosen to be 80% or 90%. Furthermore, the use of a one- or two-sided test should be decided upon. Here the conservative choice is the two-sided test. Finally, the allocation ratio for the two treatment arms must be specified, but the standard, and optimal, choice is to have an equal number of patients in each arm. The really critical factor is the specified treatment effect. Not only does this have a profound influence on the resulting size of the trial, but it is most often a manipulable quantity for which an objective choice is not available.

Regarding the effect of treatment acceleration, the most optimistic estimates are from single-institution series showing a median loss of local control per week of 12%. At the other extreme, the parameters estimated in the analysis by HENDRY (1992) (see Sect. 2.5.1.1) result in an expected gain in local control from a 1-week shortening of treatment time of 4% if the control arm has a 60% local control probability. Taking the large amount of variability in multi-institutional data into consideration, this estimate is probably on the low side. In between these two extremes, the split-course trials (Table 2.4) suggest a gain of about 7% for a 1-week acceleration. Taking the larynx data from OVERGAARD et al. (1988) as a typical example, the expected improvement is 8% for a 1-week acceleration and 14% for a 2-week acceleration. Figure 2.4 shows the calculated sample size in a randomized trial as a function of the difference in overall treatment time. The calculations are done using the arcsin approximation (see for example MEINERT and TONASCIA 1986), but even though more optimal statistical tests are available for analyzing time-to-recurrence data (e.g., the logrank test) the basic features of these sample-size curves are the same. Many biological and practical aspects are involved in devising an optimal accelerated fractionation schedule. However, some interesting features are revealed by the sample size calculation (Fig. 2.4). As expected, a steep increase

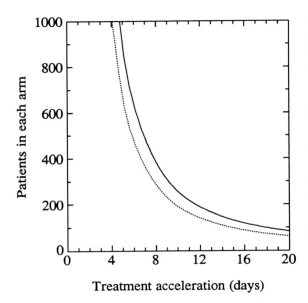

Fig. 2.4. Number of patients in each treatment arm as a function of the treatment acceleration in days. Total dose and dose per fraction were assumed to be identical in the two arms. The expected change in control rate is estimated from the time factor derived from the experience with split-course radiotherapy in laryngeal carcinoma (see Fig. 2.1). The locoregional control in the conventional arm was 74%. The two curves correspond to an 80% (*broken line*) and a 90% (*solid line*) power of the test. The significance level was 5%

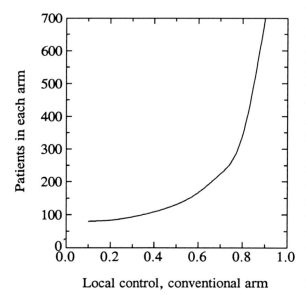

Fig. 2.5. Dimensioning a trial of a 10-day shortening of radiotherapy with unchanged total dose and dose per fraction. The graph shows the number of patients in each treatment arm as a function of the local control rate in the control arm. Significance level 5% and power of the test 90%. The expected change in control rate is estimated from the time factor derived from the experience with split-course radiotherapy in laryngeal carcinoma (see Fig. 2.1)

in the number of patients needed is seen as the shortening of treatment gets below 1 week. On the other hand, further acceleration beyond 10-14 days does not reduce the required size very much.

Furthermore, as discussed in Sect. 2.3.1, the expected gain from a 1-week shortening depends on the control rate of the standard arm. This is illustrated in Fig. 2.5. A steep rise in the sample size is seen when the local control rate in the control arm approaches 0.7-0.8. Loosely speaking: the more failures are seen, the more room there is for improvement. This, of course, presumes that the effect of treatment acceleration is described by the same time factor in the various cases. Patients with a very poor local control rate may not necessarily show the same benefit from treatment acceleration because other factors, like intrinsic radioresistance, may limit the success rate.

2.8.3 Selecting Candidates for Accelerated Radiotherapy

Patient-to-patient variability in tumor characteristics is most likely a main cause of the shallow dose-response and time-response relationships observed in the clinic. This hypothesis was explored by BENTZEN (1992a), who forced variability in the in vitro intrinsic radiosensitivity into a direct analysis of tumor control data for oropharyngeal carcinomas. The in vitro data were kindly provided by W.A. Brock, Houston. A dose-modifying factor was needed in the fit to correct for the apparent difference between in vitro and clinical radiosensitivities. Using this method, the shallow clinical dose-response curve could be resolved in a spectrum of quite steep curves for tumors of a specific radiosensitivity (BENTZEN 1992b). The target cell doubling time during treatment was estimated at 3.2 days. This means that after stratification for intrinsic radiosensitivity, the subgroup of patients who were on the steep part of the dose-response curve at the dose level used (the stochastic fraction in the terminology of ZAGARS et al. 1987) would have a dramatic benefit from a 1-week acceleration of treatment, the local control probability increasing from 20% to 65% in favorable cases. If these patients could be reliably identified by some predictive assay, the eventual advantage of treatment acceleration could be demonstrated in a very small trial comprising only 23 patients in each arm (significance level 5%, power 90%).

2.9 Conclusion

At present the most convincing clinical demonstration of the importance of treatment time comes from the studies in which split-course radiotherapy was instituted as a new standard treatment. Although it remains to be clarified whether it is the extension of the overall time per se or the length of the treatment-free interval that is the biologically important factor, the experience from split-course radiotherapy in head and neck cancer shows unequivocally that treatment-free intervals should be avoided as they cause a diminished probability of local control. This is a very important message in itself as significant treatment protractions are experienced by a sizeable proportion of radiotherapy patients even among those treated with a curative intent. WHELDON and BARRETT (1990) have suggested that attempts should be made to catch up with any unplanned treatment interruption by giving two fractions per day (with unchanged fraction size). Provided that repair of sublethal damage is complete between the two fractions given in one day, this strategy would be expected to produce an unchanged probability of late reactions and an essentially unchanged early reaction, and to maintain the tumor control probability of the planned treatment schedule.

Current radiobiological models focus on the importance of overall treatment time, disregarding the distribution in time of the dose fractions (as long as repair of sublethal damage can be assumed to be complete between fractions), but the fact that a treatment-free interval of some weeks reduces the local control rate does not logically imply a gain from shortening the treatment time. Therefore prospective randomized trials of accelerated radiotherapy are needed.

At present, it is uncertain what gain we should expect from a moderate treatment acceleration of 1–2 weeks. Yet, the experience from studies in which split-course radiotherapy was instituted as a standard treatment suggests that, without compromising the statistical power, the potential gain could be sought in intermediate sized studies (300–1000 patients) depending on the exact design of the treatment arms. Some literature studies have shown very large losses of local control with treatment prolongation, but it is indisputable that these estimates are inflated by selection bias. The danger in over-optimistic expectations is that this will lead to too small clinical trials that might overlook a potentially important—but less dramatic—benefit from acceleration. False-negative trials create frustrations that will backfire on the proponents of treatment acceleration.

References

Amdur RJ, Parsons JT, Mendenhall WM, Million RR, Cassisi NJ (1989) Split-course versus continuous course irradiation in the post-operative setting of squamous cell carcinoma of the head and neck. Int J Radiat Oncol Biol Phys 17: 279–285

Amdur RJ, Parsons JT, Fitzgerald LT, Million RR (1990) The effect of overall treatment time on local control in patients with adenocarcinoma of the prostate treated with radiation therapy. Int J Radiat Oncol Biol Phys 19: 1337–1382

Barton MB, Keane TJ, Gadalla T, Maki E (1992) The effect of treatment time and treatment interruption on tumour control following radical radiotherapy of laryngeal cancer. Radiother Oncol 23: 137–143

Bataini JP, Bernier J, Asselain B, Lave C, Jaulerry C, Brunin F, Pontvert D (1988) Primary radiotherapy of squamous cell carcinoma of the oropharynx and pharyngolarynx: tentative multivariate modelling system to predict the radiocurability of neck nodes. Int J Radiat Oncol Biol Phys 14: 635–642

Bataini JP, Asselain B, Jaulerry C, Brunin F, Bernier J, Pontvert D, Lave C (1989) A multivariate primary tumour control analysis in 465 patients treated by radical radiotherapy for cancer of the tonsillar region: clinical and treatment parameters as prognostic factors. Radiother Oncol 14: 265–277

Bentzen SM (1992a) Steepness of the clinical dose-control curve and variation in the in vitro radiosensitivity of head and neck squamous cell carcinoma. Int J Radiat Biol 61: 417–423

Bentzen SM (1993) Quantitative clinical radiobiology. Acta Oncol (to be published)

Bentzen SM, Overgaard J (1992) Time-dose relationships in radiotherapy. In: Steel GG (ed) ESTRO book of basic clinical radiobiology. ESTRO, Leuven, pp 47–54

Bentzen SM, Thames HD (1991) Clinical evidence for tumor clonogen regeneration: interpretations of the data. Radiother Oncol 22: 161–166

Bentzen SM, Thames HD (1992) Overall treatment time and tumor control dose for head and neck tumors: the dog leg revisited. Radiother Oncol 25: 143–144

Bentzen SM, Thames HD, Overgaard M (1989a) Latent-time estimation for late cutaneous and subcutaneous radiation reactions in a single-follow-up clinical study. Radiother Oncol 15: 267–274

Bentzen SM, Overgaard J, Thames HD, Overgaard M, Hansen PV, von der Maase H, Meder J (1989b) Clinical radiobiology of malignant melanoma. Radiother Oncol 16: 169–182

Bentzen SM, Johansen LV, Overgaard J, Thames HD (1991) Clinical radiobiology of squamous cell carcinoma of the oropharynx. Int J Radiat Oncol Biol Phys 20: 1197–1206

Budihna M, Skrk J, Smid L, Furlan L (1980) Tumor cell repopulation in the rest interval of split-course radiation treatment. Strahlentherapie 156: 402–408

Cohen L (1949) Clinical radiation dosage, part II. Br J Radiol 22: 706–713

Cohen L (1971) A cell population kinetic model for fractionated radiation therapy. I. Normal tissues. Radiology 101: 419–427

Dische S, Saunders MI (1989) Continuous, hyperfractionated, accelerated radiotherapy (CHART): an interim report upon late morbidity. Radiother Oncol 16: 65–72

Edsmyr F, Anderson L, Esposti PL, Littbrand B, Nilsson B (1985) Irradiation with multiple small fractions per day in urinary bladder cancer. Radiother Oncol 4: 197–203

Ellis F (1969) Dose, time and fractionation: a clinical hypothesis. Clin Radiol 20: 1–7

Feinstein AR, Sosin DM, Wells CK (1985) The Will Rogers phenomenon: stage migration and new diagnostic techniques as a source of misleading statistics for survival in cancer. N Engl J Med 312: 1604–1608

Fowler JF (1991) The effect of overall treatment time in radiotherapy for localized prostate carcinoma. Int J Radiat Oncol Biol Phys 21: 1097–1098

Fowler JF, Lindstrom M (1992) Loss of local control with prolongation in radiotherapy. Int J Radiat Oncol Biol Phys 23: 457–467

Fowler JF, Morgan MA, Silvester JA, Bewley DK, Turner BA (1963) Experiments with fractionated X-ray treatment of the skin of pigs. I. Fractionation up to 28 days. Br J Radiol 36: 188–196

Fyles A, Keane TJ, Barton M, Simm J (1992) The effect of overall treatment duration in the local control of cervix cancer. Radiother Oncol 25: 273–279

Hendry JH (1992) Treatment acceleration: the relative time factors and dose-response slopes for tumours and normal tissues. Radiother Oncol 25: 308–312

Hendry JH, Roberts SA (1991) The sensitivity of human tissues to changes in dose fractionation: deductions from the RCR survey among UK radiotherapists. Clin Oncol 3: 22–27

Hjelm-Hansen M (1980) Laryngeal carcinoma. IV. Analysis of treatment results using the Cohen model. Acta Radiol Oncol 19: 3–12

Hoekstra CJM, Levendag PC, Van Putten WLJ (1990) Squamous cell carcinoma of the supraglottic larynx without clinically detectable lymph node metastases: problem of local relapse and influence of overall treatment time. Int J Radiat Oncol Biol Phys 18: 13–21

Holsti LR, Mäntylä M (1988) Split-course versus continuous radiotherapy. Analysis of a randomized trial from 1964 to 1967. Acta Oncol 27: 153–161

Kleineidam M, Dubben HH (1992) Overall treatment time in the radiotherapy of transitional cell cancer of the bladder. Radiother Oncol 23: 270

Lai PP, Perez CA, Shapiro SJ, Lockett MA (1990) Carcinoma of the prostate stage B and C: lack of influence of duration of radiotherapy on tumor control and treatment morbidity. Int J Radiat Oncol Biol Phys 19: 561–568

Lai PP, Pilepich MV, Krall JM, Asbell SO, Hanks GE, Perez CA, Rubin P, Sause WT, Cox JD (1991) The effect of overall treatment time on the outcome of definitive radiotherapy for localized prostate carcinoma: the Radiation Therapy Oncology Group 75-06 and 77-06 experience. Int J Radiat Oncol Biol Phys 21: 925–933

Lindberg RD, Jones K, Garner HH, Jose B, Spanos WJ Jr, Bhatnagar D (1988) Evaluation of unplanned interruptions in radiotherapy treatment schedules. Int J Radiat Oncol Biol Phys 14: 811–815

Lindstrom M, Fowler JF (1991) Re-analysis of the time factor in local control by radiotherapy of T_3 T_4 squamous cell carcinoma of the larynx. Int J Radiat Oncol Biol Phys 21: 813–817

Maciejewski B, Majewski S (1991) Dose fractionation and tumour repopulation in radiotherapy for bladder cancer. Radiother Oncol 21: 163–170

Maciejewski B, Preuss-Bayer G, Trott KR (1993) The influ-ence of the number of fractions and of overall treatment time on local control and late complication rate in squamous cell carcinoma of the larynx. Int J Radit Oncol Phys 9: 321–328

Marks LB (1992) Treatment time in bladder cancer. Radiother Oncol 23: 269–270

Meinert CL, Tonascia S (1986) Clinical trials. Oxford University Press, New York, pp 71–89

Mendenhall WM, Parsons JT, Stringer SP, Cassissi NJ, Million RR (1989) T2 oral tongue carcinoma treated with radiotherapy: analysis of local control and complications. Radiother Oncol 16: 275–281

Overgaard J, Hjelm-Hansen M, Johansen LV, Andersen AP (1988) Comparison of conventional and split-course radiotherapy as primary treatment in carcinoma of the larynx. Acta Oncol 27: 147–152

Pajak TF, Laramore GE, Marcial VA et al. (1991) Elapsed treatment days—a critical item for radiotherapy quality control review in head and neck trials: RTOG report. Int J Radiat Oncol Biol Phys 20: 13–20

Parsons JT, Bova FJ, Million RR (1980) A re-evaluation of split-course technique for squamous cell carcinoma of the head and neck. In J Radiat Oncol Biol Phys 6: 1645–1652

Parsons JT, Mendenhall WM, Cassisi NJ, Isaacs JH, Million RR (1988) Hyper-fractionation for head and neck cancer. Int J Radiat Oncol Biol Phys 14: 649–658

Parsons JT, Mendenhall WM, Million RR, Cassisi NJ, Stringer SP (1992) Twice-a-day irradiation of squamous cell carcinoma of the head and neck. Sem in Radiat Oncol 2: 29–30

Pedersen D, Bentzen SM, Overgaard J (1992) Continuous versus split-course brachytherapy and external radiotherapy in locally advanced cervical cancer. In: Mould RF (ed) Brachytherapy in the Nordic Countries. Nucletron, Leersum, pp. 114–116

Sambrook DK (1962) Clinical trial of a modified ("split-course") technique of x-ray therapy in malignant tumors. Clinical Radiology 13: 1–18

Slevin NJ, Hendry JH, Roberts SA, Agren-Cronqvist A (1992) The effect of increasing the treatment time beyond three weeks on the control of T2 and T3 laryngeal cancer using radiotherapy. Radiother Oncol 24: 215–220

Strandqvist M (1944) Studien über die kumulative Wirkung der Röntgenstrahlen bei Fraktionierung. Acta Radiol 55 [Suppl]: 1–300

Taylor JMG, Kim DK (1989) The poor statistical properties of the Fe-plot. Int J Radiat Biol 56: 161–167

Taylor JMG, Withers HR, Mendenhall WM (1990) Dose-time considerations of head and neck squamous cell carcinomas treated with irradiation. Radiother Oncol 17: 95–102

Taylor JMG, Mendenhall WM, Lavey RS (1991) Time-dose factors in positive neck nodes treated with irradiation only. Radiother Oncol 22: 167–173

Thames HD, Bentzen SM, Turesson I, Overgaard M, van den Bogaert W (1990) Time-dose factors in radiotherapy. Radiother Oncol 19: 219–235

Wang CC (1988) Local control of oropharyngeal carcinoma after two accelerated hyperfractionation radiation therapy schemes. Int J Radiat Oncol Biol Phys 14: 1143–1146

Wheldon TE, Barrett A (1990) Radiobiological rationale for compensation for gaps in radiotherapy regimes by post-gap acceleration of fractionation. Br J Radiol 63: 114–119

Withers HR, Taylor JMG, Maciejewski B (1988) The hazard of accelerated tumor clonogen repopulation during radiotherapy. Acta Oncol 27: 131–146

Zagars GK, Schultheiss TE, Peters LJ (1987) Inter-tumor heterogeneity and radiation dose-control curves. Radiother Oncol 8: 353–362

3 Limitations of the Bromodeoxyuridine Technique for Measurement of Tumour Proliferation

G.D. WILSON

CONTENTS

3.1 Introduction

The study of cell kinetics is proving to be a cyclical phenomenon. A brief history shows a pattern of interest and activity similar to a percent labelled mitosis (plm) curve (Fig. 3.1). Interest rose with the first description of the cell cycle by HOWARD and PELC (1951). A zenith was reached in the 1960s following the development of tritiated thymidine (^{3}H-TdR) to label cells actively engaged in DNA synthesis (TAYLOR et al. 1957) and of cell kinetic quantitation techniques such as the plm analysis (QUASTLER and SHERMAN 1959) in which cell kinetic parameters could be quantitated by counting the passage of ^{3}H-TdR labelled cells through the "mitotic window" on tissue sections. This led to a rapid proliferation of studies in which the cell growth kinetics of normal and neoplastic tissues was described. During this period in the 1960s and early 1970s, clinicians and biologists began to attempt to therapeutically exploit the features of cell population kinetics of normal and malignant tissues. The relationship between tumour growth kinetics and therapeutic response was studied and the utility

G.D. WILSON, PhD, CRC Gray Laboratory, Mount Vernon Hospital, P.O. Box 100, Northwood, Middlesex, HA6 2JR, England

of using cell kinetic concepts to plan cancer therapy was investigated.

The impact of these studies on the management of patients with cancer was disappointing. The failure to influence treatment was due to the limitations of the technology used to measure cell kinetic parameters and to the realisation that, although proliferation is undoubtedly a factor in determining the response of tumour to various forms of cancer therapy, it is not the only cause of failure. Interest in cell kinetics waned but was never lost, with several groups repeatedly demonstrating that the ^{3}H-TdR labelling index (LI) gave important prognostic information in a variety of tumours (see TUBIANA and COURDI 1989 for review). The nadir for cell kinetics was to be found in the late 1970s and early 1980s.

The advent of flow cytometry to study cell proliferation has renewed interest in this field of research. The technique of measuring S-phase fractions from flow cytometry-derived DNA profiles was analogous to LI measurement but quantitative and universally applicable (BARLOGIE et al. 1983).

A battery of techniques and markers became available in the 1980s to measure proliferation. Long before monoclonal antibodies were developed that recognised bromodeoxyuridine (BUdR), it was recognised that this halogenated pyrimidine could suppress or quench the binding of thymidine-specific dyes, such as Hoechst 33342 or 33258, to newly synthesized DNA (LATT 1973). Flow cytometry techniques were developed to measure simultaneously BUdR-quenched Hoechst fluorescence and ethidium bromide, whose binding is not compromised by BUdR substitution of thymidine (BÖHMER and ELLWART 1981). This technique allowed cell divisions to be followed for up to three cell cycles. In the field of flow cytometry, there have been several other techniques to dissect the cell cycle, including the use of fluorochromes with differing accessibilities to DNA under normal or acid conditions or of fluorescent dyes with metachromatic properties such as acridine orange (DARZYNKIEWICZ et al. 1977).

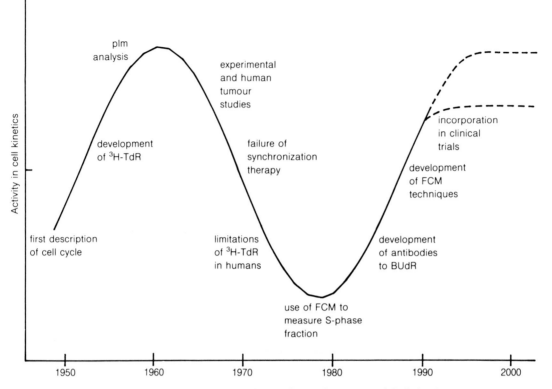

Fig. 3.1. Cyclical variation in cell·kinetic studies in the form of a percent labelled mitosis (plm) curve. *FCM*, flow cytometry

Flow cytometry and immunohistochemistry share the ability to detect expression of a whole series of proliferation-associated proteins (such as Ki-67, proliferating cell nuclear antigen, etc.), which may give prognostic information (HALL and LEVISON 1990; DANOVA et al. 1990).

The significant resurgence in interest in human tumour cell kinetics was the result of a sequence of three events. First, the production of monoclonal antibodies recognising halogenated pyrimidines incorporated into DNA by GRATZNER (1982). This was followed by the development of flow cytometry techniques which simultaneously measured the uptake of halogenated pyrimidines as a function of DNA content (DOLBEARE et al. 1983). In many respects, these two events were as significant, if not more so, than the development of ^{3}H-TdR autoradiography and plm analysis. The third event was the development, at the Gray Laboratory, of a flow cytometric analysis to obtain a measure of LI and duration of the S phase (T_s) from a single observation. From these parameters the potential doubling time (T_{pot}) of the cell population can be calculated (BEGG et al. 1985).

This led to a steep increase in the use of cell kinetic information, because for the first time, temporal measurements could be made in vivo rapidly, quantitively and with minimum inconvenience to the patient (WILSON et al. 1985). Many groups are now actively involved in applying the in vivo administration of bromo- or iododeoxyuridine (IUdR) to patients being treated by surgery, chemotherapy and in particular radiotherapy. In terms of the activity curve in Fig. 3.1, we are now approaching a second zenith in the life cycle of cell kinetics but it remains to be seen whether the second peak will be "damped" as is the case for many plm curves of tumours or whether it will become a plateau in which cell kinetics will become established as an important clinical parameter.

The purpose of this chapter is to take stock of where the methodology of measuring cell kinetics has reached and what are, and may be, the limitations of the technology and its application in the clinical setting.

3.2 How to Measure Potential Doubling Time

3.2.1 The Halogenated Pyrimidines

A limiting factor in the study of human tumour proliferation has been the lack of supply of BUdR or IUdR suitable for human use. There are several alternative avenues to the acquisition of a preparation which can be injected into patients. BUdR and IUdR had been available as radiosensitizers for many years and could be obtained from the Investigational Drugs Branch of the National Cancer Institute. The supply of these drugs for a use which was not strictly therapeutic presented problems. However, it is possible to obtain a lyophilized preparation from this source and is probably the most common supply of the halogenated pyrimidines. Commercial sources of a ready-made human preparation were available in the past from companies such a Takeda in Japan, but the demise of BUdR as a commonly used radiosensitizer led to the closure of production.

Many groups simply obtain BUdR or IUdR from the major chemical suppliers and have a suitable preparation formulated by in-house pharmacies. This usually only involves filtration and freedom from pyrogens. This route depends on the individual hospital and pharmacy taking responsibility for the safety of the preparation. It has the disadvantage that a solution of BUdR is not as stable as a powder and so has to be used within a short period of time.

There is a real need for a reliable commercial source of the halogenated pyrimidines suitable for human use. Increasing usage will surely make this a viable concern.

Having obtained the preparation, a single bolus intravenous injection of either 100 mg/m^2 or, in our case, 200 mg is given to the patient. In the interests of pulse labelling, the shorter the injection period the better. Our practice has been to administer 200 mg in 20 ml normal saline over 5 min.

There has been no report of any acute toxicity associated with the injection of BUdR for cell kinetic investigations. However, it should be remembered that halogenated pyrimidines can be mutagenic, teratogenic, oncogenic and cytotoxic depending on the dose (Goz 1978).

The cell kinetic dosage should produce plasma concentrations below the level required for any of these contra-indications. However, it has been our policy to restrict the usage of the drug in younger patients and not to use it in pregnant women.

3.2.2 The Time Between Injection and Surgical Procedures

The technique to measure T_{pot} from a single observation depends on a time gap being left between the injection of BUdR and the surgical removal of the specimen, whether it be biopsy or resection. In the time between these events, the S-phase cells which initially incorporated BUdR will progress through the cell cycle (Fig. 3.2). The staining procedure depends on being able to recognise the BUdR-labelled cells as a function of their position

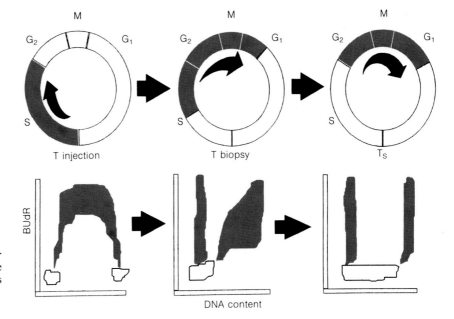

Fig. 3.2. Measurement of T_s and LI and computation of T_{pot} from one observation using flow cytometry. The *upper panel* shows the cell cycle position of a cohort of BUdR-labelled cells at the time of injection, the time of a putative biopsy and the duration of S phase. The *lower panel* shows stylised bivariate BUdR/DNA staining profiles which would be obtained at those times

in the cell cycle (DNA content). Enough time must be left to be able to detect movement of cells through their cycle but the time period should not be so long that all the BUdR-labelled cells have divided. The choice of time period will depend on the duration of the S phase of each tumour. This is, of course, an unknown entity prior to the measurement.

As a general rule, a time period of 0.5 T_s is ideal to produce a profile with sufficient redistribution of the BUdR label with minimal error in the calculation of T_{pot}. This is problematical as our studies (WILSON et al. 1988), as well as those of others (BEGG et al. 1988; REW et al. 1991), show a large variation in T_s both within a group of tumours and between different groups of tumours. The median T_s of tumours from the oral cavity is about 10 h whilst bronchial tumours have a median T_s of about 15 h. Based on the median value, a choice of 5 h and 8 h may be envisaged to result in optimal profiles for most tumours within these two groups. However, as can be seen from Table 3.1, there is a range of T_s within both groups, with some as short as 5–6 h and some longer than 30 h. Undoubtedly the choice of time period will be suboptimal for some tumours.

The other consideration and limitation is how the time period between injection and biopsy can be incorporated into a working day without disrupting clinical practice. Clearly, times exceeding 8 h cannot easily be accomplished unless the injection is given at midnight and patients are dealt with early the next morning. This would normally be restricted to resection patients as these measurements are made prior to treatment in patients who are being biopsied. Our practice is to use a delay period of 4–6 h unless we are dealing with tumour groups such as lung, oesophagus and cervix, which have a longer median T_s. In these cases, some patients are injected at night and the specimen removed the following day. Time intervals

less than 4 h are not recommended as there may not be enough cell progression, whilst time intervals greater than 12 h may result in too few cells remaining undivided.

3.2.3 Tissue Handling and BUdR Staining

Flow cytometry is dependent on presenting suspended cells or nuclei in single file to an excitation source (usually a laser beam). There has long been a maxim in flow cytometry that "garbage in—garbage out", the point being that the final result is dependent on the quality of the original suspension made from the specimen.

In most early studies, including our own (WILSON et al. 1985), enzymes such as collagenase, trypsin or pronase or mechanical methods were used to produce cell suspensions. This meant that surgical specimens had to be collected fresh from the operating theatre and, ideally, a cell suspension made immediately.

This method has been superceded in most studies of BUdR by a modification of the method reported by SCHUTTE et al. (1987). In this procedure, solid pieces of material are fixed in 70% ethanol. This means that there is no requirement for specimens to be collected and processed immediately. A representative sample of the biopsy or resection can be fixed in theatre or in the pathology department. The specimen can be stored at 4 °C and can even be sent by post to a flow cytometry facility. This has opened up the possibility of multicentre studies and the inclusion of the measurement in clinical trials or routine clinical use.

The basis of the flow cytometric staining procedures is to produce a nuclei suspesion from the solid material using pepsin digestion. This method has been discussed in detail elsewhere (WILSON 1992). There are several major advantages involved in the

Table 3.1. Summary of proliferation parameters for six of the major groups of tumours studied at the Gray Laboratory (numbers in parentheses are the total number of tumours studied in each groups; CVs are coefficients of variation expressed as a percentage)

Tumour group	LI			T_s(h)			T_{pot} (days)		
	Median	Range	CV	Median	Range	CV	Median	Range	CV
Head/neck (130)	4.9	0.6–20.3	76	9.9	5.4–21.9	45	6.4	1.8– 66.6	101
Lung (38)	8.0	0.3–28.5	70	15.1	5.6–37.6	66	7.3	1.4–132.5	167
Oesophagus (30)	7.8	0.4–27.5	64	12.4	6.9–28.6	46	5.2	1.6– 56.8	156
Cervix (22)	11.6	2.8–23.4	52	15.8	10.6–30.4	35	4.5	2.9– 15.8	61
Melanoma (24)	4.2	1.3–13.6	67	10.7	6.3–20.5	28	7.2	3.5– 41.3	82
Colorectal (98)	9.0	0.7–25.5	61	13.1	4.0–28.6	52	3.9	1.7– 21.4	68

preparation of a nuclei suspension:

1. The procedures at the clinic are minimal: simple fixation in 70% ethanol.
2. The digestion procedure with pepsin can be standard for all the different tumour groups where as preparation of cell suspensions would often employ different enzyme cocktails or mechanical modes of disaggregation depending on the tumour type.
3. The yield of nuclei per gram of tissue using pepsin is usually much greater than could be achieved with enzymes producing cell suspensions. The result of this is that measurements can be obtained on very small amounts of tissue (< 20 mg).
4. The detection of BUdR incorporation and the quality of DNA staining are improved by using nuclei as opposed to cell suspensions owing to the abolition of non-specific staining by removal of the cytoplasm.

There are few disadvantages to using the pepsin method. However, the production of nuclei negates any possibility of extending the staining procedures to include a marker, such as a cytokeratin (as will be discussed in Sect. 3.4.1), which may help to identify tumour cells from stromal or infiltrating cells.

The major questions that arise with any flow cytometric technique are: How representative is the final cell suspension compared to the original tissue? Is the yield good and has there been any cell selection? These question are difficult to answer. The yield is certainly improved by the use of pepsin (typically by 10%–40%). Cell selection will be addressed later in this chapter, when the results from flow cytometry are compared with immunohistochemical staining for BUdR incorporation (Sect. 3.4.2).

A limitation within the staining procedure is the necessity to find a balance during the denaturation procedure with hydrochloric acid, to produce sufficient unwinding of DNA for optimal antibody access without disturbing the stoichiometry of propidium iodide intercalation into double-stranded DNA. The final result is dependent on the quality of both aspects of the staining procedure. Over denaturation may produce optimal BUdR detection but it may also result in the profiles being uninterpretable due to poor DNA staining. Under-denaturation might result in underestimation of the BUdR-labelled cells, giving a low LI. There is also the possibility that different cell types may denature differently under the same conditions. Again, a compromise must be made to denature all tumours under the same conditions.

3.2.4 Flow Cytometry

There are several areas in the actual running of samples on the flow cytometer which may influence the measurement of T_{pot}. First, the hardware itself: There are basically three different manufacturers of flow cytometers with a variety of models on which measurements may be made. It is often assumed that the same answer may result from a sample run on different machines. This may not be the case.

A recent study by the Bladder Cancer Flow Cytometry Network (WHEELESS et al. 1991) compared known samples amongst six laboratories. The measurements and flow cytometry required in the study were much simpler than a BUdR measurement. They were asked to calculate the DNA index and percentage of hyperdiploid cells in each of the four specimens run on three separate days. The results showed significant inter- and intralaboratory differences. Variation was broken down into four components termed specimen, runs, interaction and error. These could be attributed to systematic differences in the operation of the laboratory, lack of consistency among specimen types or the way measurements were made or samples prepared and finally, variability between replicate measurements within the same run. The conclusion from the study was that prediction intervals were quite good for the DNA index but were troublesome for the hyperdiploid fraction, such that results from a single sample may not be sufficiently precise to allow comparison with results obtained in other laboratories.

The problems are compounded for measurement of T_{pot} as more computer-generated regions are required for data analysis. Figure 3.3 shows an aneuploid tumour and the regions that are required to calculate all of the parameters. Typically, eight regions are set and subjective decisions have to be made as to their exact location. The first problem is to delineate the boundary between BUdR-labelled and non-labelled cells. Ideally, this decision should be based on a control sample in which the monoclonal antibody has been omitted from the otherwise complete staining procedure. In practice, this is often not possible due to the paucity of material that may be available from a biopsy specimen. The setting of the lower limit for detection then becomes a subjective decision based on each individual staining profile and observer experience. The use of a

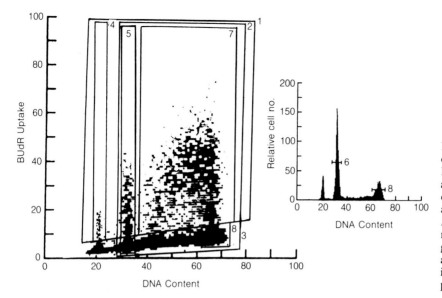

Fig. 3.3. The bivariate distribution of BUdR versus DNA content obtained from a squamous cell cancer biopsy of the cervix removed 5.8 h after an injection of BUdR. *Boxes* have been drawn to represent the computer-generated regions required for analysis of this specimen. The inset shows the single parameter DNA profile

nuclei suspension helps this decision as non-specific staining is almost completely abolished owing to removal of the cytoplasm. In a recent interinstitutional and interobserver comparison between the Gray Laboratory and the Paterson Insititute, no significant differences were recorded in the estimation of LI or DNA index in a series of 139 colorectal cancer specimens run at the two centres and analysed by three observers (one analysing at both the Gray Laboratory and the Paterson Institute) (M. WILSON et al. 1993).

However, there is still a need for this decision to be taken out of the responsibility of individual observers. Recently, WHITE and TERRY (1992) have described a method to attempt to do this using landmark features of the bivariate distributions. These are based on the ratio of green fluorescence of the G_1 and G_2 populations, which would appear to be relatively constant. The procedure enables a line to be drawn between the landmarks, which can then be shifted upwards a certain number of standard deviations based on the coefficients of variation (CV) of the green fluorescence of these two populations. This will undoubtedly be the way to standardise the separation of the BUdR-labelled cells but it will require either convincing manufacturers to write software for this purpose or to have a universal off-line analysis package. This procedure is far beyond the capabilities of currently used bench-top flow cytometers.

Having defined the region separating labelled cells, the LI can be calculated. This is not simply a proportion of labelled to total cells as some cells will have divided and shared their BUdR between their progeny. These cells can be seen as the BUdR-labelled cells emanating from the G_1 population of the diploid and aneuploid populations at channels 21 and 33, respectively, and defined by regions 4 and 5 in Fig. 3.3. These regions are relatively simple to set based on the CV of the DNA profile (see inset in Fig. 3.3). How the LI is corrected will be dealt with in the next section.

The calculation of T_S depends on three regions designated 6, 7 and 8 in Fig. 3.3. These regions were defined by BEGG et al. (1985) to measure the mean DNA content of the G_1 and $G_2 + M$ population and the cohort of BUdR-labelled cells that remain undivided in the time between injection and biopsy. There is usually no problem in defining the G_1 and G_2 populations, regions 6 and 8, as they can be obtained from either the bivariate cytogram or more readily from the single parameter DNA profile as shown in the inset of Fig. 3.3. If the G_2 population is poorly defined, an alternative calculation is to assume that G_2 is twice G_1. This might, however, introduce errors if the actual ratio of G_2:G_1 is not 2 on the flow cytometer; this can sometimes be the case. The region defining the undivided BUdR-labelled cells can be difficult to define in some aneuploid tumours but should be relatively straightforward in diploid tumours or aneuploid tumours with higher DNA indices or few diploid cells, such as that shown in Fig. 3.3. Estimation of T_S will be inaccurate unless two labelled populations can be seen (divided and undivided). Whenever possible, the left-hand edge of this region should be set at the right-hand edge of the region defining the G_1 population, i.e. regions 5 and 6, and should be extended to the right-hand edge of the G_2 region. Problems can arise where the aneuploid population may be the minor component of the tumour specimen or where diploid cells are proliferating in addition to the aneuploid cells, usually indicating that both populations contain tumour stemlines. In these situations a decision has to be made whether the left-hand edge of region 7 can be moved further to the right to exclude overlapping S and G_2 cells from the diploid population. In cases such as this, it would be advantageous to leave a longer time between injection and biopsy such that movement of the BUdR-labelled cells through the cell cycle towards G_2 were greater and would alleviate a subjective decision.

In the interinstitutional study mentioned above (M. WILSON et al. 1993) it was the placement of this region which produced the variation both between observers and between institutions. This results in variation in the calculation of relative movement and thus T_S and T_{pot}.

3.2.5 Calculation of T_{pot}

The calculation of T_{pot}, from a single observation, has received much attention in recent years. In particular, WHITE and colleagues in Houston (WHITE and MEISTRICH 1986; WHITE et al. 1990; TERRY et al. 1991) have sought ways to improve the method of calculation.

The original description by BEGG et al. (1985) described an algorithm based on several assumptions. First, the distribution of BUdR-labelled cells, immediately after pulse labelling, is uniform throughout the S phase (see Fig. 3.2). This defines that the mean DNA content of this population will be in the middle of the S phase. The term "relative movement" (RM) was used to describe the position of this population relative to G_1 and G_2 by:

$$RM = \frac{Fl_{(BUdR)} - Fl_{(G_1)}}{Fl_{(G_2)} - Fl_{(G_1)}}, \qquad (3.1)$$

where $Fl_{(BUdR)}$, $Fl_{(G_1)}$ and $Fl_{(G_2)}$ represent the mean relative red fluorescence values of these populations of cells. Thus the RM at time zero (RM_0) is 0.5. With time, the RM (RM_t) will increase (see Fig. 3.2) as the BUdR-labelled cohort progresses to G_2. Eventually the RM_t value will equal 1.0 when the only BUdR-labelled cells which remain undivided reside in G_2.

The second assumption is that progression of labelled cells through the S phase is linear. By definition, the labelled cells in G_2 when the $RM_t = 1.0$ must represent those cells that were in early S phase at time zero. Therefore the progression of cells from an RM value of 0.5 to 1.0 describes the T_S. Thus from a single observation the T_S could be calculated by:

$$T_S = \frac{1.0 - 0.5}{RM_t - 0.5} \times t, \qquad (3.2)$$

where t is the time between injection and biopsy and RM_t is the relative movement value computed at that time. For Fig. 3.3, an RM of 0.78 was obtained with a time interval of 5.8 h, which results in a T_S of 10.4 h.

The correction of LI for cell division is accomplished by halving the number of BUdR-labelled cells residing in G_1 at the time of biopsy, i.e. regions 4 and 5, and subtracting these from the total number of labelled cells and the total cell number and recalculating the LI. This can be done for the complete cell population or for aneuploid cells only. No correction for dividing $G_2 + M$ cells is made for reasons outlined later. The corrected LIs were 10.8% and 13.3% for the total of aneuploid-only cells in Fig. 3.2. The T_{pot} can then be calculated according to the method of STEEL (1977):

$$T_{pot} = \lambda \cdot \frac{T_S}{LI}, \qquad (3.3)$$

where λ is a function of the age distribution of the cell population and can vary between the limits of 0.693 and 1.38. It is a parameter that can be calculated for any given population but only if the complete growth characteristics are known. We have chosen to assign a value of 0.8 to this parameter based on observations in experimental tumours (WILSON et al. 1992). BEGG et al. (1988) have chosen a value of 1.0 for λ. This is only an operational difference, as the ranking of tumours will remain unaltered.

In his original publication, Begg pointed out that the assumptions may not be entirely true and that certain situations may profoundly influence the calculation of T_S using the RM method. In particular Begg drew attention to the fact that, theoretically, the RM plot is not linear as there should be an inflection at $G_2 + M$ and that cell populations with long $G_2 + M$ durations will bias the T_S result to a faster value owing to their persistence in the region used to define the BUdR-labelled cohort.

WHITE and MEISTRICH (1986) addressed some of these problems by attempting to derive RM_0 rather than assume 0.5. Using a complex series of derivations they showed that:

$$RM_0 = \frac{P_S - Z}{Z(P_S + P_{G_2 + M})},$$ (3.4)

where

$$Z = \ln\left(\frac{1 + P_S + P_{G_2 + M}}{1 + P_{G_2 + M}}\right),$$

where P_S and $P_{G_2 + M}$ represent the proportion of cells in S phase and $G_2 + M$ and could be derived from the DNA profile. The slope (M) of the relative movement plot was shown to equal 0.5 T_S such that using Eq. 3.4, the T_S was:

$$RM_t = RM_0 + \frac{t}{2T_S}.$$ (3.5)

There are problems associated with this modification; in particular, the $G_2 + M$ population may not always be well defined and may require computer modelling to extract it from the DNA profile. Secondly, it is our experience that a large proportion of G_2 cells in solid tumours (up to 50%) do not appear to divide even though cells labelled in S phase have done so (see Fig. 3.3). This latter phenomenon is also the reason why we do not attempt to calculate the $G_2 + M$ population and include it in our correction of LI.

The most recent derivation from the Houston group (WHITE et al. 1990) has put the computation of T_{pot} on a much more rigorous mathematical footing. This method introduced the parameter v, which is a function of the fraction of labelled divided cells (F^{1d}) and fraction of labelled undivided cells (F^{1u}). This value relates T_S to T_{pot} and is only weakly dependent on the time following labelling. It is calculated using the same regions as with RM except that fractions of cells are used rather than mean DNA contents:

$$v = \ln\left[\frac{1 + F^{1u}}{1 - \dfrac{F^{1d}}{2}}\right].$$ (3.6)

Using v, it is also possible to obtain an independent estimate of RM_0 making the assumption that $T_{G_2 + M}$ is approximately 0.3 T_S. Thus for the most common situation in human tumours where the observation is made at times greater that $T_{G_2 + M}$

but shorter that $T_S + T_{G_2 + M}$:

$$RM_0 = \left[\frac{1 - e^{-v} - ve^{-1.3v}}{v(1 - e^{-1.3v})}\right].$$ (3.7)

The T_S can be calculated using the RM-type analysis but using Eqs. 3.7 and 3.5.

The T_{pot} was shown to be:

$$T_{pot} = \ln(2)\frac{T_S}{v}.$$ (3.8)

This method, although more complicated, has several advantages: (a) it is not necessary to correct LI for cell division, (b) linear S-phase progression does not need to be assumed and (c) assumptions regarding the values of RM_0 (i.e. 0.5) and λ (i.e. 0.8 or 1.0) are unnecessary.

3.3 What Derivation of T_{pot} Should We Use?

The work of White and colleagues now leaves us in a quandary as to which method we should be using to calculate T_{pot}. The problem is that the absolute value of T_{pot} is different when measured using the Begg method and the White method. To illustrate the differences, Fig. 3.4 shows the results obtained in 148 squamous cell cancers from the head and neck region which have been calculated using our standard method and the v function.

In Fig. 3.4A, it can be seen that the v function and the corrected LI are almost exactly correlated. This is not surprising as they are derived in virtually the same way, based on correcting for the appearance of BUdR-labelled cells that have divided. The median v and corrected LI (expressed as a proportion) were identical with a value of 0.049.

The discrepancy between the two methods arises in the calculation of T_S. The median T_S using the standard Begg method was 9.7 h for this group of tumours whilst it was 16.3 h using the White method. The results are highly significantly different both by paired and by unpaired analysis. However, it can be seen from Fig. 3.4B that the results are correlated. The closeness of the correlation depends on the RM_t; the higher the RM_t, the better the correlation. This arises because of the RM_0 value. In the Begg method it is assumed to be 0.5, whilst in the White method it is derived as in Eq. 3.7. It would appear that the derived RM_0 could also be regarded as a constant. In the 148 tumours described above, the mean RM_0 was 0.608 with a standard deviation of 0.005 and a range of 0.593–0.615.

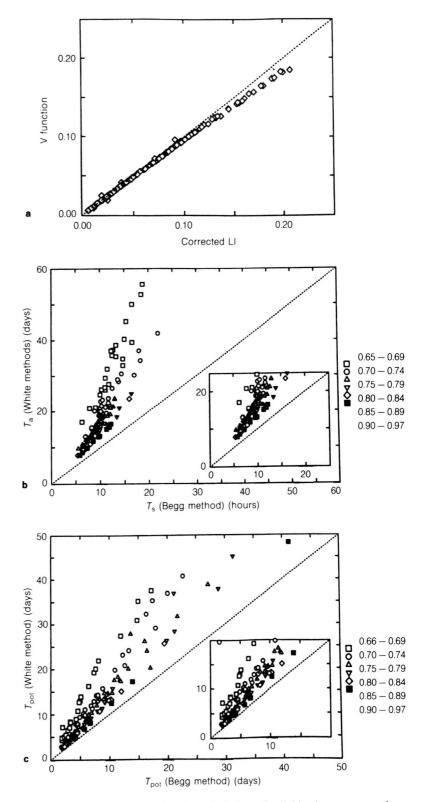

Fig. 3.4. Comparison of the Begg method and the White method for the calculation of cell kinetic parameters from BUdR/DNA staining profiles of head and neck tumours. The comparison of T_s and T_{pot} has been subdivided according to the observed RM value at the time of biopsy. The *insets* show the correlation over a restricted range at the faster end of T_s and T_{pot}. The *dotted lines* represent the line of exact correlation

The difference in T_S between the two methods of analysis translates into a difference in the ultimate parameter, the T_{pot}. However, through the vagaries of the two methods, the differences are reduced. They are reduced because v and corrected LI are almost identical and because White introduces an exponential term (0.693) into the calculation of T_{pot} from T_S and v whereas we use a factor of 0.8 for λ. Again the median T_{pot} values are highly significantly different on both paired and unpaired analysis. The median T_{pot} using the Begg method was 6.3 days but it was 9.9 days with the v function. However, the results were highly correlated with a Spearman's correlation of 0.90. When the data were log transformed the Pearson correlation coefficient (r^2) was 0.897, which has a P value greater than 0.0001. This means that discrimination of "fast" and "slow" proliferating populations based on medians or log-transformed means would not be compromised by the choice of method of analysis of T_{pot}. However, if an absolute value of T_{pot} has biological significance for selection of tumours that may benefit from altered treatment schedules, then the two methods do not give the same information.

Which is the right method? This still remains unanswered and can only be answered fully in the clinical setting. This will be discussed later in conjunction with results obtained with histological evaluation of BUdR LIs. These data sets can be transformed to give almost equivalent T_{pot} values by employing the suggestion made by Begg in 1985 that an RM_0 of 0.6 may be better than 0.5 when the $G_2 + M$ is relatively long. Using on RM_0 of 0.6 in the Begg method gives the results obtained in Fig. 3.5, where T_{pots} are now even more highly

correlated and almost, but not quite, the same, the median values being 9.9 and 8.8 for the White and Begg methods respectively.

Without the final proof of clinical significance there are several factors which may influence the choice of method of analysis. First, the simplicity of the procedure. There is no doubt that the Begg method is simpler and easier to understand, which can be factor influencing the use of such measurements. Although the White method does not make the same assumptions as the Begg method, some assumptions are still made, e.g.: (a) that there is an exponentially growing population with a steady-state distribution of cells with quiescent cells in G_1 (to introduce the exponential term in Eq. 3.8) and (b) that $T_{G_2 + M}$ is 0.3 T_S (for calculation of RM_0). Intuitively, the T_S values obtained by the White method appear a little long in relation to the profile obtained on the flow cytometer. A simple visual check can be made by measuring, with a ruler, the distance between G_1 and the trailing left-hand edge of the BUdR-labelled cohort and the distance to $G_2 + M$. This gives T_S values higher than Begg but lower than White.

In conclusion, this section remains with a question mark until clinical results are obtained. However, the data should be generated using both methods as exactly the same regions of analysis are used for the flow cytometry.

3.4 The Problem of "Normal" Cells

Although flow cytometry has many advantageous attributes for the study of proliferation, precision

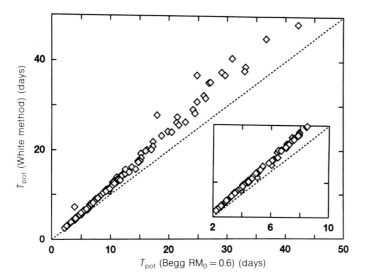

Fig. 3.5. Convergence of results using the Begg method and the White method using the assumption that RM_0 equals 0.6. The *inset* shows the relationship over the clinically meaningful range of proliferation rate

of measurement, speed and quantitative power, there is a major problem with the standard BUdR/DNA staining technique. The problem is the difficulty in distinguishing malignant cells from normal cells in biopsy or resection material. There can only be true separation of non-malignant cells when the DNA index is greater than tetraploid.

In tumours where the DNA index is greater than 1 but less than 2, an approximation of the true tumour cell proliferation can be made by excluding cells to the left of aneuploid G_1 peak from the calculation. This has been done in Fig. 3.3, where the total cell population LI was 10.8% but that in the aneuploid population (defined by regions 2 and 3) was 13.3%. As in this case, the procedure usually results in a higher LI by removing the diluting influence of non-proliferating normal cells. In some tumours both the diploid and aneuploid cells and proliferating, suggesting two tumour stem lines. In these hypotetraploid tumours, there will be some diploid S and G_2 cells overlapping into the aneuploid population which cannot be discriminated on the basis of DNA content.

The greatest problems are found in diploid tumours, where there is no possibility of accurately predicting proliferation in the tumour cell component with two-parameter flow cytometry.

There are two approaches to overcome these problems, i.e. three-parameter flow cytometry or immunohistochemistry.

3.4.1 Three-Colour Flow Cytometry

Three-colour flow cytometry exploits one of the other main attributes of flow cytometry: the ability to make several simultaneous measurements on the same object. A recent report (BEGG and HOFLAND 1991) has employed an antibody (CAM5.2) specific for cells of epithelial origin, in conjunction with the detection of BUdR and staining of DNA. With such an approach, non-malignant tumour cells which consist of mainly lymphocytes, macrophages, fibroblasts and endothelial cells can be discriminated by their lack of staining with the cytokeratin and on the basis of their DNA content.

In the past, this type of three-colour analysis would have been restricted to the more powerful and less user-friendly flow cytometers, but now it is relatively straightforward with the modern bench-top machine.

There is one major disadvantage with the use of antibodies to cytoplasmic antigens in that it pre-cludes the use of pepsin. As mentioned previously, the use of fixation in alcohol and dissociation in pepsin has been a major source of improvement in the technique of using BUdR for human tumour studies. Not only are the staining profiles improved, but the amount of material required is less due to both the improvement in yield and, probably more importantly, the ease of use in the clinical setting. There is no need for cell suspensions to be made when the biopsy is removed and so no need for specialist facilities or prompt collection. The production of cell suspensions of good quality is an art in itself whilst the use of pepsin is less fraught with problems and means that all specimens can be handled in a similar way.

In summary, this method can be applied to human tumours, with the assumption that good cell suspensions can be made, and should improve the accuracy of cell kinetic measurements on clinical material using a flow cytometric-only approach.

3.4.2 Immunohistochemistry

The other procedure to overcome the problem of discriminating non-malignant and malignant cells is to use immunohistochemical localisation of BUdR and the skills of the pathologist.

In many respects, this is a retrograde step for flow cytometry and is similar to the approach of using ^{3}H-TdR and autoradiography. However, when used in combination with the in vivo administration of BUdR and flow cytometry, it is a very powerful technique. In the past, studies with ^{3}H-TdR were often carried out on either cell suspensions or tissue fragments such that the true tissue architectural information was lost. There were often problems associated with artefacts of in vitro staining techniques due to DNA precursor penetration and viability of the tissue. The administration of BUdR in vivo overcomes these problems although it will be subject to variation due to poor diffusion and transient alteration in vascular perfusion. The advantage is that the complete specimen can be studied and this is particularly important in resection material where the growing edge can be discriminated from the necrotic core tissue and microscopic heterogeneity studies.

We have used this approach in a study of head and neck cancer (BENNETT et al. 1992) in which the problem of discrimination of non-malignant cells was particularly acute due to the relatively low

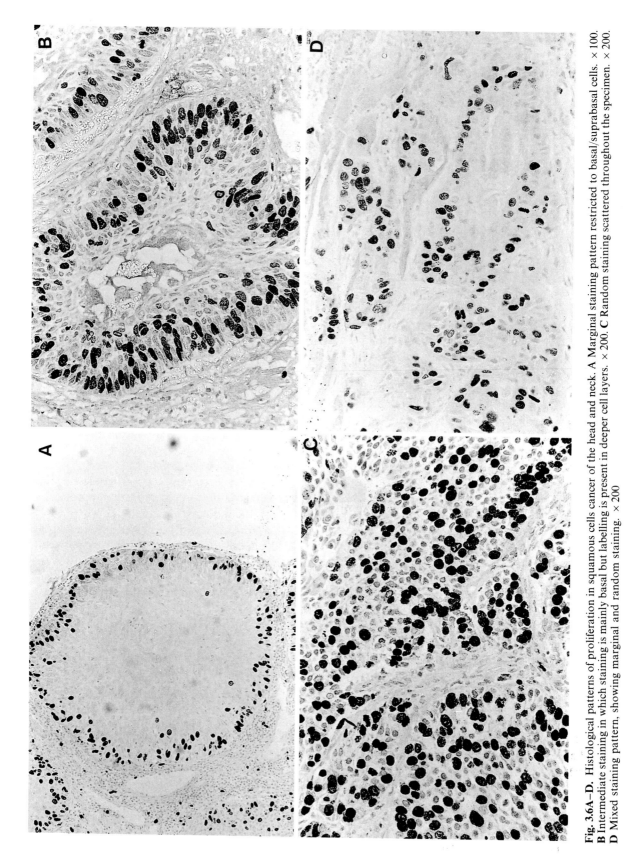

Fig. 3.6A–D. Histological patterns of proliferation in squamous cells cancer of the head and neck. A Marginal staining pattern restricted to basal/suprabasal cells. × 100. B Intermediate staining in which staining is mainly basal but labelling is present in deeper cell layers. × 200. C Random staining scattered throughout the specimen. × 200. D Mixed staining pattern, showing marginal and random staining. × 200

incidence of aneuploidy (40%). In this study, representative samples were taken for both flow cytometry and histopathology. Using flow cytometry, we measured DNA index, LI, T_S and T_{pot}. With immunohistochemistry, the average tumour cell LI and a maximum tumour cell LI were quantitated, the type of staining pattern was classified and the number of BUdR-labelled mitoses counted and the standard histopathological parameters reported (e.g. grade). The information from flow cytometry regarding the proportion of BUdR-labelled divided and undivided cells was used to correct the histological LI as there will obviously be daughter cells produced between injection and biopsy in the tissue section. The flow cytometry-generated T_S was then used in conjunction with the histological LIs to produce a hybrid T_{pot}.

The results from this study draw into question any statements made about proliferation in diploid tumours and how they compare with aneuploid tumours. Prior to this analysis I highlighted the differences between diploid and aneuploid tumours in terms of their BUdR proliferation characteristics (WILSON 1991). In every group of tumours we have studied, the median LI and median T_S have been lower or shorter in the diploid tumours found within each tumour group. These observations would fit into the generally held belief that progression to aneuploidy is associated with a proliferative advantage.

In head and neck cancer, we have measured a median LI of 4.6% for diploid tumours and 10.7% for aneuploids, whilst the T_S was 9.0 and 11.7 h respectively. These values result in very different T_{pots} of 6.8 and 3.9 days, emphasising the apparent proliferative differences between diploid and aneuploid cancer.

Histological evaluation revealed a very different picture. The average corrected histological LI was actually higher in diploid tumours, at a value of 17%, than it was in aneuploid tumours (14%). The latter value was quite similar to the 11% measured by flow cytometry for the same aneuploid tumours and suggests there is no cell selection problem using the flow cytometry techniques. The small discrepancy between the two can be accounted for by the presence of non-malignant S and G_2 cells in many of the flow cytometry staining profiles as none of the aneuploid tumours had a DNA index greater than 2. It should also be pointed out that there was no difference in the presence of "normal" and malignant cells in the make-up of diploid and aneuploid squamous cell cancers. The median percentage of

tumour cells was 45% in both groups, determined on histopathological criteria.

The combination of histological LI and flow cytometry T_S produces the surprising finding that the median T_{pot} was shorter in diploid (2.1 days) than in aneuploid tumours (2.8 days). We have now extended these studies to lung, oesophagus, cervix, and colorectal cancers and in each case the apparent proliferative difference between diploid and aneuploid cancers has been drastically reduced or abolished.

The key to the difference in proliferation between diploid and aneuploid cancers may lie in the modes of cell death and cell loss. The study by BENNETT et al. (1992) classified four staining patterns based on their BUdR localisation: marginal, intermediate, random and mixed (Fig. 3.6). Marginal staining (Fig. 3.6A) was restricted to the basal and suprabasal layer whilst intermediate staining (Fig. 3.6B) showed that presence of labelled cells in the next few layers as well. Tumours with the random staining pattern (Fig. 3.6C) showed labelled cells scattered throughout the specimen. The mixed pattern (Fig. 3.6D) could be a combination of the three distinct patterns, one of which was usually random. These patterns were related, but not identical, to histological grade. When the proliferative organisation is marginal or intermediate it is possible to conceive a "normal" pathway of cell death by proliferation, migration, differentiation, maturation and exfoliation as well as apoptosis and necrosis. When the staining pattern is mixed and random, the differentiation pathway to cell loss will not be in operation. This may well result in cell loss not only being different but less in tumours of this type; in general, aneuploidy is more frequent in the higher grade tumours.

The result of the histological studies may have a profound influence on the selection of patients who might be considered for treatment regimens such as accelerated fractionation. Table 3.2 shows that the percentage of primary squamous cell

Table 3.2. The percentage of tumours with T_{pots} less than 1, 2, 3, 4 or 5 days measured using flow cytometry alone or a combination of flow cytometry T_s and average LI of tumour cells only

Days	T_{pot} (days)	
	Flow cytometry	Average histology
< 1	0	8
< 2	4	38
< 3	19	63
< 4	31	80
< 5	46	84

cancers with T_{pots} less than 5 days was only 46% when assessed by flow cytometry but 84% when histological information was used. There were 63% of tumours with T_{pots} less than 3 days using the hybridised T_{pot} measurement. In every tumour studied, irrespective of the overall proliferation rate, there were areas where the LI was very high (30%–50%). The T_{pots} in foci of proliferating cells such as these were less than 1 day. The significance of these rapidly proliferating zones has yet to be established.

In summary, immunohistochemical quantitation of BUdR can overcome the shortcomings of flow cytometry in analysing proliferation in diploid tumours as well as add information on heterogeneity and organisation of proliferation. Tritiated thymidine and autoradiography were never used clinically to determine treatment because they were slow and laborious, but modern immunohistochemistry can achieve results within 1 or 2 days and quantitation by a trained pathologist or biologist or, better still, by image analysis can be rapid.

3.5 The Biological Significance of T_{pot}

The potential doubling time is defined as the doubling time taking into account the presence of dividing and non-dividing cells (the growth fraction) in the absence of cell loss (STEEL 1977). It is undoubtedly a more complete and better measurement of proliferation than LI or S-phase fraction, but the question remains as to whether it can predict repopulation potential or response to therapy. The key cell in determining response to therapy is the surviving clonogenic cell, of which little is known biologically. Although treatment will perturb the proliferation of surviving tumour cells, there is some support from radiobiology that T_{pot} may indicate the potential for proliferation during radiotherapy. These data come from analysis of clinical data on cure dose (TCD_{50}) for different overall treatment times (WITHERS et al. 1988) and split-course radiotherapy schedules (AMDUR et al. 1989; TAYLOR et al. 1990). In studies such as these, estimates of the effective doubling times of surviving clonogenic cells during the period without treatment can be made by making assumptions about the loss of local tumour control or the extra dose required to achieve the same local control compared to a schedule without a split. FOWLER (1986) calculated that head and neck tumours have effective doubling times in the region of 3–6 days, assuming that a 10%–15% increase in local control is equivalent to a 10% increase in total dose and that a log increase in dose represents 3.3 cell doublings. These effective doubling times, and others that have been calculated (BUDIHNA et al. 1980), are similar to the measurements of pretreatment T_{pot} the have been made in these groups of tumours (WILSON et al. 1988; BEGG et al. 1988). There is also evidence from experimental tumours that pretreatment T_{pot} may give a good indication of the proliferation rate of surviving cells measured using growth delay and local control assays (KUMMERMEHR and TROTT 1982; BEGG et al. 1991).

The test of BUdR or any prognostic parameter is whether it will be important enough to play a role in determining which treatment modality or schedule is the most appropriate for a particular patient or group of patients. This can only be fully answered in a controlled, randomised clinical trial. In general, proliferation measurements have failed to surmount this final hurdle. The combination of in vivo administration of halogenated pyrimidines and flow cytometric evaluation of T_{pot} is being used in two important multicentre trials of accelerated versus conventional fractionation.

The EORTC trial number 22851 is a phase III study of accelerated fractionation in the radiotherapy of advanced head and neck cancer. Conventional fractionation (70–72 Gy in 7–8 weeks, 1.8–2.0 Gy/fraction, 35–40 fractions) is being compared with accelerated fractionation (72 Gy in 5 weeks, 1.6 Gy/fraction, 3 fractions/day, 45 fractions) given with a split of 2 weeks after the first week of treatment. In this trial, there is the option to participate in cell kinetic measurements using IUdR. There have been two interim reports of the value of T_{pot} measurements in this trial (BEGG et al. 1990). The number of patients is still small, 60, with sufficient follow-up to be included in survival and local control analyses. The success rate for the cell kinetic analysis from biopsy material was 85%. However, there is a trend for tumours with short T_{pots} (less than 4.6 days) to do worse than those with longer T_{pots} in the conventional arm whilst there is no discernible effect of proliferation in the accelerated arm. The most recent results from this trial, as yet unpublished, have prompted the clinicians to attempt to study all remaining patients entered into the trial with IUdR.

In Great Britain, the success of CHART [continuous, hyperfractionated, acceleration radiation treatment (54 Gy in 36 fractions, 1.6 Gy/fraction,

3 fractions/day) (SAUNDERS et al. 1991)] in a pilot study has prompted the establishment of a multicentre phase III trial. In this trial, we are making measurements of T_{pot} using BUdR. We have no results, as yet, from the randomised trial but do have data from patients treated in the pilot study (LOCHRIN et al. 1992). In this study can be seen that, as described for the EORTC trial, there is no profound influence of proliferation on the response of tumours to accelerated radiotherapy (Fig. 3.7). There was a trend for the more slowly proliferating tumours to do worse that the fast when categorised above and below the median value but these differences were far from significant. There was also no influence of aneuploidy; this supports the histological evidence that there is no difference in proliferation between diploid and aneuploid tumours. It remains to be seen whether the data generated from histological analysis of proliferation will influence the outcome of radiotherapy. These analyses are underway.

In both sets of clinical data presented above, the median or close to median value has been used to stratify the patients to assess the influence of proliferation on clinical outcome. It remains to be seen whether tumours need to be subclassified into "fast", "slow" or "intermediate" proliferation using cut-offs such as less than 3 days, more than 7 days and the grey area in between. It may also be that several biopsies need to be taken and individual coefficients of variation (CVs) calculated to properly classify tumours into appropriate subgroups. However, data for head and neck tumours (BENNETT et al. 1992; BEGG et al. 1988) suggest that intratumour heterogeneity in T_{pot} was not very large: CVs of 30% and 23% respectively. This may not be the case for all tumours considered for radiotherapy. HAUSTERMANS et al. (1992) showed that at least three biopsies were necessary in oesophageal cancers to obtain representative results. Similarly, in colorectal cancer, considerable variation in T_{pot} was seen (REW et al. 1991) such

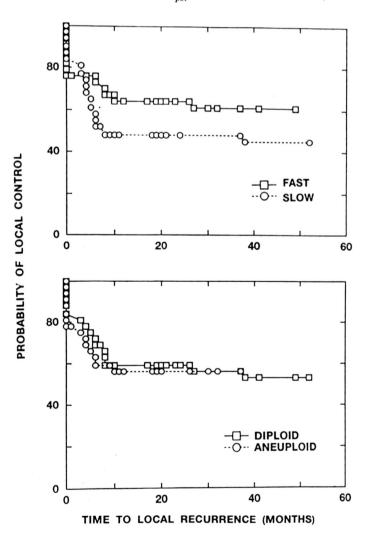

Fig. 3.7. The influence of proliferation and DNA aneuploidy on the local tumour control rate of patients with squamous cell cancer of the head and neck region treated by CHART. The data have been subdivided based on the median value where fast and slow are below or above a flow cytometry-derived T_{pot} value of 4.3 days or as diploid and aneuploid

that one biopsy was insufficient to correctly classify tumours. Clearly, it is not always possible to take more than one biopsy in patients who will undergo radiotherapy; the validity of the results will then depend on the skill of the clinician in selecting the appropriate biopsy site.

Only when a large body of biological data have been established on T_{pot} in clinical trials will its significance be established, and only then will we be able to answer the question of what cut-off should be used for selecting patients for appropriate schedules. Calculations suggest that the faster the doubling times of clonogenic cells, the shorter the optimal treatment time (FOWLER 1990), and that CHART may only benefit patients in which the tumour cell doubling time is less that 3 days (TUCKER and CHAN 1990). Clearly, the combination of histology and flow cytometry would indicate that many patients may benefit from shorter treatment schedules.

The momentum is gathering for BUdR studies. For all its potential problems, as outlined in this chapter, it is still the best available method to measure proliferation in the clinical setting. Only time will tell whether the plm curve shown in Fig. 3.1 will reflect a new dawn in the history of cell kinetics where these measurements finally achieve clinical significance or whether the interest in cell kinetics will again wane, to await the next development.

Acknowledgement. This work was supported by the Cancer Research Campaign. I acknowledge the help and inspiration of my colleagues Chris Martindale at the Gray Laboratory and Professor Stanley Dische and Dr. Michele Saunders at the Marie Curie Research Wing. I also acknowledge the part played in these studies by my late colleagues Dr. Nicolas McNally and Dr. Mike Bennett, to whom I dedicate this chapter. I thank Paula Reynolds for preparation of the manuscript.

References

Amdur RJ, Parsons JT, Mendenhall WM, Million RR, Cassisi NJ (1989) Split-course versus continuous-course irradiation in the post-operative setting for squamous cell carcinoma of the head and neck. Int J Radait oncol Biol Phys 17: 279–285

Barlogie B, Raber NM, Schumann J et al. (1983) Flow cytometry in clinical cancer research. Cancer Res 43: 3982–3997

Begg AC, Hofland I (1991) Cell kinetic analysis of mixed populations using three colour fluorescence flow cytometry. Cytometry 12: 445–454

Begg AC, NcNally NJ, Shrieve DC, Karcher H (1985) A method to measure the DNA synthesis and the potential doubling time from a single sample. Cytometry 6: 620–626

Begg AC, Moonen L, Hofland I, Dessing M, Bartelink H (1988) Human tumour cell kinetics using a monoclonal antibody against iododeoxyuridine: intratumour sampling variations. Radiother Oncol 11: 337–347

Begg AC, Hofland I, Moonen L et al. (1990) The predictive value of cell kinetic measurements in a European trial of accelerated fractionation in advanced head and neck tumours: an interim report. Int J Radiat Oncol Bio Phys 19: 1449–1453

Begg AC, Hofland I, Kummermehr J (1991) Tumour cell repopulation during fractionated radiotherapy: correlation between flow cytometric and radiobiological data in three murine tumours. Eur J Cancer 27: 537–543

Begg AC, Hofland I, van Glabekke M, Bartelink H, Horiot JC (1992) Predictive value of potential doubling time for radiotherapy of head and neck tumour patients: results from the EORTC co-operative trial 22851. Semin Radiat Oncol 2: 22–25

Bennett MH, Wilson GD, Dische S et al. (1992) Tumour proliferation assessed by combined histological and flow cytometric analysis: implications for therapy in squamous cell carcinoma in the head and neck. Br J Cancer 65: 870–878

Böhmer R-M, Ellvart J (1981) Combination of BrdUrd-quenched Hoechst fluorescence with DNA-specific ethidium bromide fluorescence for cell cycle analysis with a two parametrical flow cytometer. Cell Tissue Kinet 14: 653–658

Budihna M, Skrk M, Smid L, Furlan L (1980) Tumour cell repopulation in the rest interval of split-course radiation treatment. Strahlentherapie 156: 402–408

Danova M, Riccardi A, Mazzini G (1990) Cell cycle-related proteins and flow cytometry. Haematologica 75: 252–264

Darzynkiewicz Z, Traganos F, Sharpless T, Melamed MR (1977) Cell cycle related changes in nuclear chromatin of stimulated lymphocytes as measured by flow cytometry. Cancer Res 37:4635–4640

Dolbeare F, Gratzner HG, Pallavicini M, Gray JW (1983) Flow cytometric measurment of total DNA content and incorporated bromodeoxyuridine. Pro Soc Natl Acad Sci 80: 5573–5577

Fowler JF (1986) Potential for increasing the differential response between tumours and normal tissues: can proliferation rate be used? Int J Radiat Oncol Biol Phys 12: 641–645

Fowler JF (1990) How worthwhile are short schedules in radiotherapy? A series of exploratory calculations. Radiother Oncol 18:165–181

Goz B (1978) The effects of incorporation of 5-halogenated deoxyuridines into the DNA of eukaryotic cells. Pharmacol Rev 29: 249–272

Gratzner HG (1982) Monoclonal antibody to 5-bromo and 5-iododeoxyuridine: a new reagent for detection of DNA replication. Science 218: 474–475

Hall PA, Levison DA (1990) Assessment of cell proliferation in histological material. J Clin Pathol 43: 184–192

Haustermans K, Geboes K, Lerut T, Vam Thillo J, Coasemans W, Waer M, van der Schueren E (1992) Tumour cell kinetics and EGFr expression in oesophageal cancer and cancer of the gastro-oesophageal junction. Radiother Oncol 24: abstract 349

Howard A, Pelc SR (1951) Nuclear incorporation of ^{32}P as demonstrated by autoradiographs. Exp Cell Res 2: 178–187

Kummermehr J, Trott KR (1982) Rate of repopulation in a slow and fast growing mouse tumour. In: Karcher KH (ed) Progress in radio-oncology II. Raven, New York

Latt SA (1973) Microfluorometric detection of deoxyribonucleic acid replication in human metaphase chromosomes. Proc Soc Natl Acad Sci USA 70: 3395–3402

Lochrin D, Wilson GD, McNally NJ, Dische S, Saunders MI (1992) Tumour cell kinetics, local tumour control and accelerated radiotherapy: a preliminary report. Int J Radiat Oncol Biol Phys 24: 87–91

Quastler H, Sherman FG (1959) Cell population kinetics in the intestinal epithelium of the mouse. Exp Cell Res 17: 420–428

Rew DA, Wilson GD, Taylor I, Weaver PC (1991) The in vivo proliferation of human colorectal cancer. Br J Surg 78: 60–66

Saunders MI, Dische S, Grosch EJ, Fermont DC, Ashford RFU, Maher EJ, Makepeace AR (1991) Experience with CHART. Int J Radiat Oncol Biol Phys 21: 871–878

Schutte B, Reynders MM, van Assche CL, Hupperets PS, Bosman FT, Blijham GH (1987) An improved method for the immunocytochemical detection of bromodeoxy-uridine labelled nuclei using flow cytometry. Cytometry 8: 372–376

Steel GG (1977) Growth kinetics of tumours. Clarendon, Oxford

Taylor JH, Woods PS, Hughes WL (1957) The organisation and duplication of chromosomes using tritiated thymidine. Proc Soc Natl Acad Sci USA 43: 122–128

Taylor JMG, Withers HR, Mendenhall WM (1990) Dose-time considerations of head and neck squamous cell carcinomas treated with irradiation. Radiother Oncol 17: 95–102

Terry NHA, White RA, Meistrich ML, Calkins DP (1991) Evaluation of flow cytometric methods for determining population potential doubling times using cultured cells. Cytometry 11: 234–241

Tubiana M, Courdi A (1989) Cell proliferation kinetics in human solid tumours; relation to probability of meta-static dissemination and long term survival. Radiother Oncol 15:1–18

Tucker SL, Chan K-S (1990) The selection of patients for accelerated radiotherapy on the basis of tumour growth kinetics and intrinsic radiosensitivity. Radiother Oncol 18: 197–211

Wheeless LL, Coon JS, Cox C et al. (1991) Precision of DNA flow cytometry in inter-institutional analyses. Cytometry 12: 405–412

White RA, Meistrich ML (1986) A comment on: a method to measure the duration of DNA synthesis and the potential doubling time from a single sample. Cytometry 7: 486–490

White RA, Terry NHA (1992) A quantitative method for evaluating bivariate flow cytometric data obtained using monoclonal antibodies to bromodeoxyuridine. Cytometry 13: 490–495

White RA, Terry NHA, Meistrich ML, Calkins DP (1990) An improved method for computing the potential doubling time using monoclonal antibodies to bromo-deoxyuridine. Cytometry 11: 314–317

Wilson GD (1991) Assessment of human tumour prolifera-tion using bromodeoxyuridine: current status. Acta Oncol 30: 903–910

Wilson GD (1992) Cell kinetic sudies using a monoclonal antibody to bromodeoxyuridine. In: Manson M (ed) Methods in molecular biology, vol 10. Immunochemical Protocols. Humana, New Jersey, pp 387–393

Wilson GD, McNally NJ, Dunphy E, Pfragner R, Karcher H (1985) The labelling index of human and mouse tumours assessed by bromodeoxyuridine staining in vivo and in vitro and flow cytometry. Cytometry 6: 641–647

Wilson GD, McNally NJ, Dische S, Saunders MI, des Rochers C, Lewis AA, Bennett MH (1988) Measurement of cell kinetics in human tumours in vivo using bromo-deoxyuridine incorporation and flow cytometry. Br J Cancer 58: 423–431

Wilson GD, Martindale CA, Soranson JA, Carl UM, McNally NJ (1992) Proliferative changes in two murine tumours in response to single or fractionated doses of X-rays. Cell Proliferation 25: 415–430

Wilson MS, West CML, Wilson GD, Roberts SA, James RD, Schofield PF (1993) The reliability and reproducibility of measurements of potential doubling times (T_{pot}) on human colorectal cancers. Br J Cancer 67: 754–759

Withers HR, Taylor JMG, Maciejewski B (1988) The hazard of accelerated tumour clonogen repopulation during radio-therapy. Acta Oncol 27: 131–146

4 Hyperfractionation

H.R. WITHERS

CONTENTS

4.1 Introduction

Hyperfractionation involves the administration of a larger number of smaller dose fractions, resulting in an increased total dose given in approximately the same overall time as in conventional therapy. Its purpose is to increase the biological dose to the tumor without an increase in the biological dose to late-responding normal tissues. Although there are variations among centers in what is "conventional," for present purposes it is assumed to be 1.8–2 Gy per fraction, five times per week. In practice, hyperfractionation is usually given as more than one treatment per day, although administering treatment 7 days per week could permit a modest reduction in dose per fraction.

One of the initial rationales for this departure was that increasing the number of interfraction intervals increases the frequency of cell cycle redistribution among surviving tumor clonogens, without a similar phenomenon occurring in the nonproliferative, late-responding, dose-limiting normal tissues (WITHERS 1975; SHUKOVSKY et al. 1976). A second rationale was that the oxygen enchancement ratio was found to be lower at low doses and therefore, if a proportion of the cells in a tumor were hypoxic, they would be less radioresistant if the dose per fraction was lowered (REVESZ et al. 1975; LITTBRAND

H.R. WITHERS, MD, DSc, Professor, Department of Radiation Oncology, UCLA Medical Center, Los Angeles, CA 90024-1714, USA

et al. 1975; EDSMYR et al. 1985). Furthermore, the higher the dose per fraction, the more a hypoxic subpopulation of tumor cells will limit the effectiveness of each treatment (POWERS and TOLMACH 1963). With effective reoxygenation, a small proportion of hypoxic cells within the tumor would have little influence on the response to sequential small dose fractions whereas they could affect responses to high doses (WITHERS and PETERS 1980). More recently, after trials of hyperfractionation had actually begun, a third, more powerful rationale emerged: dose fractionation provides greater sparing for all late-responding tissues which have been studied, relative to both acute effects and most of the small number of tumors whose responses to clinically relevant dose fractions have been assessed (THAMES et al. 1982; BARENDSEN 1982; WITHERS et al. 1983b; THAMES and HENDRY 1987). Thus, by reducing dose per fraction, it is possible to increase the total dose without any increase in the incidence of late effects provided interfraction intervals are sufficiently long for complete repair of sublethal damage. Because the dose required for the same rate of response of tumors is not comparably increased by hyperfractionation, the therapeutic ratio between the tumor and late sequelae can be improved.

The differential in sparing between late-responding and early-responding tissues and, by analogy, most tumors, is interpreted, in radiobiological terms, as reflecting differences in the shapes of the survival curves for the respective target cells. The late-responding tissues are characterized by a curvy survival curve whereas early-responding tissues and most tumor cells have a survival curve which is more closely exponential over the dose ranges of clinical interest (Fig. 4.1). Changes in dose per fraction will have little effect on acute responses and a larger effect on late responses (THAMES et al. 1982; WITHERS et al. 1982a; BARENDSEN 1982). This characteristic difference in the x-ray response of early- and late-responding tissues is highlighted by the lack of a similar sparing effect on late-

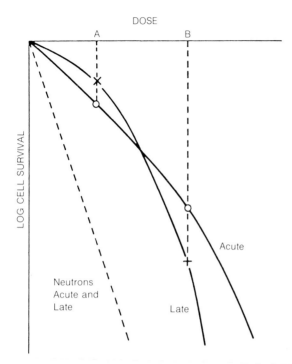

Fig. 4.1. Hypothetical cell survival curves showing a systematic difference in the responses to x-rays of the target cells for early- and late-responding normal tissues. The curviness of the response of the target cells for late-responding tissues illustrates the greater change in response of these tissues to change in dose per fraction in a multifraction regimen. The differential is not apparent at clinically relevant neutron doses. (From WITHERS et al. 1982b)

responding tissues in clinical trials of fractionated dose neutron therapy (WITHERS et al. 1982b), reflecting the linearity of cell survival curves for both early- and late-responding tissues exposed to neutrons (Fig. 4.1). It has become popular to describe the shape of survival curves in terms of a linear-quadratic survival equation (LEA 1956; DOUGLAS and FOWLER 1976; THAMES et al. 1982). The linear component of cell killing, and thus the initial slope of the survival curve, is described by α and the curvature is introduced by the quadratic relationship for cell killing, with a coefficient β, which causes a continuous bending of the survival curve. The lower the α/β ratio, the curvier the survival curve and the greater the capacity for recovery when the radiation dose is fractionated. Tissues characterized by high α/β ratios show little fractionation response. Some representative values for α/β are shown in Table 4.1.

The ratio of the α and β coefficients can be used to describe the slopes of isoeffect curves without knowing their absolute values (THAMES et al.1982). Thus, it is possible to determine the α/β ratio from comparisons of total doses needed for gross isoeffects in vivo as a function of size of dose per fraction. Conversely, the ratios of total doses necessary for an isoeffect as a function of the size of dose per fraction can be described by a simple formula (WITHERS et al. 1983a):

$$\frac{D_1}{D_2} = \frac{\alpha/\beta + d_2}{\alpha/\beta + d_1},$$

D_1 and D_2 being total doses for a constant effect using dose fractions of d_1 and d_2, respectively, all doses being expressed in Gy.

4.2 Exploratory and Nonrandomized Studies

A series of exploratory studies using hyperfractionation were initiated in the early 1970s, based, as mentioned above, on the concept of exploiting cell cycle redistribution or reduced oxygen enhancement ratios, with increasing interest during the 1980s in exploiting differentials in α/β ratios between late-responding normal tissues and tumors. These initial studies involved a variety of tumor sites: bladder (BACKSTROM et al. 1973; LITTBRAND et al. 1975; EDSMYR et al. 1985; COX et al. 1988), head and neck (SHUKOVSKY et al. 1976; JAMPOLIS et al. 1977; MEOZ et al. 1984; MARCIAL et al. 1987; PARSONS et al. 1988, 1993; WENDT et al. 1989; COX et al. 1990), brain (DOUGLAS et al. 1982), brain stem

Table 4.1. Some representative α/β values for normal tissues and tumors

α/β ratio (Gy)[a]	Normal tissues	Tumors[b]
> 10	Epithelia: Jejunum Skin Testis	Epitheliomas: Oropharynx Lung Cervix Murine fibrosarcomas
5–10	Melanocytes Bone marrow Colonic mucosa	Skin epitheliomas
2–5	Connective tissues Bone Lung Kidney	Breast carcinomas Sarcomas
< 2	Spinal cord	Melanoma Liposarcoma

[a] Broad categorization of α/β values synthesized from Tables 2–1 and 3–2 in PEREZ and BRADY (1992)
[b] Hypoxia and reoxygenation in tumors would raise estimates of α/β ratios relative to values for the euoxic state. α/β ratios for tumors are discussed elsewhere in this volume (TROTT, Chap. 7)

(PACKER et al. 1987; FREEMAN et al. 1988; EDWARDS et al. 1989), and lung (SEYDEL et al. 1985; COX et al. 1990). Dose fractions ranged from 1 to 1.25 Gy. Total doses were ultimately about 15%–30% higher than the standard for 2-Gy fractions. In some cases, total doses began at lower levels than the standard for 2-Gy fractions (e.g., MARCIAL et al. 1987; SEYDEL et al. 1985) and escalated (COX et al. 1990). Even when total doses were not increased, or even lowered slightly, the local control rates were never worse than with standard regimens, and, in the larger head and neck series (PARSONS et al. 1988, 1993; WENDT et al. 1989), local failure rates were decreased by 25% to 50%. Acute reactions were also increased, as expected, but late sequelae were comparable with those from conventional treatment. In some clinics, hyperfractionation has become the standard treatment in many head and neck cancer sites (PARSONS et al. 1988, 1993).

Hyperfractionation improved the median survival times for patients with glioblastomas and brain stem tumors. A comparison of normal brain and brain stem responses to hyperfractionated and standard regimens is difficult, but there was no definite increase in late central nervous system toxicity, even though, in one series (EDWARDS et al. 1989), the total dose was about 30% higher than the standard for 1.8-Gy regimens.

The RTOG studies on head and neck (COX et al. 1990), bladder (COX et al. 1988), and lung (SEYDEL et al. 1985; COX et al. 1990) have progressed into randomized trials, the results of which are not yet available.

4.3 Randomized Studies

Randomized studies of hyperfractionation in head and neck cancer (Table 4.2) have been reported by the EORTC (HORIOT et al. 1993), and from India (DATTA et al. 1989). Studies by the RTOG are also in progress. The large EORTC study shows a significant reduction in local failure for T2–T3 squamous carcinomas of the oropharynx, from a 5-year actuarial failure rate of 60% to 42%, a 30% reduction. There was improved survival, with only a 1 in 12 chance that the improvement was not the result of the altered fractionation.

An important finding in the EORTC study was that late sequelae, plotted actuarially, were the same in the control and the experimental protocols. Using the linear-quadratic formula to interpret the results, it can be calculated that if 80.5 Gy given in 70

Table 4.2. Randomized studies of hyperfractionation

Site	Dose/dose per fraction/weeks	Local control	Author
Oropharynx T2–3	80.5/1.15/7 70/2/7	58% vs 40% (actuarial)	HORIOT et al. 1993
Head and neck T2–3	79.2/1.2/6.5 66/2/6.5	63% vs 33% (2 yr, absolute)	DATTA et al. 1989
Oropharynx T3–4	70.4/1.1/6.5 66/2/6.5	84% vs 64%[a] (3.5 yr, actuarial)	PINTO et al. 1991
Bladder T2–4	84/1/8[b] 64/2/8[b] (split course)	34% vs 22% (5-yr survival)	EDSMYR et al. 1985

[a] Primary tumor response only
[b] These doses were not isoeffective for late complications: the improvement may not be the result of hyperfractionation

fractions of 1.15 Gy is equivalent to 70 Gy given as 35 fractions of 2 Gy, then the α/β value for late-responding tissues in the head and neck would be about 4.5 Gy. Because of the difficulty in proving, with statistical significance, that two results are the same, the EORTC trial is *definitive* evidence neither for an α/β estimate of 4.5 Gy, nor that the doses used in the two arms were isoeffective for late sequelae (BENTZEN 1992): but it could not be shown that such assumptions are wrong.

Values greater than 10 Gy for the α/β ratio have been found for squamous cell carcinomas of the head and neck (MACIEJEWSKI et al. 1989). If the value were 25 Gy, it may be calculated that the total dose to achieve the same tumor control rate as 70 Gy in 2-Gy fractions would be only about 72.25 Gy in 1.15-Gy fractions. Since the total dose was increased to 80.5 Gy, the therapeutic gain factor, expressed as the ratio of the dose actually given and the dose which would have been necessary to yield a constant rate of tumor control, is 80.5/72.25 = 1.11. If the tumor α/β ratio was infinity, no adjustment of total dose for change in fraction size would be necessary, and the ratio of "biological" doses would be 80.5/70 = 1.15. Obviously, the lower the α/β value chosen for tumor response, the more similar the "biological" doses to tumor and late-responding normal tissues would be until, for a value of 4.5 Gy (as determined for the late-responding tissues), there would be no therapeutic differential between conventional and hyperfractionated regimens. However, using a reasonable α/β ratio of 25 Gy for tumor response, hyperfractionation should result in a biological dose to the tumor which is about 11% higher than 70 Gy in 2-Gy fractions: in contrast, the biological dose to late-responding tissues would be unchanged. The escalation in relative biological dose by about 11% resulted in about an 18 percentage point improvement in local control (HORIOT et al. 1993). This is consistent with calculations that a 1% increase in tumor dose would yield a 1.5%–2% increase in tumor control rate at around the 50% control level (BRAHME 1984; SUIT and WALKER 1988; TAYLOR and WITHERS 1993; THAMES et al. 1992).

The results of other randomized trials are shown in Table 4.2. The details of the randomized trial by DATTA et al. (1989) have not been fully published. PINTO et al. (1991) reported a single institutional trial in which the total dose in the hyperfractionated arm was only 7% higher than in controls. The local failure rate was more than halved, from 36% to 16% ($P < 0.02$). Locoregional results were not different in the two arms and survival was not improved with statistical significance. The trial in bladder cancer (EDSMYR et al. 1985) showed improved 5-year survival (from 22% to 34%, a 15% reduction in failure rate) but normal tissue sequelae were much more severe. Therefore, in a biological sense, the total dose of 84 Gy in 1-Gy fractions in the hyperfractionated arm was higher than the standard dose of 64 Gy in 2-Gy fractions. (For 84 Gy in 1-Gy fractions to be equivalent to 64 Gy in 2-Gy fractions would require the tissues to be characterized by an α/β value of 2.2 Gy.) Thus, although the trial was randomized, it does not establish that hyperfractionation is useful in bladder cancer.

4.4 Unresolved Problems

4.4.1 α/β Ratios

It is not established that all tumors are characterized by high α/β ratios. Some analyses have shown very low α/β ratios for some tumors and most human tumors studied to date have shown a greater fractionation response than squamous cell carcinomas of the head and neck (THAMES and SUIT 1986; BENTZEN et al. 1989; THAMES et al. 1990; PETERS et al. 1992). Thus, there may be categories of tumors, or subgroups within a given category, which would be more spared by hyperfractionated radiation therapy than the critical late-responding tissues within the treatment volume. Although α/β values for normal tissues do vary significantly, they would vary more for tumors because of greater heterogeneity in proliferation kinetics, oxygenation, and intrinsic radiosensitivity. At present, there are no sufficiently reliable prospective assays based on

estimating the α/β ratio for individual tumors which could permit selection of patients for inclusion or exclusion from hyperfractionated regimens: in fact, the data for whole classes of tumors are inadequate for reliable prognostication of the result of hyperfractionation (Table 4.1).

4.4.2 Repair Kinetics

The initial assumption that a 3- to 4-h interfraction interval was sufficient for essentially complete repair of sublethal cellular injury was wrong (WITHERS 1975). The kinetics of repair varies among tissues (THAMES and HENDRY 1987). Intervals shorter than 6 h should not be used if tissue tolerance is being threatened by high total doses. This is especially important with administration of more than two fractions per day and if the spinal cord is in the treatment volume (GUTTENBERGER et al. 1993). There is still a need for more detailed research on repair, especially since the addition of a slow component to a fast component introduces major complexities into its quantitation.

An unexplained increase in the incidence of myelopathy has been observed in a continuous hyperfractionated accelerated radiation therapy (CHART) protocol (DISCHE and SAUNDERS 1989; SAUNDERS et al. 1991). Five cases have been observed in the pilot study with fewer than 100 patients at risk (SAUNDERS, personal communication, 1992). The problem may reflect incomplete repair of sublethal damage within the target cells in the spinal cord during the 6-h daytime fractionation intervals (THAMES et al. 1988). However, given that one of every three fractionation intervals is 12 h, even this explanation is only plausible if half-times for repair in the spinal cord are assumed to be considerably longer than in any other tissue studied (GUTTENBERGER et al. 1993). The present experimental evidence from animal studies also does not support this explanation (ANG et al. 1993; SCALLIET et al. 1989; WITHERS et al. 1993; WONG et al. 1992), and nor do the results of hyperfractionated radiotherapy for brain stem gliomas (EDWARDS et al. 1989; PACKER et al. 1987; FREEMAN et al. 1988). That myelopathy should occur at all after total doses of less than 50 Gy in 1.5-Gy fractions is even more surprising in view of the reduction in severity of late sequelae reported from the same regimen for other tissues, such as the parotid gland (LESLIE and DISCHE 1992; THAMES et al., Chap. 1, this volume).

4.5 Future Directions

Recent evidence suggests that faster treatments for at least a proportion of tumors would provide a therapeutic advantage (see THAMES et al., Chap. 1, this volume). It has become common to combine acceleration and hyperfractionation. For example, CHART employs 1.5-Gy fractions in an overall treatment duration of only 12 days (SAUNDERS 1991; DISCHE and SAUNDERS 1989). Split-course accelerated regimens (WANG et al. 1986; WANG 1987; BEGG et al. 1990, 1992) employ 1.5- to 1.6-Gy fractions given twice per day in both parts of split-course regimens which may be as short as 5 weeks. These accelerated treatments are discussed in detail elsewhere in this volume (THAMES et al., Chap. 1, this volume).

Pure hyperfractionation probably has a limited place in radiation therapy. It should always be considered whenever high doses are needed in situations where late tolerance has been compromised, e.g., by prior radiation therapy. However, in standard curative treatment situations, it may be superseded by a combination of hyperfractionation and accelerated treatment (BEGG et al. 1990, 1992; PETERS et al. 1992; SAUNDERS et al. 1991; THAMES et al., Chap. 1, this volume; WANG et al. 1986; WANG 1987). It should be remembered, however, that even in "pure" hyperfractionation there is an element of acceleration because the biological dose to the tumor (although not the late-responding normal tissues) is increased by about 11% without any prolongation of overall treatment duration.

Acknowledgements. This investigation was supported by PHS grant number CA-31612 awarded by the National Cancer Institute, DHHS. The author thanks Dr. Hans-Peter Beck-Bornholdt for useful suggestions and Jan Haas for typing the manuscript.

References

Ang KK, Jiang G-L, Guttenberger R et al. (1992) Impact of spinal cord repair kinetics on the practice of altered fractionation schedules. Radiother Oncol 25: 287–294

Backstrom A, Jakobsson DA, Littbrand B, Wersall J (1973) Fractionation scheme with low individual doses in irradiation of carcinomas of the mouth. Acta Radiol Ther Phys Biol 12: 401–406

Barendsen GW (1982) Dose fractionation, dose rate and isoeffect relationships for normal tissue responses. Int J Radiat Oncol Biol Phys 8: 1981–1997

Begg AC, Hofland J, Moonen L et al. (1990) The predictive value of cell kinetic measurements in a European trial of accelerated fractionation in advanced head and neck tumors. Int J Radiat Oncol Biol Phys 19: 1449–1453

Begg AC, Hofland J, van Glabbeke et al. (1992) Predicive value of potential doubling time for radiotherapy of head and neck tumor patients: results from the EORTC trial. Semin Radiat Oncol 2: 22–25

Bentzen SM (1992) Radiobiological considerations in the design of clinical trials. Radiother Oncol 24 (Suppl): abstract 376

Bentzen SM, Overgaard J, Thames HD et al. (1989) Clinical radiobiology of malignant melanoma. Radiother Oncol 16: 169–182

Brahme A (1984) Dosimetric precision requirements in radiation therapy. Acta Oncol 23: 379–391

Cox JD, Azarnia N, Byhardt RW et al. (1990) Hyperfractionated radiation therapy (1.2 Gy b.i.d.) with 69.6 Gy total dose increases survival in favorable patients with stage III non-small cell carcinoma of the lung: report of RTOG 83-11. J Clin Oncol 8: 1543–1545

Cox JD, Guse C, Asbell S et al. (1988) Tolerance of pelvic normal tissues to hyperfractionated radiation therapy: results of protocol 83-08 of the Radiation Therapy Oncology Group. Int J Radiat Oncol Biol Phys 15: 1331–1336

Cox JD, Pajak T, Marcial VA et al. (1990) Dose-response for local control with hyperfractionated radiation therapy in advanced carcinomas of the upper aerodigestive tracts: preliminary report of the Radiation Therapy Oncology Group protocol 83-13. Int J Radiat Oncol Biol Phys 18: 515–521

Datta NR, Choudhry AD, Gupta S (1989) Twice a day versus once a day radiation therapy in head and neck cancer (abstract). Int J Radiat Oncol Biol Phys 17: 132 Suppl 1

Dische S, Saunders MI (1989) Continuous hyperfractionated, accelerated radiotherapy (CHART): an interim report upon late morbidity. Radiother Oncol 16: 65–72

Douglas BG, Fowler JF (1976) The effect of multiple small doses of x-rays on skin reactions in the mouse and a basic interpretation. Radiat Res 66: 401–421

Douglas BG, Worth A (1982) Superfractionation in glioblastoma multiforme: results of a phase II study. Int J Radiat Oncol Biol Phys 8: 1787–1794

Edsmyr F, Andersson L, Esposti PL et al. (1985) Irradiation therapy with multiple small fractions per day in urinary bladder cancer. Radiother Oncol 4: 197–203

Edwards MSB, Wara WM, Urtasun RC et al. (1989) Hyperfractionated radiation therapy for brain-stem gliomas: a phase I–II trial. J Neurosurg 70: 691–700

Freeman CR, Krischer J, Sanford RA et al. (1988) Hyperfractionated radiotherapy in brain stem tumors: results of a Pediatric Oncology Group study. Int J Radiat Oncol Biol Phys 15: 311–318

Guttenberger R, Thames HD, Ang KK (1992) Is the experience with CHART compatible with experimental data? A new model of repair kinetics and computer simulations. Radiother Oncol 25: 280–286

Horiot JC, LeFur R, Nguyen T et al. (1992) Hyperfractionation versus conventional fractionation in oropharyngeal carcinoma: final analysis of a randomized trial of the EORTC Cooperative Group of Radiotherapy. Radiother Oncol 25: 231–241

Jampolis S, Pepard G, Horiot JC et al. (1977) Preliminary results using twice a day fractionation in the radiotherapeutic management of advanced cancers of the head and neck. AJR 129: 1091–1093

Lea DEA (1956) Actions of radiations on living cells, 2nd edn. Cambridge University Press, Cambridge, England

Leslie MD, Dische S (1992) Changes in serum and salivary amylase during radiotherapy for head and neck cancer: a comparison of conventionally fractionated radiotherapy with CHART. Radiother Oncol 24: 27–31

Littbrand B, Edsmyr F, Revesz L (1975) A low dose fractionation scheme for the radiotherapy of the carcinoma of the bladder. Experimental and preliminary results. Bull Cancer 62: 241–248

Maciejewski B, Withers HR, Taylor JMG et al. (1989) Dose fractionation and regeneration in radiotherapy for cancer of the oral cavity and oropharynx: tumor dose-response and repopulation. Int J Radiat Oncol Biol Phys 16: 831–843

Marcial V, Pajak T, Chang C et al. (1987) Hyperfractionated photon radiation therapy in the treatment of advanced squamous cell carcinoma of the oral cavity, pharynx, larynx, and sinuses, using radiation therapy as the only planned modality: preliminary report by the Radiation Therapy Oncology Group (RTOG). Int J Radiat Oncol Biol Phys 13: 41–47

Meoz R, Fletcher GH, Peters LJ et al. (1984) Twice-daily fractionation schemes for advanced head and neck cancer. Int J Radiat Oncol Biol Phys 10: 831–836

Packer R, Littman P, Sposto R et al. (1987) Results of a pilot study of hyperfractionated radiation therapy for children with brain stem gliomas. Int J Radiat Oncol Biol Phys 13: 1647–1651

Parsons J, Mendenhall W, Cassisi N, Million RR (1988) Hyperfractionation for head and neck cancer. Int J Radiat Oncol Biol Phys 14: 649–658

Parsons J, Mendenhall W, Cassisi N (1993) Twice a day treatment for head and neck cancer. In: Johson JT, Didolkar MS (eds) Head and neck cancer. Proceedings of the International Meeting of Head and Neck Cancer 1992. Elsevier, Amsterdam, vol 3, pp 171–178

Perez CA, Brady LW (eds) (1992) Principles and practice of radiation oncology, 2nd edn. J.B. Lippincott, Philadelphia

Peters LJ, Ang KK, Thames HD (1992) Altered fractionation schedules. In: Perez CA, Brady LW (eds) Principles and practice of radiation oncology, 2nd edn. J.B. Lippincott, New York, p 97

Pinto LHJ, Canary PCV, Araujo CMM et al. (1991) Prospective randomized trial comparing hyperfractionated versus conventional radiotherapy in stages II and IV oropharyngeal carcinoma. Int J Radiat Oncol Biol Phys 21: 557–562

Powers WE, Tolmach LJ (1963) A multicomponent x-ray survival curve for mouse lymphosarcoma cells irradiated in vivo. Nature 197: 710–711

Revesz L, Littbrand B, Midander J et al. (1975) Oxygen effects in the shoulder region of cell survival curves. In: Alper T (ed) Proceedings of the 6th LH Gray Conference. John Wiley, London, p 141

Saunders MI, Dische S, Grosch EJ et al. (1991) Experience with CHART. Int J Radiat Oncol Biol Phys 21: 871–878

Scalliet P, Landuyt W, van der Schueren E (1989) Repair kinetics as a determining factor for late tolerance of central nervous system to low dose rate irradiation. Radiother Oncol 14: 345–353

Seydel H, Diener-West M, Urtasun R et al. (1985) Radiation Therapy Oncology Group (RTOG): hyperfractionation in the radiation therapy of unresectable non-oat cell carcinoma of the lung. Preliminary report of a RTOG pilot study. Int J Radiat Oncol Biol Phys 11: 1841–1847

Shukovsky L, Fletcher GH, Montague ED et al. (1976) Experience with twice-daily fractionation in clinical radiotherapy. AJR 126: 155–162

Suit HD, Walker AM (1988) Predictors of radiation response in use today: criteria, new assays and methods of verification. In: Chapman JD, Peters LJ, Withers HR (eds) Prediction of tumor treatment response. Pergamon, Oxford, p 3

Taylor JMGT, Withers HR (1992) Dose-time factors in head and neck data. Radiother Oncol 25: 313–315

Thames HD, Hendry JH (eds) (1987) Fractionation in radiotherapy. Taylor and Francis, London

Thames HD, Suit HD (1986) Tumor radioresponsiveness versus fractionation sensitivity. Int J Radiat Oncol Biol Phys 12: 687–691

Thames HD, Withers HR, Peters LJ et al. (1982) Changes in early and late radiation responses with altered dose fractionation: implications for dose-survival relationships. Int J Radiat Oncol Biol Phys 8: 219–226

Thames HD, Ang KK, Stewart F (1988) Does incomplete repair explain the apparent failure of the basic LQ model to predict spinal cord and kidney response to low doses per fraction? Int J Radiat Biol 54: 13–19

Thames HD, Bentzen SM, Turesson I et al. (1990) Time-dose factor in radiotherapy: a review of the human data. Radiother Oncol 19: 219–235

Thames HD, Schultheiss TE, Hendry JH et al. (1992) Can modest escalations of dose be detected as increased tumor control? Int J Radiat Oncol Biol Phys 22: 241–246

Wang CC (1987) Accelerated fractionation. In: Withers HR, Peters LJ (eds) Innovations in radiation oncology. Springer, Berlin Heidelberg New York, p 239

Wang CC, Suit HD, Blitzer PH (1986) Twice-a-day radiation therapy for supraglottic carcinoma. Int J Radiat Oncol Biol Phys 12: 3–7

Wendt CD, Peters LJ, Ang KK et al. (1989) Hyperfractionated radiotherapy in the treatment of squamous cell carcinomas of the supraglottic larynx. Int J Radiat Oncol Biol Phys 17: 1057–1062

Withers HR (1975) Cell-cycle redistribution as a factor in multifraction irradiation. Radiology 114: 199–202

Withers HR, Peters LJ (1980) Biological aspects of radiation therapy. In: Fletcher GH (ed) Textbook of radiotherapy, 3rd edn. Lea & Febiger, Philadelphia, p 103

Withers HR, Thames HD, Peters LJ (1982a) Differences in the fractionation response of acute and late-responding tissues. In: Karcher KH, Kogelnik HD, Reinartz G (eds) Progress in radio-oncology II. Raven, New York, p 287

Withers HR, Thames HD, Peters LJ (1982b) Biological bases for high RBE values for late effects of neutron irradiation. Int J Radiat Oncol Biol Phys 8: 2071–2076

Withers HR, Thames HD, Peters LJ (1983a) A new isoeffect curve for change in dose per fraction. Radiother Oncol 2: 187–192

Withers HR, Thames HD, Peters LJ et al. (1983b) Normal tissue radioresistance in clinical radiotherapy. In: Fletcher GH, Nervi C, Withers HR (eds) Biological bases and clinical implications of tumor radioresistance. Masson, New York, p 139

Withers HR, Mason KA, Taylor JMG et al. (1993) Response of guinea pig spinal cord to fractionated radiotherapy. Int J Radiat Oncol Biol Phys (submitted)

Wong CS, Minkin S, Hill RP (1992) Linear-quadratic model underestimates sparing effect of small doses per fraction in rat spinal cord. Radiother Oncol 23: 176–184

5 The Limitation of the Linear-Quadratic Model at Low Doses per Fraction

M.C. JOINER, B. MARPLES, and H. JOHNS

CONTENTS

5.1 Introduction

The Linear-Quadratic (LQ) equation is used widely to model and predict the increase in total dose with decreasing dose per fraction needed for an isoeffective response to radiotherapy in normal tissues and tumours (reviewed by JOINER 1989). It is thought that this relationship reflects the gradual decrease in radiation effectiveness ("per unit dose") with lowered doses due to these doses being further and further back "on the shoulder" of an underlying

survival curve for the cells at risk in tissues. A considerable amount of work has been devoted to defining the operational limits of this model in a range of normal tissues and tumours during the last 10 years although these studies have been largely done on animal models for ethical reasons. What information there is on human dose-fractionation characteristics and repair kinetics *does* indicate that the animal systems predict the apparent situation in man reasonably accurately (THAMES et al. 1990).

There has been an indication in these experimental studies in vivo that the LQ model may not predict changes in the effect of radiation with fractionation as reliably as expected in certain specific situations although in the majority of cases it works very well. For doses greater than 1 Gy per fraction, the LQ model probably does reasonably describe the *fundamental* radiation response of normal tissues, but identifiable factors operating between fractions like incomplete repair of sublethal damage, changes in oxygen tension, cellular proliferation or redistribution of cells around their cycle may modify this so that the LQ model may appear to be deficient in summarising the *overall* fractionation response. The issue of incomplete repair is now largely understood and is relevant in explaining some responses of both late- and acutely-responding normal tissues and tumours. For example, it was thought initially that the LQ model was underpredicting late effects of radiation in mouse kidney and rat spinal cord, for doses per fraction in the range 1–2 Gy relative to higher doses per fraction; this now appears to be due to incomplete repair between successive doses in experiments with 3- or 4-h intervals between the low but not the high doses per fraction (THAMES et al. 1988). However, the influence of other factors which affect primarily *acute* tissue and tumour responses like oxygenation, proliferation and redistribution between fractions is generally more poorly understood at the present time in specific cases although the principles have been defined by classical radiobiology. For example, studies on pig skin have suggested that the LQ model can "over-

M.C. JOINER, PhD, CRC Gray Laboratory, P.O. Box 100, Mount Vernon Hospital, Northwood, Middlesex HA6 2JR, UK
B. MARPLES, PhD, B.C. Cancer Research Centre, 601 West 10th Ave., Vancouver, B.C. V5Z 1L3, Canada
H. JOHNS, BSc, CRC Gray Laboratory, P.O. Box 100, Mount Vernon Hospital, Northwood, Middlesex HA6 2JR, UK

predict" radiation effect in the range 2–6 Gy, but this has been attributed to a combination of cellular repopulation and cell-cycle redistribution both affecting the fundamental radiation response in a complex manner to determine the *net* tissue response (HOPEWELL and VAN DEN AARDWEG 1991). What is emerging from these more recent studies is a need to understand the way in which all the "R's" of radiobiology and radiotherapy interact together in determining the overall response of individual tumours and normal tissues to fractionated radiotherapy.

Of potentially greater significance, since it implies mechanisms as yet unknown, is the possibility that even if the above modifying factors are accounted for, the LQ model may still fail to describe adequately the observed relationship between total isoeffective radiation dose and the dose per fraction in the case of radiation responses in vivo, and the shape of cell survival curves at a more basic level in vitro. This article focuses on this issue and describes data we have obtained on radiation responses to low doses and doses per fraction in some normal tissue and cell systems. We have evaluated the effect of very low doses per fraction, less than 2 Gy and typically down to 0.1 Gy, on skin and kidney (JOINER et al. 1986; JOINER and JOHNS 1988). Lung has also been tested down to 0.15 Gy per fraction by Gray Laboratory workers (PARKINS and FOWLER 1986). These studies have been possible by utilising an experimental design in which only a part of the underlying damage equivalent to full tissue tolerance is produced by the x-ray fractions of interest, and the balance is supplied by a "top-up" dose of low-energy (high-LET) neutrons available in our laboratory (JOINER 1987; JOINER et al. 1989, 1992) and generated by the reaction of 4-MeV deuterons on beryllium. These neutrons are ideal for use as top-up doses because the biological effect they produce is hardly influenced at all by factors which would normally be expected to modulate *x-ray* sensitivity, such as the position of cells in the cell cycle and the cellular oxygen tension. Additionally, there is little or no sparing effect of fractionation for neutrons of this low energy and to a first approximation, the amount of underlying damage contributed by the top-up dose is directly proportional to the neutron dose given, enabling the effect of the x-ray treatment of interest to be easily deduced from the top-up dose needed to produce measurable tissue reactions: the smaller the top-up dose needed, the larger is the effect of the x-ray treatment. The top-up technique enables the

effect of very low doses per fraction to be assessed after 20 or 30 fractions for example, since even though this may generate less than 10% of the underlying damage which is necessary to produce measurable functional loss, the balance ($> 90\%$) is supplied by the neutron top-up dose. If a complete "full-course" treatment were given wholly with low x-ray doses per fraction, this would need 100 or more fractions and such an experiment would be extremely difficult to carry out.

This work is now being extended to enable us to compare these data obtained in vivo with direct measurements of survival made on established lines of mammalian cells in vitro exposed to very low *single* doses of x-rays. Accurate measurement of cell survival in the low-dose, high-survival region has been possible by using a computerized microscope (Dynamic Microscopic Image Processing Scanner: DMIPS) to locate and record the positions of single cells on a growth surface, and monitoring these cells individually to determine whether or not each produces a colony indicative of cell survival (PALCIC and JAGGI 1986; SPADINGER and PALCIC 1992; MARPLES and JOINER 1993).

5.2 Summary of Experimental Techniques

5.2.1 Irradiation

For studies in vivo, mice received fractionated treatments with 240 kVp x-rays (half-value layer = 1.3 mm Cu) at a "high" dose rate of 2.3 Gy min^{-1} for skin irradiations and 2.5 Gy min^{-1} for kidney irradiations. For the lung studies quoted from the literature, the dose rate used in the irradiations was 1.8 Gy min^{-1}. In the special top-up type of experiment described above, the top-up doses were d(4)-Be neutrons produced by the reaction of 4-MeV deuterons with a thick beryllium target; this gives neutrons with a mean energy of 2.3 MeV (FOLKARD 1986).

For studies in vitro, cells attached to plastic were irradiated with single doses of 250 kVp x-rays (half-value layer = 1.46 mm Cu) at dose rates of 0.016 Gy min^{-1} (0.01–0.5 Gy), 0.44 Gy min^{-1} (0.2–5 Gy) or 1.7 Gy min^{-1} (1–10 Gy). The dose rate was selected according to the dose delivered so that exposure times were always greater than 35 s in order to maintain dosimetric accuracy; however, it was confirmed that for doses less than 1 Gy, the dose rate did not significantly affect the cell survival (MARPLES and JOINER 1993).

5.2.2 Normal Tissue Studies

In the skin studies, acute reactions were scored on the left hind feet of mice during the period 10–32 days after irradiation, and an average value of skin reaction was calculated (DENEKAMP 1973; DOUGLAS and FOWLER 1976; JOINER 1989). The skin-scoring system uses a series of arbitrary scores of erythema, dry desquamation and moist desquamation, within a scale ranging from 0 to 3. A single x-ray dose of ~ 23 Gy is required for an average skin reaction of 1.5, which corresponds to transient moist desquamation at about day 20 post irradiation.

Late renal damage in mice was assessed from typically 25 to 40 weeks post irradiation, using decreased clearance of radiolabelled ethylenediamine tetraacetic acid (EDTA) from the plasma, reduction in haematocrit and increased urine output as endpoints (JOINER and JOHNS 1988). At 29 weeks post irradiation, equivalent mid-range responses are typically 3% residual EDTA per millilitre plasma, 40% haematocrit and 15 urination events per day for an x-ray dose of ~ 21.5 Gy delivered in two fractions (JOINER and JOHNS 1988), compared to values of ~ 0.4% residual EDTA, ~ 50% haematocrit and ~ 6.3 urination events per day in unirradiated age-matched animals (STEVENS et al. 1991).

The studies on mouse lung by PARKINS and FOWLER (1986), cited in Fig. 5.4, used breathing frequency to assess an acute phase of lung damage at about 28 weeks post irradiation and mortality as an endpoint for a late phase of damage by about 48 weeks post irradiation. Typically in this system, for single-dose schedules the ED_{50} (dose at which 50% of animals exhibited breathing frequency > 1.2 times that in unirradiated animals) at 28 weeks and $LD_{50/48\ weeks}$ are both ~ 11 Gy. These values of *functional* damage, and the other values given above for skin and kidney, have been used as the specification of "full tissue tolerance" in these three experimental systems.

Analysis of these top-up experiments has been carried out using the methods described in detail by JOINER et al. (1986), JOINER and JOHNS (1988), JOINER et al. (1989) and JOHNS and JOINER (1991). In particular, the "extrapolated total" x-ray doses were calculated; these are the x-ray doses that would be needed to reach full tissue tolerance if the treatment had all been given with x-ray fractions alone instead of partially with x-ray fractions plus a subsequent top-up; this calculation has been described by JOINER and DENEKAMP (1986).

5.2.3 In Vitro Studies

Samples of Chinese hamster V79–379A cells, maintained routinely in suspension culture in the logarithmic phase of growth (WATTS et al. 1986), were allowed to attach to the bottom surface of tissue culture flasks which were then filled completely with culture medium, sealed and irradiated with either x-rays or neutrons at room temperature (21°–25°C). Following irradiation, a DMIPS cell analyser (PALCIC and JAGGI 1986; SPADINGER and PALCIC 1992; MARPLES and JOINER 1993) was used to locate and record the positions of ~ 300 cells in each flask, which were then incubated at 37°C for 3.5 days to allow six or seven divisions, producing colonies of greater than 50 cells from a single surviving cell. After this time, the location of each recorded cell was revisited automatically to determine whether a colony was present and, if so, to measure its size. The fraction of surviving cells at each dose level was determined in the conventional way as the plating efficiency (irradiated cells) divided by the plating efficiency (unirradiated cells). The full protocol for these experiments has been described by MARPLES and JOINER (1993).

5.3 Studies of Normal Tissues and Tumours In Vivo

5.3.1 Skin

Figure 5.1 shows the relationship between extrapolated total dose needed to achieve full tisse tolerance and dose per fraction, for an experiment using 20 initial fractions of x-rays as low as 0.1 Gy, followed by a single neutron top-up dose (JOINER et al. 1986). Additionally, Fig. 5.1 includes data from experiments using eight higher-dose x-ray fractions plus top-up and full courses of x-ray fractions (no top-up) for comparison. The LQ model has been used successfully in previous studies to describe this relationship in mouse skin but only at doses per fraction greater than 1 Gy (DOUGLAS and FOWLER 1976). In this formulation, the survival of the notional underlying target cell population is given by

$$E' = -\log(\text{SF}) = n(\alpha d + \beta d^2), \quad (5.1)$$

where SF is the surviving fraction, d is the dose per fraction given in n fractions and α and β are constants in the model which together describe the shape of the survival curve: a higher ratio of α/β

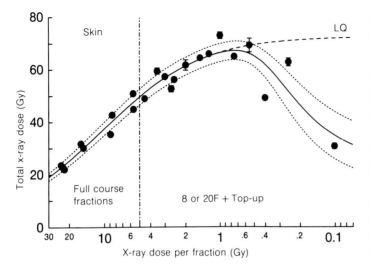

Fig. 5.1. Total dose required to achieve full acute skin tolerance (see text) in mice feet as a function of dose per fraction in the range 0.1–20 Gy. Experiments used either a full course of fractions (no top-up) or 8 or 20 x-ray fractions followed by a neutron top-up dose. Data points are mean ± SEM, within the data points if not shown. The data are well-fitted by a Linear-Quadratic (LQ model (*dashed line*) in the dose per fraction range above 1 Gy. Below 0.6 Gy per fraction, the LQ model under-predicts the effect of x-rays and total dose decreases with decreasing dose per fraction. Total dose is better predicted over the complete range of dose per fraction by a modified LQ model which includes induced repair, shown by the *solid line*; 95% confidence limits on the mean (expected) values of the fit are shown by *dotted lines*. Data from JOINER et al. (1986)

indicates a more "linear" survival curve and correspondingly less effect of fractionation. This may be seen by rearranging Eq. 5.1 to give the relationship between total dose $D = nd$ and dose per fraction, for a fixed level of damage E. Thus,

$$D = \frac{E/\alpha}{1 + d/(\alpha/\beta)}. \tag{5.2}$$

This equation is shown in Fig. 5.1 as a solid/dashed line (marked LQ). Even down to doses per fraction as low as 0.6 Gy, the data fit the LQ model very well but below this dose there is a significantly reduced total dose compared with the LQ prediction: the LQ model *underestimates* the true effect of these low doses per fraction, which is better described by the solid line.

Figure 5.2 summarises a further experiment on mouse skin, using 30 initial fractions of x-rays as low as 0.07 Gy, plus a single neutron top-up dose.

In this study, we also tested the influence of giving the neutron top-up dose either before or after x-rays (closed and open symbols respectively); we found there was no significant difference in the effect of x-rays measured using these two protocols. However, again there is evidence of an increased effect of low x-ray doses per fraction (< 0.2 Gy) compared with the simple LQ model, as indicated by a reduction in total dose needed for full tolerance (skin reaction = 1.5). In these 30-fraction x-ray experiments, the increased sensitivity at low doses per fraction is not as marked as in the 20-fraction study shown in Fig. 5.1; additionally the deviation from the LQ model occurs at a lower dose per fraction so that the maximum total dose measured is higher at about 100 Gy in Fig. 5.2 compared with about 70 Gy in Fig. 5.1. We do not yet understand the reason for this difference between these two skin studies.

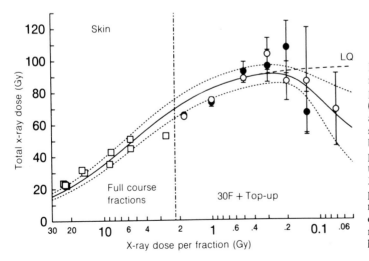

Fig. 5.2. Experiments similar to those summarised in Fig. 5.1, but using 30 x-ray fractions plus neutron top-up doses given either before (●) or after (○) the x-ray schedule. Data points are mean ± SEM, within the data points if not shown. There is no significant difference between these two protocols, and at low doses per fraction the LQ model again underpredicts the effect of x-ray treatment. However, in this 30-fraction study, the phenomenon is not as pronounced as shown in Fig. 5.1, and the maximum value of total dose occurs at a lower dose per fraction. *Solid line*: fit of the induced-repair model; *dotted lines*: 95% confidence limits on mean (expected) values of this fit

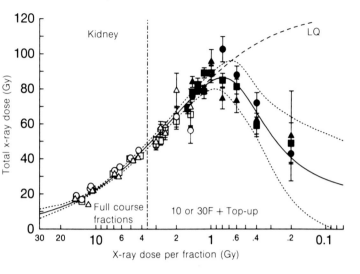

Fig. 5.3. Relationship between total dose and dose per fraction for equal late renal damage in the mouse assayed at 29 weeks post-irradiation by EDTA clearance (■, □), haematocrit (●, ○) and urination frequency (▲, △). Irradiation was with 10 (*open symbols*) or 30 (*closed symbols*) x-ray fractions followed by a neutron top-up treatment, and is compared with the response to a full course of x-ray fractions (no top-up). Data points are mean ± SEM, within the data points if not shown. The LQ model underpredicts the effect of x-ray treatment with doses per fraction less than 0.8 Gy; however, the induced-repair model fits all the data well (*solid line* with *dotted lines* as 95% CL). Data from JOINER and JOHNS (1988)

5.3.2 Kidney

In this typical late-reacting tissue, we have tested the effect of x-ray doses per fraction down to 0.2 Gy in an experiment using 30 x-ray fractions followed by a neutron top-up treatment (JOINER and JOHNS 1988). Figure 5.3 summarises the data obtained in this study; data from three assays of renal damage (see above) are included. Additionally, for comparison, we have included data from experiments using ten higher-dose x-ray fractions (1.5–3.5 Gy per fraction) plus a top-up dose, and full courses of x-ray fractions which received no top-up dose. All these data are in close agreement and show clearly an increased effect of small x-ray dose fractions, with total dose reaching a maximum average of about 92 Gy at 1 Gy per fraction, decreasing by a factor of 1.9 to about 49 Gy at 0.2 Gy per fraction.

5.3.3 Lung

We examined further the data published previously on the dose-fractionation response of mouse lung (PARKINS et al. 1985; PARKINS and FOWLER 1985, 1986). These experiments used 1–40 fractions in a full course of treatment with no top-up dose, and 20 low-dose fractions plus a neutron top-up dose. These data are shown in Fig. 5.4 in the same format as in Figs. 5.1–5.3. Also shown on Fig. 5.4 are unpublished data from an experiment using 40 low-dose x-ray fractions plus neutron top-up. These data were kindly supplied by Dr. C.S. Parkins at the Gray Laboratory. The lines drawn in Fig. 5.4 show the fit of the LQ model to only the full-course

fractionation data (open symbols, dose per fraction > 1 Gy). The ratio of α/β from this fit was 2.8 Gy, similar to the values quoted previously for these studies (PARKINS et al. 1985; PARKINS and FOWLER 1985). In these experiments, the data from both the early and the late phases of response indicate a trend for x-rays to become more effective as the dose per fraction is reduced below 0.8 Gy, in agreement with the data for skin and kidney. Unfortunately, however, the large errors on the total dose estimates below 1 Gy per fraction do not permit a firm conclusion to be drawn and it would be useful to repeat these experiments.

5.3.4 Evidence of Tumour Radiosensitivity to Low Doses per Fraction

To our knowledge, there has only been one study on tumours irradiated in vivo which has assessed the response to doses per fraction less than 0.6 Gy. This was the study of BECK-BORNHOLDT et al. (1989), who irradiated the R1H rhabdomyosarcoma of the rat with full-course schedules of 6 up to 126 fractions of 200 kVp x-rays. No top-up doses were used. The schedules were given in the same overall time of 6 weeks so that the influence of proliferation was expected to be the same and interfraction intervals were at least 8 h in all schedules to allow complete repair between the successive doses. This was achieved even with the 126-fraction schedule, by irradiating three times per day 7 days per week. Tumours were irradiated in unanaesthetised animals breathing air, and assuming a constant pattern of reoxygenation throughout each schedule one would expect the total radiation dose in each schedule

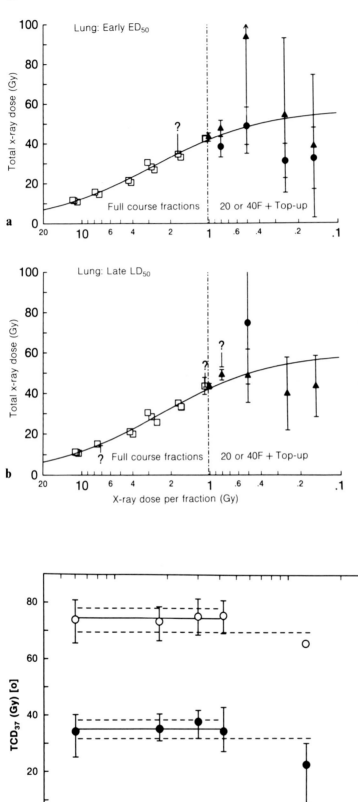

Fig. 5.4. Total dose to the mouse lung needed to cause an increase in breathing rate by 20% compared with controls in half the subjects measured at 28 weeks (ED_{50}, **a**), or total dose needed for mortality in half the subjects at 44–48 weeks (LD_{50}, **b**). Irradiations were full-course x-ray fractionation (□), 20 x-ray fractions + neutron top-up (●) and 40 x-ray fractions + neutron top-up (▲). Data points are mean ± SEM, within the data points if not shown. For data points designated with?, only lower or upper limits on the possible range of ED_{50} or LD_{50} could be computed. Although not significant in these studies, there is a trend towards a greater effect of low-dose x-ray fractionation compared with the LQ model fitted to the data at ≥ 1 Gy per fraction (*solid line*). Data from Parkins et al. (1985); Parkins and Fowler (1985, 1986) and Dr. C.S. Parkins (personal communication)

Fig. 5.5. Dose required to locally control 37% of R1H tumours (*left vertical axis*) or net growth delay per unit dose (*right vertical axis*) for radiotherapy using different numbers of fractions given in a similar overall time. *Error bars* indicate 95% confidence intervals on mean values. Confidence intervals on the mean value for 6–42 fractions (*solid line*) are shown as *dashed lines*. The effect of radiotherapy is similar for schedules with 6–42 fractions, but is greater for the schedule with 126 fractions, where doses per fraction are less than 0.5 Gy. (Redrawn from Beck-Bornholdt et al. 1989)

required for local tumour control to be determined only by the shape of the survival curve of the tumour cells, in other words their "fundamental" radio-sensitivity versus dose relationship. Figure 5.5 shows that the same total dose was needed for cure and the net growth delay per gray was similar, in schedules using 6 to 42 fractions. This could reflect a high α/β ratio for the tumour cells which is not unusual for tumours irradiated in animals breathing air. However, Fig. 5.5 also shows that curative doses were lower, and net growth delay per gray higher, for the 126-fraction schedule (dose per fraction < 0.5 Gy) compared with the schedules using 6–42 fractions (dose per fraction > 1 Gy). Although the cellular basis for tumour response to radiotherapy is well understood, the interpretation of radiation effects on tumours in vivo can be subject to more uncertainty than in the case of normal tissues due to the varying (and in most cases unknown) pattern of tumour oxygenation throughout treatment. However, the qualitative agreement of increased sensitivity at very low doses per fraction in both the R1H tumour and mouse skin and kidney (and possibly lung) is interesting and if this reflects a phenomenon that is more fundamental and widespread, then it suggests that low-dose radio-sensitivity of this order should be detectable in vitro under the right conditions.

5.4 Studies of Cells In Vitro

5.4.1 Survival of V79 Cells

To investigate this phenomenon further, we carried out a large series of 56 experiments in which we measured the survival of V79 hamster cells after exposure to *single* doses of 250 kVp x-rays or d(4)-Be neutrons. These experiments comprised a total of 364 separate assessments of cell survival after x-ray doses in the range 0–10 Gy, with 84% of the measurements made at doses less than 1 Gy, 76% made at less than 0.5 Gy and 57% made at less than 0.25 Gy. For neutrons, 146 separate assessments of cell survival were made after doses ranging from 0.02 to 3 Gy. Figure 5.6 shows the cell survival measured in this large series of experiments. The response to x-ray doses above 1 Gy is well-described by a conventional downward-bending survival curve; in Fig. 5.6 the solid line in the main panel and dotted line in the magnified inset show the LQ model (Eq. 5.1 with $n = 1$) fitted to the x-ray data at doses ≥ 1 Gy. The α/β ratio is quite large at 25 Gy even

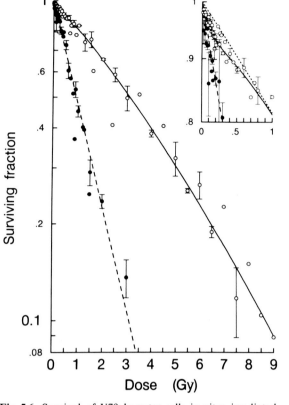

Fig. 5.6. Survival of V79 hamster cells in vitro irradiated with single doses of x-rays or neutrons. Data points are mean $\pm$ SEM. At x-ray doses > 1 Gy, the dose-survival relationship conforms to a conventional LQ model (*dotted line in inset*). At x-ray doses < 0.6 Gy, the LQ model substantially underpredicts the effect of x-rays, which is better fitted by the induced-repair model (*solid line, see text*). The response to neutrons is described by a simple exponential survival curve (*dashed line*) and there is no indication of increased sensitivity at low doses

though V79 cells are relatively radioresistant, with a surviving fraction at 2 Gy (SF$_2$) of 0.65. However, for x-ray doses below 0.5 Gy, the data deviate from the expected response extrapolated from higher doses. The solid line in the magnified inset shows the fit of an induced-repair model (see Sect. 5.5) to the x-ray data and this clearly shows the increased effectiveness of low x-ray doses compared with the prediction from the LQ model. For neutrons, V79 cell survival was always reduced exponentially with dose with an SF$_2$ of 0.23; the straight dashed line indicates this in Fig. 5.6. Just as in the systems in vivo described above, low x-ray doses are more effective than predicted. Indeed, in this example, x-ray doses < 0.2 Gy were almost as effective as neutrons.

To further magnify the differences in radiosensitivity at low doses, it is also useful to express each measurement of surviving fraction at a particular dose as $-$ dose/$\log_e$(SF). This may be thought of as an "effective D_0" and is the inverse slope of a line joining the origin of the survival curve (plotted on log-linear coordinates as in Fig. 5.6) to each data point. Lower values of effective D_0 indicate a greater average effect of the radiation per unit dose, just as with the traditional D_0. This approach is useful because it is a normalised measure of the radiation effect, and therefore provides a magnified picture of the low-dose region compared with Fig. 5.6. Effective D_0 is shown in Fig. 5.7 for all survival measurements made after both neutrons and x-rays. Figure 5.7a confirms that over the dose range studied (0.02–3 Gy), neutrons appear to be equally effective per unit dose at killing cells so that effective D_0 is, on average, constant, reflecting a survival curve for V79 cells that is single exponential as shown in Fig. 5.6. In contrast, x-rays (Fig. 5.7b) are maximally effective per gray (with minimum effective D_0) at doses approaching zero, becoming less effective as the dose increases from 0.01 to 1 Gy, being *minimally* effective per gray (with maximum effective D_0) at about 1 Gy and then becoming more effective again as the dose increases above 1 Gy and the survival is more and more influenced by the βd^2 term in the LQ formulation. This pattern over the whole dose range of 0.01–10 Gy reflects the complex low-dose shape of the x-ray survival curve shown in Fig. 5.6 and

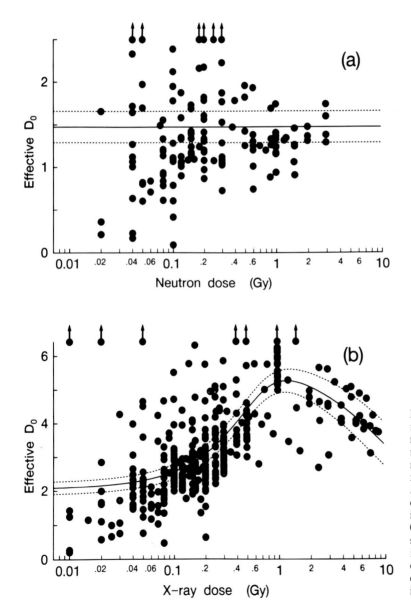

Fig. 5.7a,b. Data from the 56 experiments (Fig. 5.6) where each of 146 measurements of survival after single neutron doses (**a**) and each of 364 measurements of survival after single x-ray doses (**b**) is expressed as an effective D_0 (see text). Effective D_0 is, on average, constant for neutron treatments but increases with x-ray dose over the range 0.01 to 1 Gy, reflecting the shape of the survival curve at low doses shown in Fig. 5.6. *Solid lines* with 95% confidence limits (*dotted*) show the mean effective D_0 for neutrons or the fit of the induced-repair model to the x-ray data

shows clearly the increased effectiveness of low x-ray doses compared with the traditional expectation.

Each of the 56 experiments summarised in Figs. 5.6 and 5.7 included both neutron and x-ray responses. This strategy had been adopted so that as well as measuring x-ray cell survival directly, a comparison could be made between neutron and x-ray survival. As a result of this, we can now say that it is less likely that the apparent increase in x-ray sensitivity at low doses shown in Fig. 5.6 could be an artefact of the specialised DMIPS procedure that we used to measure cell survival, since (on average) dose-related changes were not seen in the sensitivity to neutrons. Therefore, at similar high levels of cell survival in excess of 95%, the x-ray and neutron doses required to give these small amounts of cell kill were similar. By taking advantage of the exponential neutron survival curve in each experiment, this comparison was expressed as relative biological effectiveness (RBE) by relating each x-ray survival point to the neutron survival line, and calculating the ratio of x-ray to neutron dose required to achieve this level of cell survival. Figure 5.8 summarises the 364 RBE values calculated in this way from all the experiments. Since the response to neutrons was exponential, an increasing RBE corresponds directly to increasing x-ray resistance, as we have already shown in Fig. 5.7. Thus a low RBE at low x-ray doses indicates high x-ray sensitivity and the RBE is well below the prediction which is made with the LQ model extrapolated from doses above 2 Gy, shown by the dashed line. As the x-ray dose increases, RBE increases (reflecting increasing x-ray resistance) to reach a peak at about 1–1.5 Gy, after which RBE

decreases with increasing dose, which is the conventional picture due to the downward bending of the x-ray survival curve. For example, at an x-ray dose of 0.1 Gy, RBE was 2.1 corresponding to an effective x-ray D_0 of 2.6 Gy; for 1 Gy x-rays, RBE was 3.9, corresponding to an effective x-ray D_0 of 5.2 Gy. Thus x-ray radioresistance increased by a factor of 2 as x-ray dose increased from 0.1 to 1 Gy. This is a substantial change although not as large as the changes seen in x-ray effectiveness in kidney over the same dose range.

Of course, an RBE approach gives results which look similar to results obtained by analysing with the effective D_0 approach (compare Figs. 5.7b and 5.8) because both techniques express x-ray effect in terms of an x-ray dose needed to produce a specific effect. This is also true of the skin and kidney data, which we have also presented previously in terms of RBE (JOINER et al. 1986; JOINER and JOHNS 1988). However, we have found that an advantage of the RBE technique is that interexperimental variations in the x-ray survival response are reduced in the RBE data, presumably because slight changes in radiosensitivity from time to time affect both the x-ray and the neutron responses similarly. This can be checked by calculating a mean coefficient of variation (CV) as the standard deviation of regression ÷ median RBE or effective D_0, from the fit of the induced-repair model to the data (see Sec. 5.5). This CV is 43% for the data expressed as effective D_0 in Fig. 5.7 compared with 35% for the data expressed as RBE in Fig. 5.8.

The cell survival data obtained with V79 hamster cells in vitro seem to leave no doubt that low (< 1 Gy) single x-ray doses, or doses per fraction in vivo, are

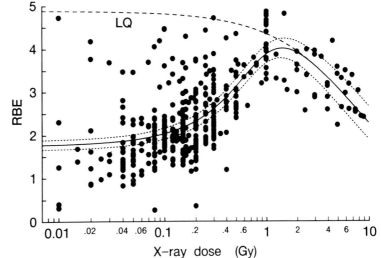

Fig. 5.8. Data from the 56 experiments (Fig. 5.6) where each of 364 measurements of cell survival after a single x-ray dose is expressed as an RBE value relative to the line fitted to survival after neutrons measured in the same experiment (see text). These data show how the increased effect of low-dose x-rays is mirrored by a decreasing RBE with decreasing dose; the LQ model (*dashed line*) substantially overpredicts the RBE at low x-ray doses, which is better described by the induced-pair model (*solid line*)

much more effective than expected, or predicted from any reasonable extrapolation (e.g., with the LQ model) from high-dose data. We are now confirming that low single x-ray doses are also hyper-effective in a *human* tumour cell line (HT29) and in this system the low-dose sensitivity appears even more marked than in V79 cells (LAMBIN et al. 1993).

5.4.2 Mutation of V79 Cells

If low doses of low-LET radiations are more effective than expected at *killing* cells, then there is also a possibility that low doses might be more effective at causing mutation (and by implication cancer induction) since both cell killing and mutation result from DNA damage caused by radiation which is either repaired incorrectly or not repaired at all.

In one system, there is indeed evidence that suggests this may be the case. CROMPTON et al. (1990) have measured mutation at the *hprt* locus, which confers resistance to growth in 6-thioguanine, in three sublines of V79-S cells which are in turn a subline of the V79–379 Chinese hamster fibroblasts used in the cell survival work described in Sect. 5.4.1. Figure 5.9, redrawn from CROMPTON et al. (1990), summarises some of these data in terms of the number of mutant cells per million survivors induced by a 4-Gy dose of cobalt-60 γ-rays, at low dose rates varying from $4.5\,\text{mGy}\,\text{h}^{-1}$ to acute dose rates of $1.4\,\text{Gy}\,\text{min}^{-1}$. Overall, a decrease in muta-

tion induction occurred as the dose rate was decreased from acute to low values of about $0.05\,\text{Gy}\,\text{h}^{-1}$. However, further reduction in the dose rate below $0.05\,\text{Gy}\,\text{h}^{-1}$ resulted in a "reverse dose-rate" effect with an *increase* in mutation frequency.

A low-dose-rate exposure may be thought of as a schedule of increasingly small acute doses per fraction which are taken to the zero limit. This equivalence has been well known for many years and a formula for equating a low-dose-rate exposure with a series of acute dose fractions to the same total dose giving the same effect, has been described by LIVERSAGE (1969). We have used this formula to add a scale of acute dose per fraction to the top of Fig. 5.9, so that the data may be compared with those described in the previous sections. This calculation just requires the half-time for repair of "sublethal" radiation injury to be supplied; we used a value of 1.5 h. The conclusion is that the point at which a substantial increase in the mutational effectiveness of radiation occurs is equivalent to doses per fraction of the same order as we have found for the increased cell-killing effect in normal tissues and V79 cells. This suggests (but does not confirm) that at least in V79 hamster cells, a similar mechanism may be responsible for increased mutational and lethal effects (per unit dose) of small radiation exposures and that hypersensitivity to low doses of radiation (at least for low-LET radiations) could result at the fundamental level from the increased accrual per unit dose of either misrepaired or unrepaired DNA lesions.

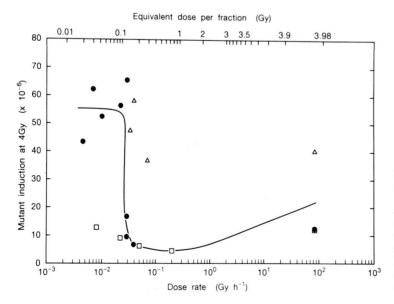

Fig. 5.9. Mutation frequency in three sublines of V79-S cells ($\triangle$, S_{80}; $\bullet$, S_{83}; $\square$, S_{85}) irradiated with single doses of 4 Gy given at low-dose rates. Exposures at dose rates $< 0.05\,\text{Gy}\,\text{h}^{-1}$ are more effective at causing mutation than higher dose rate treatments. This dose-rate "threshold" is equivalent to a dose per fraction of about 0.2 Gy (see text). (Redrawn from CROMPTON et al. 1990)

5.5 An Induced-Repair Model of the Low-Dose Radiation Response

How, then, can these data both in vivo and in vitro be explained? One possibility would be that a sensitive response at low doses is a consequence of a small subpopulation of cells (for example in a particular position or positions within the cell cycle) with exquisite radiosensitivity. When such a model was fitted to the in vitro data, it predicted that this hypothetical population would comprise about 4% of the total cells, but would have an increased sensitivity to x-rays by a factor of about 60 compared with the rest of the cell population (MARPLES and JOINER 1993). This seems unlikely; for example the work of SINCLAIR (1972) indicates a maximum difference of about tenfold between the radiosensitivity in the different phases of the cell cycle. Additionally, further experiments in vitro (MARPLES and JOINER 1993) appear to rule out the existence of a stable genetic subpopulation of sensitive cells and also indicate that low-dose sensitivity and the relationship shown in Figs. 5.7 and 5.8 occur regardless of the phase of the cell cycle at the time of irradiation. It is also hard to reconcile a mechanism based on cell cycle progression with the data on mouse kidney described in Sect. 5.3.2, where estimates of labelling index are generally less than 0.5% (WILSON et al. 1987).

An alternative explanation is that low-dose sensitivity represents a baseline or "resting" response to radiation, and that higher doses become less effective at killing cells per unit dose because they produce increased amounts of DNA damage which stimulates or induces repair systems, stress proteins or other protective mechanisms within a few hours, which can then increase either the absolute rate of DNA damage repair or its fidelity. Such radiation induced systems that protect against chromosomal damage have been documented in human lymphocytes (TUSCHL et al. 1980; SHADLEY and WOLFF 1987; SHADLEY and WIENCKE 1989) and in hamster cells (IKUSHIMA 1987, 1989), and an induced-repair mechanism such as this has been proposed to explain the shapes of highly radio-resistant lepidopteran cell survival curves (KOVAL 1984, 1986, 1988) which bear more than a passing resemblance to the x-ray survival curve shown in Fig. 5.6. As a necessary part of an induced-repair hypothesis, it is now clear that ionising radiation can indeed induce expression of certain genes, for example the *gadd45* system (PAPATHANASIOU et al.

1991), as well as proteins (BOOTHMAN et al. 1989), although of course there is no actual evidence that the particular gene or proteins induced in these two studies are specifically involved in the phenomenon described here.

We propose, therefore, that the data presented here could reflect repair induction as the x-ray dose is increased. Since this is essentially an effect on survival restricted to the first gray of x-radiation, such a mechanism would have to affect predominantly the α term in the LQ equation (Eq. 5.1). A simple modification of the LQ model is to make α in Eq. 5.1 decrease with dose; thus

$$\alpha = \alpha_{RES}[1 + g\exp(-d/d_c)], \tag{5.3}$$

where two new parameters are defined: d_c represents the dose at which 63% $(1 - e^{-1})$ of induction has occurred and g is the amount by which α at very low doses (α_{SENS}) is larger than α at high doses (α_{RES}). Thus $\alpha_{SENS} = \alpha_{RES}(1 + g)$. Equation 5.2 therefore becomes

$$D = \frac{E/\alpha_{RES}}{1 + g\exp(-d/d_c) + d/(\alpha_{RES}/\beta)} \tag{5.4}$$

The solid lines in Figs. 5.1–5.3 represent this equation fitted to the data for skin and kidney, using non-linear least-squares regression. In all these cases, the fit of this simple model is very good. To fit the data in Fig. 5.7, Eqs. 5.1 and 5.3 are expressed as the effective D_0; thus

$$\text{Effective } D_0 = \frac{1/\alpha_{RES}}{1 + g\exp(-d/d_c) + d/(\alpha_{RES}/\beta)}. \tag{5.5}$$

To fit the data in Fig. 5.8, Eqs. 5.1 and 5.3 are expressed as the RBE compared with an exponential response to neutrons given by $E' = n(\alpha_N d_N)$ in analogy with Eq. 5.1. Thus

$$\text{RBE} = \frac{\alpha_N/\alpha_{RES}}{1 + g\exp(-d/d_c) + d/(\alpha_{RES}/\beta)}. \tag{5.6}$$

The solid lines in Figs. 5.7b and 5.8 show the excellent fit of these equations to the data. It appears, therefore, that a concept of induced repair, as implemented simply in Eq. 5.3, can adequately account for the phenomenon of unexpected radiosensitivity to low x-ray doses, which we have seen both in vivo and in vitro.

Table 5.1 summarises the values of g and d_c obtained from the fits of Eqs. 5.4 and 5.5 to the data from the different systems. Interestingly, g appears to be largest in the kidney; this tissue is

Table 5.1. Parameters g and d_c in the simple induced repair model. Data from [1]JOINER et al. (1986) (Fig. 5.1), [2]JOINER et al. (unpub.) (Fig. 5.2), [3]JOINER & JOHNS (1988) (Fig. 5.3) and [4]MARPLES & JOINER (1992) (Fig. 5.6)

Parameter	Lower 95% conf. limit	Value	Upper 95% conf. limit
[1]Skin in vivo			
g	0.62	2.02	3.42
d_c	0.07	0.16	0.26
[2]Skin in vivo			
g	− 0.07	1.88	3.83
d_c	0.01	0.07	0.12
[3]Kidney in vivo			
g	− 2.92	5.66	14.2
d_c	0.04	0.19	0.34
[4]V79 cells in vitro			
g	1.06	2.14	3.22
d_c	0.11	0.21	0.31

late reacting, with the lowest value of α/β of these systems. Values of d_c, the dose needed to cause significant "induction", are all less than 0.25 Gy but do vary between systems and even, in the skin, between experiments. At usual values of dose per fraction used clinically, therefore, tissues are all "fully induced" and the radiation response appears conventional and is reasonably described by the LQ model. However, these data suggest that the effect of much smaller doses in penumbrae or in multiple-field treatments outside the target volume may need to be re-assessed in critical cases, for example where the target volume is adjacent to spinal cord (see Sect. 5.6.2).

If induced repair *is* the explanation of the substructure we have observed in the V79 survival curve at low doses, and the corresponding decrease in isoeffective total dose in normal tissues exposed to very low doses per fraction, then the modified induced-repair LQ model (Eq. 5.3) and the rough range of values of d_c and $g + 1$ from Table 5.1 predict that radioprotection can be triggered in these systems over the dose range 0.05–0.25 Gy and that low doses ($\ll 1$ Gy) of x-rays can be up to three to seven times more effective per unit dose at killing cells than high doses of x-rays (> 1 Gy), due to *lack* of repair. The value of g may be even higher for particularly radioresistant human tumour cells like HT29 (LAMBIN et al. 1993). Interestingly, the value of d_c, the dose required for 63% induction of radio-resistance, is similar in the normal tissue and cell systems we have studied (Table 5.1) although much larger than the doses used to induce radio-protection in lymphocytes (WOLFF et al. 1989).

Low-dose sensitivity does not appear to be a feature of the response to neutrons of either cells in vitro (e.g. Figs. 5.6 and 5.7a) or the normal tissues in vivo (data not shown; see JOINER et al. 1986; JOINER and JOHNS 1988). However, even with x-ray doses as high as 0.5 Gy, GOODHEAD (1989) has calculated that in each cell only about 20 initial DNA double-strand breaks are produced with perhaps 25 times this number of single-strand breaks (SSB). It therefore seems more likely that "repair induction" is triggered by types of damage (e.g. SSB) which predominate after low- rather than high-LET irradiation and this might explain the lack of substructure in the response to low neutron doses. Alternatively, highly effective irreparable damage dominates the response to d(4)-Be neutrons to such an extent, producing essentially a linear survival curve, that any substructure due to repair phenomena would be extremely difficult to detect even if it were present. Therefore inducible effects of low doses of high-LET radiation cannot be ruled out and it would be of interest in the future to study low doses of radiation of intermediate LET which, although more effective than x-rays, still produce downward-bending survival curves in which low-dose substructure might be seen.

It is also interesting to note that in extreme cases, values of the parameters in the induced-repair model can be chosen so that there is actually a small *increase* in cell survival as dose increases over the range 0.2–0.7 Gy. In this case, higher doses of radiation would actually kill less cells than smaller doses. In spite of the amazing nature of this proposal there is some evidence that this may really occur in human HT29 cells treated with very low radiation doses (LAMBIN et al. 1993).

5.6 Clinical Implications of Low-Dose Sensitivity

5.6.1 Significance for Radiosensitivity Measurements

If induced repair is the correct explanation for the increased radiosensitivity which we have seen at low doses, then an implication is that radiosensitivity may be governed largely by the amount of repair, with variations in initial DNA damage and tolerance to residual DNA injury being less important (POWELL and McMILLAN 1990). This is supported by the hypersensitivity to radiation of cells and tissues of patients with genetic conditions which are characterised by a defect in an aspect of DNA repair, for example ataxia telangiectasia, Fanconi's anaemia, Cockayne's syndrome (FRIEDBERG 1985) and xeroderma pigmentosum (CLEAVER 1968). Therefore, one could suggest that the variations seen in radiosensitivity among cell lines, tumours and other tissues might be linked to differences in the degree of repair induction in response to radiation. A measurement of surviving fraction at > 1 Gy *should* therefore be an adequate predictor of clinical radiosensitivity, as this is in excess of the dose required to induce repair and clinical radiotherapy uses doses per fraction > 1 Gy. Conversely, any predictions of clinical radiosensitivity made with doses less than 1 Gy might be suspect, as would any comparison between the "true" initial slopes of survival curves, which should be much steeper than expected from examination of measurements made above 1 Gy, as illustrated in Fig. 5.6.

As reducing the dose rate and increasing the number of fractions are biologically equivalent in radiotherapy, it may be questioned whether predictions of clinical radiosensitivity made from the effect of low-dose-rate exposures of 1–5 cGy min^{-1} (e.g. STEEL et al. 1987) may be suspect in the light of our results. Although we have not yet determined whether increased cell killing per unit dose can be detected as the dose *rate* is reduced, the data of CROMPTON et al. (1990), shown in Fig. 5.9, imply that dose rates of > 1 cGy min^{-1} should be "fully inducing" and therefore *should* accurately reflect the response to acute doses of > 1 Gy.

5.6.2 Therapeutic Exposure to Very Low Doses

It is now accepted that the clinical use of doses per fraction less than 2 Gy is therapeutically beneficial because it spares radiation injury in late-reacting tissues, which allows an increase in the total dose (HORIOT et al. 1990). How would increased sensitivity at low doses per fraction modify this? As explained previously (WITHERS et al. 1989) and elsewhere in this volume, the LQ model can be used with a range of α/β values to predict the changes in isoeffective doses for late-reacting tissues, acutely-reacting tissues and tumours as the dose per fraction is reduced. Usually, one calculates an isoeffect dose (D_d), normalised to the isoeffect dose for 2-Gy fractions ($D_{2\,Gy}$), as a function of dose per fraction d. We have taken the reverse approach by calculating the ratio of isoeffect dose for 2-Gy fractions to the

isoeffect dose, as a function of dose per fraction. By incorporating the induced-repair model (Eq. 5.3) into Eq. 5.1, this is given by

$$\frac{D_{2Gy}}{D_d} = \frac{1 + ge^{-d/d_c} + d/(\alpha/\beta)}{1 + ge^{-2/d_c} + 2/(\alpha/\beta)}, \tag{5.7}$$

and by considering Eq. 5.2, this ratio can also be thought of as the "effect per unit total dose", normalised to its value for 2-Gy fractions. The major advantage of this approach is that this relationship is *linear* with dose per fraction for the standard LQ model, i.e. in the absence of any "induced repair". This can be seen in Fig. 5.10, which plots Eq. 5.7 for a range of α/β values of 1–4 Gy for late-reacting tissues, 8–15 Gy for acutely-reacting tissues and 18 Gy for tumours. In addition, $g = 5.66$ and $d_c = 0.19$ have been used for late tissues and $g = 1.95$ and $d_c = 0.115$ for acute tissues and tumours, averaged from Table 5.1. As expected, Fig. 5.10 shows that at between 1 and 2 Gy per fraction there is no conflict with the accepted strategy of hyperfractionation since effect per unit total dose is always less in late-reacting tissues than in acutely-reacting tissues or tumours. However, if doses per fraction were reduced below about 0.7 Gy, there could conceivably be some loss of therapeutic gain and at less than 0.5 Gy per fraction there could even be a therapeutic disadvantage from hyperfractionation. However, Fig. 5.10 also shows

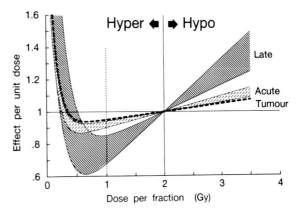

Fig. 5.10. Schematic diagram showing the dependence of the effect of a fractionated radiotherapy treatment per unit total dose on the dose per fraction. Hyperfractionated schedules with doses per fraction of 1–2 Gy are therapeutically beneficial because the effectiveness of radiotherapy is always reduced more in the late-reacting tissues than the tumour, allowing the total dose to be raised compared with a conventional 2-Gy-per-fraction schedule. However, because of the influence of low-dose hypersensitivity, the picture is complicated at doses per fraction less than 1 Gy and a therapeutic gain may not always be possible

that if dose was highly localised to the tumour, for example in interstitial or brachytherapy, then doses per fraction below 0.3 Gy given with high-dose-rate remote afterloading techniques or protracted low dose rates of less than 7 cGy h^{-1} (by comparing the horizontal axes in Fig. 5.9) could be more effective in tumours compared with conventional high-dose-rate 2-Gy fractions.

Since the effectiveness of very small does fractions could be much greater than expected, this may lead to greater subthreshold damage than previously thought at the edges or in the penumbrae of treatment plans. One has to keep this is perspective because although the effect per *unit* total dose could be much higher, the *total* doses in these regions are still very small so the final damage is still not going to exceed tolerance. However, it may be important to bear in mind the possible extra effect of low doses outside the target volume if regions in the vicinity are subsequently retreated. As an illustration of this, Fig. 5.11 shows how much of a schedule of 2-Gy fractions, as a proportion, would produce equivalent late damage to full schedules with doses per fraction less than 2 Gy, calculated

with either the LQ model or the induced-repair model. Diagrams such as this allow one to express the effect of a schedule of small doses per fraction in terms of the number of 2-Gy fractions which would give equivalent damage (see example in legend). This always decreases with decreasing dose per fraction, although not as quickly with the induced-repair model. The maximum absolute difference between the predictions of the two models occurs at a dose equal to d_c (with the constraint that $d_c \ll 2$ Gy), in this case 0.19 Gy, where the proportion of a 2-Gy schedule increases from 5% with the LQ model to 15% with the induced-repair model.

Finally, one must ask whether increased mutational effect of very low doses is likely to lead to an increased incidence of secondary cancers outside the target volume. Carcinogenic risk is a product of mutation frequency and cell kill: there is minimum risk either at very low doses because there are no mutations, or at very high doses because all mutated cells are killed. This leads to a bell-shaped relationship between risk and dose, with maximum risk normally at around 2–3 Gy. If mutation frequency *and* cell kill are both increased at low doses, as is likely since both are determined by residual DNA damage, then the maximum risk and the dose at which it occurs would probably remain the same. A net increase in low-dose risk might occur if induction of repair of lethal damage but not mutational damage occurred. Clearly this should be an area of intensive future research in the field of radiation protection.

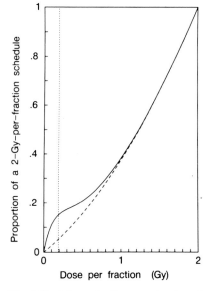

Fig. 5.11. Schematic diagram showing the effect of radiotherapy schedules with doses per fraction between 0 and 2 Gy, expressed as a proportion of a schedule with the same number of 2-Gy fractions which produces equivalent late damage. For example, 35 fractions of 1.5 Gy are equivalent to $35 \times 0.66 = 23$ fractions of 2 Gy. The relationship is calculated using $\alpha/\beta = 2$ Gy, with the LQ model (*dashed line*), or the induced-repair model (*solid line*) with $d_c = 0.19$ Gy and $g = 5.66$. The induced-repair model predicts an increased effect of low-dose fractions and deviates maximally from the LQ prediction at a dose per fraction equal to d_c (see text)

5.7 Conclusions

The aim of this article has been to highlight the following points:

1. Low x-ray doses per fraction (< 0.6 Gy) are *more* effective per unit dose compared with higher doses per fraction. This has been confirmed in skin and kidney, and is suggested in lung.
2. V79 cells also demonstrate the same pattern of sensitivity to low *single* x-ray doses in vitro.
3. An explanation is that this phenomenon reflects increasing radioresistance as x-ray dose is increased from zero to about 1 Gy, owing to the induction of repair systems or other radioprotective mechanisms.

Acknowledgements. This work was supported entirely by the Cancer Research Campaign of the UK. We are grateful to

Dr. C.S. Parkins for supplying us with the data on which Fig. 5.4 is based.

References

Beck-Bornholdt HP, Maurer T, Becker S, Omniczynski M, Vogler H, Wurschmidt F (1989) Radiotherapy of the rhabdomyosarcoma R1H of the rat: hyperfractionation—126 fractions applied within 6 weeks. Int J Radiat Oncol Biol Phys 16: 701–705

Boothman DA, Bouvard I, Hughes EN (1989) Identification and characterization of x-ray-induced proteins in human cells. Cancer Res 49: 2871–2878

Cleaver JE (1968) Defective repair replication of DNA in xeroderma pigmentosum. Nature 218: 652–656

Crompton NEA, Barth B, Kiefer J (1990) Inverse dose-rate effect for the induction of 6-thioguanine-resistant mutants in Chinese hamster V79-S cells by ^{60}Co γ rays. Radiat Res 124: 300–308

Denekamp J (1973) Changes in the rate of repopulation during multifraction irradiation of mouse skin. Br J Radiol 46: 381–387

Douglas BG, Fowler JF (1976) The effect of multiple small doses of x-rays on skin reactions in the mouse and a basic interpretation. Radiat Res 66: 401–426

Folkard M (1986) Determination of d(3)-Be and d(4)-Be neutron spectra using a recoil proton spectrometer. Phys Med Biol 31: 135–144

Friedberg EC (1985) DNA repair. W.H. Freeman, New York

Goodhead DT (1989) The initial physical damage produced by ionizing radiations. Int J Radiat Biol 56: 623–634

Hopewell JW, van den Aardweg GJMJ (1991) Studies of dose-fractionation on early and late responses in pig skin: a reappraisal of the importance of the overall treatment time and its effects on radiosensitization and incomplete repair. Int J Radiat Oncol Biol Phys 21: 1441–1450

Horiot JC, le Fur R, N'Guyen T et al. (1990) Hyperfractionated compared with conventional radiotherapy in oropharyngeal carcinoma: an EORTC randomized trial. Eur J Cancer 26: 779–780

Ikushima T (1987) Chromosomal responses to ionizing radiation reminiscent of an adaptive response in cultured Chinese hamster cells. Mutat Res 180: 215–221

Ikushima T (1989) Radio-adaptive response: characterization of a cytogenetic repair induced by low-level ionizing radiation in cultured Chinese hamster cells. Mutat Res 227: 241–246

Johns H, Joiner MC (1991) A simple method for fitting curves to dose-effect data for functional damage. Int J Radiat Biol 60: 533–541

Joiner MC (1987) The design and interpretation of top-up experiments to investigate the effects of low radiation doses. Int J Radiat Biol 51: 115–130

Joiner MC (1989) The dependence of radiation response on the dose per fraction. In: McNally NJ (ed) The scientific basis for modern radiotherapy (BIR Report 19). British Institute of Radiology, London, pp 20–26

Joiner MC, Denekamp J (1986) Evidence for a constant repair capacity over 20 fractions of x-rays. Int J Radiat Biol 49: 143–150

Joiner MC, Johns H (1988) Renal damage in the mouse: the response to very small doses per fraction. Radiat Res 114: 385–398

Joiner MC, Denekamp J, Maughan RL (1986) The use of top-up experiments to investigate the effect of very small doses per fraction in mouse skin. Int J Radiat Biol 49: 565–580

Joiner MC, Rojas A, Johns H (1989) Does the repair capacity of skin change with repeated exposure to x-rays? Int J Radiat Biol 55: 993–1005

Joiner MC, Rojas A, Johns H (1992) A test of equal effect per fraction in the kidney of the mouse. Radiat Res 130: 227–235

Koval TM (1984) Multiphasic survival response of a radio-resistant lepidopteran insect cell line. Radiat Res 98: 642–648

Koval TM (1986) Inducible repair of ionizing radiation damage in higher eukaryotic cells. Mutat Res 173: 291–293

Koval TM (1988) Enhanced recovery from ionizing radiation damage in a lepidopteran insect cell line. Radiat Res 115: 413–420

Lambin P, Marples B, Fertil B, Malaise EP, Joiner MC (1993) Hypersensitivity of a human tumour cell line to very low radiation doses. Int J Radiat Biol 63: 639–650

Liversage WE (1969) A general formula for equating protracted and acute regimes of radiation. Br J Radiol 42: 432–440

Marples B, Joiner MC (1993) The response of V79 cells to low radiation doses: evidence of enchanced sensitivity of the whole cell population. Radiat Res 133: 41–51

Palcic B, Jaggi B (1986) The use of solid state sensor technology to detect and characterise live mammalian cells growing in tissue culture. Int J Radiat Biol 50: 345–352

Papathanasiou MA, Kerr NCK, Robbins JH et al. (1991) Induction by ionizing radiation of the gadd45 gene in cultured human cells: lack of mediation by protein kinase C. Mol Cell Biol 11: 1009–1016

Parkins CS, Fowler JF (1985) Repair in mouse lung of multifraction x-rays and neutrons: extension to 40 fractions. Br J Radiol 58: 225–241

Parkins CS, Fowler JF (1986) The linear quadratic fit for lung function after irradiation with x-rays at smaller doses per fraction than 2 Gy. Br J Cancer 53 [Suppl VII]: 320–323

Parkins CS, Fowler JF, Maughan RL, Roper MJ (1985) Repair in mouse lung for up to 20 fractions of x-rays or neutrons. Br J Radiol 58: 225–241

Powell S, McMillan TJ (1990) DNA damage and repair following treatment with ionizing radiation. Radiother Oncol 19: 95–108

Shadley JD, Wiencke JK (1989) Induction of the adaptive response by x-rays is dependent on radiation intensity. Int J Radiat Biol 56: 107–118

Shadley JD, Wolff S (1987) Very low doses of x-rays can cause human lymphocytes to become less susceptible to ionizing radiation. Mutagenesis 2: 95–96

Sinclair WK (1972) Cell-cycle dependence of the lethal radiation response in mammalian cells. Curr Top Radiat Res Q 7: 264–285

Spadinger I, Palcic B (1992) The relative biological effectiveness of ^{60}Co γ-rays, 55 kVp x-rays, 250 kVp x-rays and 11 MeV electrons at low doses. Int J Radiat Biol 61: 345–353

Steel GG, Deacon JM, Duchesne GM, Horwich A, Kelland LR, Peacock JH (1987) The dose-rate effect in human tumour cells. Radiother Oncol 9: 299–310

Stevens G, Joiner MC, Joiner B, Johns H, Denekamp J (1991) Early detection of damage following bilateral renal irradiation in the mouse. Radiother Oncol 20: 124–131

Thames HD, Ang KK, Stewart FA, van der Schueren E (1988) Does incomplete repair explain the apparent failure of the basic LQ model to predict spinal cord and kidney responses to low doses per fraction? Int J Radiat Biol 54: 13–19

Thames HD, Bentzen SM, Turesson I, Overgaard M, van den Bogaert W (1990) Time-dose factors in radiotherapy: a review of the human data. Radiother Oncol 19: 219–235

Tuschl H, Altmann H, Kovac R, Topaloglou A, Egg D, Gunther R (1980) Effects of low-dose radiation on repair processes in human lymphocytes. Radiat Res 81: 1–9

Watts ME, Hodgkiss RJ, Jones NR, Fowler JF (1986) Radio-sensitisation of Chinese hamster cells by oxygen and mis-onidazole at low x-ray doses. Int J Radiat Biol 50: 1009–1021

Wilson GD, Soranson JA, Lewis AA (1987) Cell kinetics of mouse kidney using bromodeoxyuridine incorporation and flow cytometry: preparation and staining. Cell Tissue Kinet 20: 125–133

Withers HR, Maciejewski B, Taylor JMG (1989) Biology of options in dose fractionation. In: McNally NJ (ed) The scientific basis for modern radiotherapy (BIR Report 19). British Institute of Radiology, London, pp 27–36

Wolff S, Wiencke JK, Afzal V, Youngblom J, Cortes F (1989) The adaptive response of human lymphocytes to very low doses of ionizing radiation: a case of induced chromosomal repair with the induction of specific proteins. In: Baverstock KF, Stather JW (eds) Low dose radiation: biological bases of risk assessment. Taylor & Francis, London, pp 446–454

6 The Influence of the Size of Dose on the Repair Kinetics of X-ray-Induced DNA Strand Breaks Studied in CHO Cells

E. DIKOMEY

CONTENTS

6.1 Introduction

After ionizing irradiation the loss of proliferative capacity is caused by damage induced within the genetic material (MARIN and BENDER 1963a, b; BURKI and OKADA 1970; MUNRO 1970). Among the various types of damage induced, DNA strand breaks and base damage are regarded as the critical lesions leading to cell death (WARD 1985; FRANKENBERG-SCHWAGER 1989).

Most of the DNA damage induced is repaired by cellular enzymes and only a small fraction remains unrepaired (SAKAI and OKADA 1984; BLÖCHER 1988; DAHM-DAPHI et al. 1993). Out of this damage, chromosomal aberrations are formed that finally lead to cell death (HOPWOOD and TOLMACH 1979; FRANKENBERG-SCHWAGER 1989).

After low doses, when the number of damaged sites is much smaller than the number of available repair enzymes, repair of DNA damage is in an *unsaturated* state and for a certain type of damage the *relative* rate of repair is constant and independent of the number of DNA lesions present in the cell (GOODHEAD 1985). After higher doses, when the number of lesions exceeds the number of repair enzymes, repair is in a *saturated* state and the relative rate of repair is rather low at the beginning and increases with decreasing number of lesions.

The transition of the repair system from an unsaturated to a saturated state leading to a decreased repair efficiency after higher doses might have some implications for the radiotherapeutic treatment of cancer. The radiotherapeutic treatment is generally given in small fractions, whereby the interfraction interval is long enough to allow maximum recovery from damage. If one assumes that the repair efficiency decreases with increasing dose, the time interval required to obtain maximum recovery should increase with the size of dose. Then, a higher dose given per fraction would have to be accompanied by a prolonged interfraction interval in order to avoid overexposure of the normal tissue.

6.2 Repair of X-ray-Induced DNA Strand Breaks

Figure 6.1 shows the repair kinetics of DNA strand breaks as obtained for Chinese hamster ovary (CHO) cells which were exposed to single x-ray doses of 3–90 Gy. Cells were irradiated at ice temperature, in order to prevent repair during the irradiation, followed by incubation at 37°C to allow for repair. DNA strand breaks were measured using the alkaline unwinding technique (RYDBERG 1975; AHNSTRÖM and ERIXON 1981). This technique is based on a partial denaturation of the DNA in an alkaline solution, whereby the fraction of DNA remaining double-stranded after denaturation for a given time correlates with the number of strand breaks present per cell. The fraction of double-stranded DNA can be converted into the absolute number of strand breaks assuming that an x-ray dose of 1 Gy leads to 1000 strand breaks per cell (AHNSTRÖM and ERIXON 1981).

The repair curves shown in Fig. 6.1 represent the repair of single- and double-stranded breaks, since the alkaline unwinding technique is known to detect both types of breaks (DIKOMEY and FRANZKE 1988).

E. DIKOMEY, PhD, Institute for Biophysics and Radiobiology, University of Hamburg, University Hospital Eppendorf, Martinistraße 52, 20246 Hamburg 20, Germany

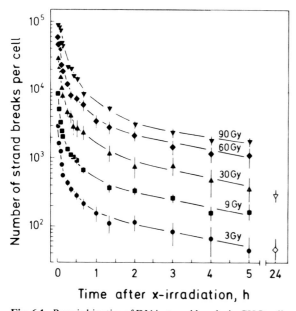

Fig. 6.1. Repair kinetics of DNA strand breaks in CHO cells exposed to x-ray doses of 3, 9, 30, 60, and 90 Gy. Cells were irradiated at 0 °C followed by an incubation at 37°C and the number of strand breaks was measured after different intervals up to 5 h (*closed symbols*) and—in order to determine the number of nonrepairable strand breaks—also after an interval of 24 h (*open symbols*). Strand breaks were measured using the alkaline unwinding technique. Data are the means ± SEM. (From DIKOMEY and LORENZEN 1993)

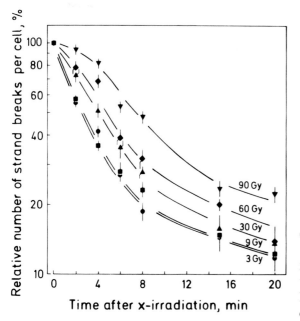

Fig. 6.2. Relative repair kinetics of x-ray-induced DNA strand breaks in CHO cells. The data plotted are obtained from the measured points shown in Fig. 6.1 after dividing the absolute numbers by the corresponding initial number. Data are the means ± SEM. (From DIKOMEY and LORENZEN 1993)

The repair curves obtained for the different doses are rather similar with a fast phase for $t = 0$–0.25 h followed by an intermediate phase for $t = 0.25$–2 h, and finally a slow phase for $t \geq 2$ h. The main difference between these curves was found to occur during the fast phase. This difference can be seen more clearly in Fig. 6.2, where the *relative* number of DNA strand breaks is plotted versus the time after irradiation. After the lower doses (3 and 9 Gy) strand breaks were initially rejoined with a relative rate which was much higher than after the higher doses (30–90 Gy). However, this difference disappears with time after irradiation.

6.2.1 Repair of DNA Double-Strand Breaks

The slow phase of the repair curve is interpreted as the repair kinetics of DNA double-strand breaks, since this phase was shown to correspond to the kinetics measured by the neutral sedimentation technique, which is considered exclusively to detect DNA double-strand breaks (BRYANT and BLÖCHER 1980, 1982; BLÖCHER et al. 1983; DIKOMEY and FRANZKE 1986a).

The repair curve of DNA double-strand breaks has to be corrected for the number of *nonrepairable* breaks in order to obtain the kinetics of those double-strand breaks which are actually repaired (FRANKENBERG-SCHWAGER et al. 1990). The number of nonrepairable breaks can be determined 24 h after irradiation (DAHM-DAPHI et al. 1993). The corresponding numbers measured after doses of 60 and 90 Gy are also shown in Fig. 6.1 (open symbols). After doses of 3, 9, and 30 Gy these numbers were not significantly different from the numbers of strand breaks measured for nonirradiated cells (DIKOMEY and LORENZEN 1993).

When the slow phase was corrected for the number of nonrepairable breaks, the resulting kinetics of repairable double-strand breaks were best described by a single exponential component (DIKOMEY and LORENZEN 1993). From the extrapolation of this component to the ordinate the initial fraction of all double-strand breaks could be derived, which on average was $f_{dsb} = 0.053 \pm 0.008$. The half-time of double-strand break repair was determined from the slope of this exponential decline and was found to be independent of the dose with a mean value of $\tau_{dsb} = 166 \pm 35$ min (Fig. 6.3). Each of these two results—first, that the kinetics of double-strand break repair are described by an exponential decline and, second, that the half-time of double-strand break repair is independent of the dose applied—indicated that the repair of double-strand breaks was unsaturated at least for doses up to 90 Gy.

6.2.2 Repair of DNA Single-Strand Breaks

The kinetics obtained after subtracting the exponential component determined for double-strand break repair from all strand breaks represents the repair of primary and secondary single-strand breaks (DIKOMEY and FRANZKE 1992). Primary single-strand breaks are induced during the irradiation, while secondary single-strand breaks are generated during the repair of damaged bases, when the sugar–phosphate bond is incised by a specific endonuclease.

Figure 6.4 shows the kinetics of single-strand break repair obtained for CHO cells after a dose of 3 or 90 Gy. For both doses the kinetics of single-strand break repair are biphasic. The initial decline mainly reflects the repair of primary single-strand breaks with the half-time τ_{rep} (Fig. 6.4, broken line), while the second phase is associated with the repair of base damage, which is converted into secondary single-strand breaks (Fig. 6.4, dotted line). These strand breaks are generated by the half-time τ_{in} and are repaired with the same half-time as primary single-strand breaks (KOW et al. 1991). Since the formation of secondary single-strand breaks is the rate-limiting step, the half-time τ_{in} is equal to the half-time at which the number of single-strand breaks declines during the second phase.

After a dose of 3 Gy the kinetics of single-strand break repair is best fitted by a sum of two exponential components (Fig. 6.4a), which indicates that the formation and the repair of primary and secondary single-strand breaks are described by constant half-times (DIKOMEY and LORENZEN 1993). Due to this result, repair of primary and secondary single-strand breaks should be in an unsaturated state after a dose of 3 Gy.

After a dose of 90 Gy the initial phase of single-strand break repair is characterized by a convex

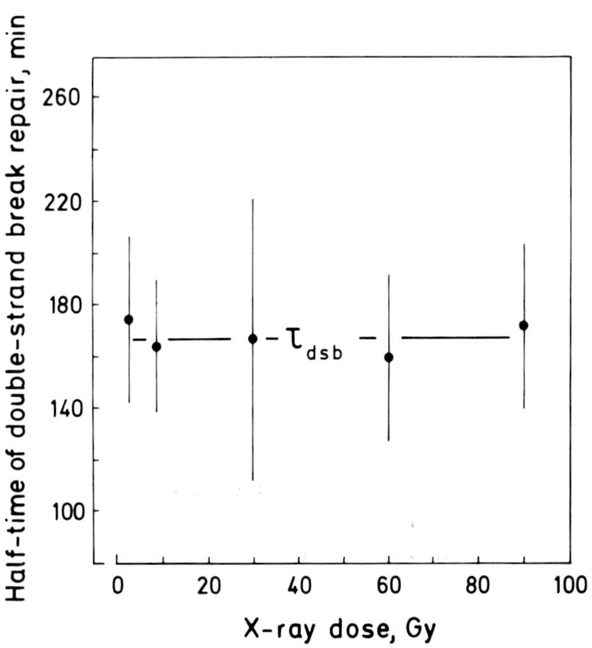

Fig. 6.4a, b. Repair kinetics of DNA single-strand breaks in CHO cells exposed to x-ray doses of 3 (**a**) or 90 (**b**) Gy. Data were obtained from Fig. 6.1 after subtracting the exponential component determined for double-strand break repair from all strand breaks. The calculated numbers of all single-strand breaks (*solid line*) of all primary single-strand breaks (*broken line*), and of all secondary single-strand breaks (*dotted line*) are shown. Data are the means ± SEM. (From DIKOMEY and LORENZEN 1993)

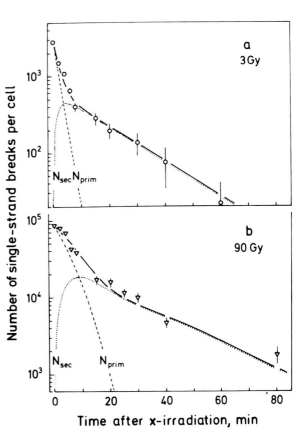

Fig. 6.3. The effect of the size of the dose on the half-time of double-strand break repair in CHO cells. The half-time was determined from the slow phase of the repair curves shown in Fig. 6.1 after subtracting the number of nonrepairable strand breaks measured 24 h after irradiation. Data are the means ± SEM. (From DIKOMEY and LORENZEN 1993)

curvature (Fig. 6.4b). This result indicates that the relative rate of repair is not constant but increases with decreasing number of single-strand breaks. An increase in the relative rate of repair with decreasing number of strand breaks suggests that the repair of single-strand breaks is saturated after an x-ray dose of 90 Gy.

For any enzymatic reaction the relation between the velocity of reaction, v, and the substrate concentration, $[S]$, is described by the Michaelis-Menten equation

$$v = \frac{v_{max} + [S]}{k_m \times [S]}, \tag{6.1}$$

where v_{max} is the maximum velocity and k_m the substrate concentration when the reaction will have half of its maximum velocity. When this equation is applied to the formation and repair of primary and secondary single-strand breaks, the half-time τ_{in} and τ_{rep} are found to be linear functions of the number of single-strand breaks or base damage, respectively (DIKOMEY and LORENZEN 1993). Figure 6.5 shows the corresponding relationships obtained, whereby τ_{in} was found to increase with a rate of 6.7×10^{-5} min per base damage with a minimum value of $\tau_{0,in} = 13$ min, and τ_{rep} to increase with a rate of 4.1×10^{-5} min per single-strand break with a minimum value of $\tau_{0,rep} = 1.4$ min.

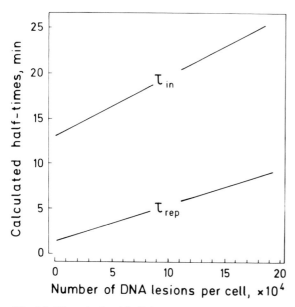

Fig. 6.5. The calculated half-times τ_{rep} and τ_{in} as a function of the number of all single-strand breaks or base damage present in the cell, respectively. The lines drawn were obtained by fitting the kinetics of single-strand break repair by the Michaelis-Menten equation. (From DIKOMEY and LORENZEN 1993)

After a dose of 3 Gy, which led to about 6.3×10^3 damaged bases and 2.9×10^3 single-strand breaks (DIKOMEY and LORENZEN 1993), incision and repair should start with a half-time of $\tau_{in} = 14$ min and $\tau_{rep} = 1.5$ min (Fig. 6.5). These values are only slightly above the corresponding minimum values so that the decline of τ_{in} and τ_{rep} during the repair incubation is negligible. As a consequence the kinetics of single-strand break repair is described by constant half-times leading to a curve which is a sum of two exponential components as shown in Fig. 6.4a.

After a dose of 90 Gy, which led to about 1.9×10^5 damaged bases and 8.6×10^5 single-strand breaks per cell, incision and repair should start with a half-time of $\tau_{in} = 2.6$ min and $\tau_{rep} = 4.9$ min. These values are longer than the corresponding minimum values by factors of 3.4 and 2.0, respectively. As a consequence, after a dose of 90 Gy both half-times, τ_{in} and τ_{rep}, are characterized by a significant decline during the repair incubation when the number of corresponding lesions declines with time after irradiation. This decline led to the convex curvature of the first and the second repair phase observed in Fig. 6.4b.

When a similar analysis is done for other doses the decline in the half-time τ_{in} with time after irradiation was negligible (i.e., with a change by a factor less than 1.3) after doses up to 30 Gy, while for τ_{rep} this was the case only after doses up to 10 Gy (see Fig. 6.5). As long as the change in the half-time τ is negligible and can be approximated by a constant value the corresponding repair process is said to be in an unsaturated state (GOODHEAD 1985). Adopting this definition, the data presented above showed that the incision and the repair step are unsaturated after x-ray doses up to 30 Gy and 10 Gy, respectively. Above these two doses both repair processes should become successively saturated. As a consequence, both the repair of primary single-strand breaks and the repair of base damage should be unsaturated only after doses up to 10 Gy, since the latter process requires both the enzymatic incision and the repair step.

6.2.3 Other Cell Lines

Dose dependence of strand break repair was also reported for some other cell lines (WOODS 1981; WHEELER and NELSON 1987, 1991; ILIAKIS et al. 1991). In these reports the kinetics of single- or double-strand break repair were described by a single or a sum of two exponential components and the half-times of these components were found to increase with the size of dose. This increase was attributed to a saturated repair system (WHEELER and NELSON 1987, 1991). However, if a repair curve is described by constant half-times, the corresponding repair process is known to be in an unsaturated state. It appears more likely that the increase in the half-time mentioned above results from an increasing amount of nonrepairable damage, which was found to cause a substantial prolongation in the *apparent* repair half-time (FRANKENBERG-SCHWAGER et al. 1990; DAHM-DAPHI et al. 1993).

So far the only data showing a saturation in strand break repair are presented for CHO cells (DIKOMEY and LORENZEN 1993). Since the kinetics of strand break repair measured for CHO cells are fairly similar to the kinetics observed for other mammalian cell lines (DIKOMEY and FRANZKE 1986b), it might be assumed that strand break repair is also saturated in other cell lines only after doses exceeding 10 Gy. As a consequence, during a fractionated regimen the time interval required to allow maximum recovery should not depend on dose as long as the dose given per fraction is below 10 Gy *and* provided that other parameters which also affect repair are not altered.

6.3 Repair of Sublethal or Potentially Lethal Damage

The recovery after ionizing irradiation can also be studied on the cellular level by split-dose irradiation or delayed plating, being termed "recovery from sublethal" or "recovery from potentially lethal damage". In most reports these processes were found to be independent of the size of the dose (see for instance: BARENDSEN 1983; ANG et al. 1987; THAMES and HENDRY 1987; VAN DEN AARDWEG and HOPEWELL 1992). However, in some reports (MCNALLY and DERONDE 1976; ZEMAN and BEDFORD 1985; ROJAS and JOINER 1989) recovery from sublethal or potentially lethal damage was found to be depressed when the size of the dose or the number of fractions was increased. These data should not be attributed to a saturated repair of DNA damage, since these effects are already observed after doses at which repair of DNA damage still can be expected to be unsaturated. Probably, these effects result from an altered supply in oxygen or adenosine triphosphate or from a change in the proliferative

status, since these parameters also affect the repair of DNA lesions (see for instance: GÄRTNER et al. 1977; DIKOMEY 1990; FRANKENBERG-SCHWAGER et al. 1991).

6.4 DNA Damage and Cell Survival

For mammalian cells the efficiency of sparsely ionizing irradiation for cell killing is known to increase with the dose and dose rate (BEDFORD and MITCHELL 1973; HALL 1972). So far, the biological mechanisms for this generally observed phenomenon are not completely understood. One explanation, which was often used in the past, is based on the assumption that the increase in radiosensitivity results from the transition of the repair system from an unsaturated to a saturated system. This concepts which was first suggested by POWERS (1962), was developed in greater detail later (HAYNES 1966; ALPER 1979; GOODHEAD 1982, 1985) and is generally termed the "repair model."

Figure 6.6 shows the dose-response curve for cell killing as obtained for CHO cells after x-irradiation. Cells were irradiated on ice and survival was determined by the colony-forming assay. The dose-response curve is characterized by a convex curvature, indicating that the efficiency of x-irradiation for cell killing increases with increasing

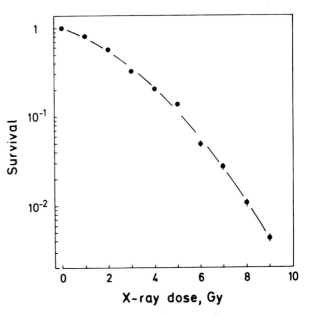

Fig. 6.6. Effect of x-irradiation on survival of CHO cells. Cells were irradiated at 0°C and survival was determined by the colony-forming assay. Data are the means ± SEM. (From DIKOMEY and JUNG 1991)

dose. This increase in radiosensitivity is already significant for doses exceeding 2 Gy. According to the repair model, this result suggests that the repair of those lesions which are relevant for cell killing is saturated after a dose as low as 2 Gy.

After ionizing irradiation, cell death is considered mainly to result from DNA double-strand breaks and probably also from base damage but not from single-strand breaks (WARD 1985, 1986; FRANKENBERG-SCHWAGER 1989). If this consideration is applied to the repair model, the repair of either double-strand breaks or base damage should be saturated in CHO cells after doses exceeding 2 Gy (Fig. 6.6). This is definitely in contrast to the results presented above. Thus, the increase in radiosensitivity found for CHO cells for doses exceeding 2 Gy cannot be attributed to a saturated repair system but has to be associated with other mechanisms. Possibly, this increase in radiosensitivity results from the enhanced number of lethal events arising from the interaction of sublethal lesions (see, for instance: BARENDSEN 1982).

6.5 Conclusion

Repair kinetics of x-ray-induced DNA strand breaks depends on the size of the dose only after doses exceeding 10 Gy.

Acknowledgements. The author is grateful to Dr. Dahm-Daphi for valuable suggestions during the preparation of this manuscript.

References

Ahnström G, Erixon K (1981) Measurement of strand breaks by alkaline denaturation and hydroxyapatite chromatography. In: Friedberg EC, Hanawalt PC (eds) DNA repair. Marcel Dekker, New York, pp 403–418

Alper T (1979) Cellular radiobiology. Cambridge University Press, London

Ang KK, Thames HD, van der Kogel AJ, van der Schueren E (1987) Is the rate of repair of radiation-induced sublethal damage in rat spinal cord dependent on the size of dose per fraction? Int J Radiat Oncol Biol Phys 13: 557–562

Barendsen GW (1982) Dose fractionation, dose rate and iso-effect relationships for normal tissue responses. Int J Radiat Oncol Biol Phys 8: 1981–1997

Bedford JS, Mitchell JB (1973) Dose-rate effects in synchronous mammalian cells in culture. Radiat Res 54: 316–327

Blöcher D (1988) DNA double-strand break repair determines the RBE of α-particles. Int J Radiat Biol 54: 761–771

Blöcher D, Nüsse M, Bryant PE (1983) Kinetics of double-strand break repair in the DNA of x-irradiated synchronised mammalian cells. Int J Radiat Biol 43: 579–584

Bryant PE, Blöcher D (1980) Measurement of the kinetics of DNA double strand break repair in Ehrlich ascites tumour cells using the unwinding method. Int J Radiat Biol 38: 335–347

Bryant PE, Blöcher D (1982) The effect of 9-β-D-arabino-furanosyladenine on the repair of DNA strand breaks in x-irradiated Ehrlich ascites tumor cells. Int J Radiat Biol 42: 385–394

Burki HJ, Okada S (1970) Killing of cultured mammalian cells by radioactive decay of tritiated thymidine at −196°C. Radiat Res 41: 409–424

Dahm-Daphi J, Dikomey E, Pyttlik C, Jeggo P (1993) Reparable and non-reparable DNA strand breaks induced by x-irradiation in CHO K1 cells and the radiosensitive mutants xrs1 and xrs5. Int J Radiat Biol (in press)

Dikomey E (1990) Induction and repair of DNA strand breaks in x-irradiated proliferating and quiescent CHO cells. Int J Radial Biol 57: 1169–1182

Dikomey E, Franzke J (1986a) Three classes of DNA strand breaks induced by x-irradiation and internal β-rays. Int J Radiat Biol 50: 893–908

Dikomey E, Franzke J (1986b) DNA repair kinetics after exposure to x-irradiation and to internal β-rays in CHO cells. Radiat Environ Biophys 25: 189–194

Dikomey E, Franzke J (1988) DNA denaturation kinetics in CHO cells exposed to different x-ray doses and after different repair intervals using the alkaline unwinding technique. Radiat Environ Biophys 27: 29–37

Dikomey E, Franzke J (1992) Effect of heat on induction and repair of DNA strand breaks in x-irradiated CHO cells. Int J Radiat Biol 61: 221–234

Dikomey E, Jung H (1991) Thermal radiosensitization in CHO cells by prior heating at 41–46°C. Int J Radiat Biol 59: 815–825

Dikomey E, Lorenzen J (1993) Saturated and unsaturated repair of DNA strand breaks after x-irradiation with doses ranging from 3 to 90 in CHO cells. Int J Radiat Biol (in press)

Frankenberg-Schwager M (1989) Review of kinetics for DNA damage induced in eukaryotic cells in vitro by ionizing radiation. Radiother Oncol 14: 307–320

Frankenberg-Schwager M, Frankenberg D, Harbich R, Adamczyk C (1990) A comparative study of rejoining of DNA double-strand breaks in yeast irradiated with 3.5 MeV α-particles or with 30 MeV electrons. Int J Radiat Biol 57: 1151–1168

Frankenberg-Schwager M, Frankenberg D, Harbich R (1991) Different oxygen enhancement ratios for induced and unrejoined DNA double-strand breaks in eukaryotic cells. Radiat Res 128: 243–250

Gärtner C, Sexauer C, Hagen U (1977) Repair of radiation-induced DNA strand breaks in thymocytes. Int J Radiat Biol 32: 293–296

Goodhead DT (1982) An assessment of the role of microdosimetry in radiobiology. Radiat Res 91: 45–76

Goodhead DT (1985) Saturable repair models of radiation action in mammalian cells. Radiat Res 104: 58–67

Hall EJ (1972) Radiation dose-rate: a factor of importance in radiobiology and radiotherapy. Br J Radiol 45: 81–97

Haynes RH (1966) The interpretation of microbial inactivation and recovery phenomena. Radiat Res [Suppl] 6: 1–29

Hopwood LE, Tolmach LJ (1979) Manifestations of damage from ionizing radiation in mammalian cells in postirradiation generations. In: Lett JT, Adler H (eds) Adavances in radiation biology, vol 8. Academic, New York, pp 317–362

Iliakis G, Blöcher D, Metzger L, Pantelias G (1991) Comparison of DNA double-strand break rejoining as measured by pulse field gel electro-phoresis, neutral sucrose gradient centrifugation and nonunwinding filter elution in irradiated plateau-phase CHO cells. Int J Radiat Biol 59: 927–939

Kow YW, Faundez G, Melamede RJ, Wallace SS (1991) Processing of model single-strands breaks in ϕX-174 RF transfecting DNA *Escherichia coli*. Radiat Res 126: 357–366

Marin G, Bender MA (1963a) Survival kinetics of HeLa S-3 cells after incorporation of ^{3}H-thymidine or ^{3}H-uridine. Int J Radiat Biol 7: 221–233

Marin G, Bender MA (1963b) A comparison of mammalian cell-killing by incorporated ^{3}H-thymidine and ^{3}H-uridine. Int J Radiat Biol 7: 235–244

McNally NJ, deRonde J (1976) The effect of repeated small doses of radiation on recovery from sub-lethal damage by Chinese hamster cells irradiated in the plateau phase of growth. Int J Radiat Biol 29: 221–234

Munro TR (1970) The relative radiosensitivity of the nucleus and cytoplasm of Chinese hamster fibroblasts. Radiat Res 42: 451–470

Powers EL (1962) Consideration of survival curves and target theory. Phys Med Biol 7: 3–28

Rojas A, Joiner MC (1989) The influence of dose per fraction on repair kinetics. Radiother Oncol 14: 329–336

Rydberg B (1975) The rate of strand separation in alkali of DNA of irradiated mammalian cells. Radiat Res 61: 274–287

Sakai K, Okada S (1984) Radiation-induced DNA damage and cellular lethality in cultured mammalian cells. Radiat Res 98: 479–490

Thames HD, Hendry JH (1987) Fractionation in radiotherapy. Taylor and Francis, London

Van den Aardweg GJMJ, Hopewell JW (1992) The kinetics of repair for sublethal radiation-induced damage in the pig epidermis: an interpretation based on a fast and a slow component of repair. Radiother Oncol 23: 94–104

Ward JF (1985) Biochemistry of DNA lesion. Radiat Res 104: 103–111

Ward JF (1986) Mechanisms of DNA repair and their potential modification for radiotherapy. Int J Radiat Oncol Biol Phys 12: 1027–1032

Wheeler KT, Nelson GB (1987) Saturation of a DNA repair process in dividing and nondividing mammalian cells. Radiat Res 109: 109–117

Wheeler KT, Nelson GB (1991) Saturation of DNA repair measured by alkaline elution. Radiat Res 125: 227–229

Woods WG (1981) Quantitation of the repair of gamma-radiation-induced double-strand DNA breaks in human fibroblasts. Biochim Biophys Acta 655: 342–348

Zeman EM, Bedford JS (1985) Loss of repair capacity in density-inhibited cultures of C3H 10T cells during multi-fraction irradiation. Radiat Res 104: 71–77

7 The Fractionation Sensitivity of Malignant Melanomas

K.R. Trott

7.1 The Radioresistance of Malignant Melanomas

Malignant melanomas have long been regarded as very radioresistant tumours. This judgement was based on the observation that contrary to other cutaneous tumours, melanomas did not respond well to radiotherapy and did not regress even if doses were escalated to levels which produced very severe skin reactions. Yet tumour regression rate is an inadequate criterion of tumour radiosensitivity, which rather should be based on local tumour control. After primary radiotherapy of stage I malignant melanomas, in-field recurrences are very rare (STORCK et al. 1972; ELSMANN et al. 1991). For more than half a century, the textbooks of radiotherapy and oncology have repeated the assertion that malignant melanomas display pronounced radioresistance, although some authors have added

K.R. TROTT, MD, Professor, Radiation Biology Department, St. Bartholomew's Medical College, Charterhouse Square, London EC1M 6BQ, England

that this is not invariably the case and have reported on some spectacular success with radiotherapy, e.g. DEL REGATO and SPJUT (1977). The first to point to the variable response of malignant melanomas to radiotherapy was MIESCHER (1926). Following radiotherapy, he observed more complete remissions of those malignant melanomas which had a higher mitotic rate before treatment. This led MIESCHER (1926) to associate the poor radiation response of some melanomas with the low proliferative activity of those melanomas.

Although complete response rates or survival rates of around 50% had been reported in the radiotherapy literature since the 1930s (reviewed by STORCK et al. 1972), malignant melanomas retained the stigma of being the paradigm of a radioresistant tumour. In Britain and the United States, radiotherapy scarcely assumed any place in the treatment of melanomas whereas in continental Europe, and particularly in Germany, radiotherapy was the preferred treatment of cutaneous malignant melanomas. Yet, since the continental Europeans also believed in the dogma of the radioresistance of melanomas, radiation doses were excessive, a typical treatment being daily doses of 1000 R of 30 to 50-kV x-rays up to about 10 000 R. Yet when megavoltage radiation with a reliable dose distribution was used for melanomas, 50 Gy in 20 fractions resulted in a high rate of local control of primary and of metastatic malignant melanomas (e.g. VON LIEVEN and SKOPAL 1976).

A fair number of experimental studies were performed to identify the causes of the presumed radioresistance of melanomas, the most interesting being that reported by ROHDE and WISKEMANN (1964). Harding-Passey melanomas of about 8 mm diameter growing in inbred mice were given single radiation doses with 40-kV x-rays. The tumours were removed 24 h later and 3 × 5 mm pieces were transplanted into new hosts. The take rate of unirradiated transplants was about 90% and it dropped to about 20% after exposure doses of 5000 or 7500 R. No transplant from tumours which had been given

10 000 R showed any active growth. This was taken as evidence for the particular radioresistance of melanomas in general. Yet because of poor penetration and poor geometry due to very short focus-target distance some parts of the irradiated tumour received less than 50% of the nominal dose. KUMMERMEHR (1978) studied the local control rate of transplanted Harding-Passey melanomas after different single doses of 300-kV x-rays and found a TCD_{50} of 4500 R, similar to that of other transplantable tumours in his laboratory. Considering the dosimetric uncertainties, the data of ROHDE and WISKEMANN (1964) are compatible with those of KUMMERMEHR (1978) and thus cannot serve as proof for a particular radioresistance of malignant melanomas.

In a prospective randomised clinical study on metastatic malignant melanomas which will be discussed below in more detail, 20 fractions of 2.5 Gy led to a 60% remission rate (SAUSE et al. 1991). Similar results have been reported in many recent retrospective studies. Therefore there is no longer any scientific justification for ascribing any particular radioresistance to malignant melanomas in general. Even if textbooks are slow to accept this fact, many radiotherapists have been revising their

attitude towards radiotherapy for malignant melanomas. But at the same time as the dogma of radioresistance has been waning, malignant melanomas have been attributed another special feature which makes them different from most or all other cancers: it is widely believed that malignant melanomas have a particular fractionation sensitivity which requires a radiotherapy schedule different from those used for other tumours. This study will explore the experimental and clinical evidence for the aforementioned claim.

7.2 The Shoulder of the Survival Curve of Melanoma Cells In Vitro

In 1971, two experimental studies on the cellular radiosensitivity of melanoma cells in vitro changed the perception of the radioresistance of melanomas and its causes. DEWEY (1971) studied cells isolated from a Harding-Passey melanoma of the mouse and determined the surviving fraction after doses up to 8 Gy. The survival curve was adequately described by a low D_0 of 0.85 Gy and a large extrapolation number of 25 (Fig. 7.1). BARRANCO et al. (1971) studied three cell lines which had been isolated from one patient with a malignant melanoma but which had different melanin contents and different growth rates. Their radiosensitivity was very similar and could be described by a single survival curve characterised by a D_0 of 1 Gy and an extrapolation number of 40 (Fig. 7.1). Both Dewey and Barranco et al. concluded that the melanoma cell survival curves were within the normal range and could not explain the perceived clinical radioresistance of melanomas. However, HORNSEY (1972) pointed out that the melanoma cell survival curves were characterised by very large shoulders and that it is not the D_0 which matters in fractionated radiotherapy but the surviving fraction after the typical fraction size of 2 Gy (SF_2). She concluded that "the poor response of some malignant melanomas to radiotherapy could well be explained" (by the large shoulder and high SF_2) "if the cell-survival parameters of these melanomas were similar to that observed from the Harding-Passey melanoma".

ELLIS (1974) used the data of DEWEY (1971) to investigate the influence of the dose per fraction on the probability of cure (at equal NSD) for tumours with different shoulders in their cell survival curves. He concluded that "with high extrapolation numbers (as in melanomas) the sterilizing effect for the same NSD values (i.e. the same normal tissue

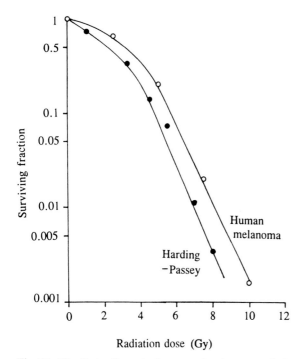

Fig. 7.1. The first cell survival curves of melanoma cells in vitro. *Open circles*: three sublines of a human melanoma (BARRANCO et al. 1971); *closed circles*: B-16 mouse melanoma cells (DEWEY 1971)

damage) of a small number of large fractions is greater than that of a large number of small fractions (the conventional schedule). The high extrapolation numbers seem to be characteristic of radioresistant types of tumours". Ellis concluded by recommending treatment of radioresistant tumours (e.g. malignant melanomas) by a few large dose fractions (of 6 Gy or more) spread over the normal treatment duration.

ZEITZ and MCDONALD (1978) extended these calculations by fitting different survival curve models to the data of DEWEY (1971). Although the absolute gain from changing the dose per fraction from 2 Gy to 6 Gy depended very much on the mathematical model, the high dose per fraction schedule always came out best. This was, however, no longer the case in the calculations made by WHELDON (1979) with the assumption that hypoxic melanoma cells do not readily reoxygenate during fractionated radiotherapy. Obviously more information is needed than just on the shoulder size of the survival curve to design an appropriate treatment protocol for melanomas.

The recommendation of ELLIS (1974) was followed by many radiotherapists and resulted in some unexpectedly favourable responses of malignant melanomas, to be discussed below.

However, not all studies on the radiosensitivity of melanoma cells in vitro produced the same wide shoulder. ZEITZ and SILAGI (1977) isolated cells from another mouse melanoma (B-16). The survival data after irradiation were fitted by a shoulder curve characterised by a D_0 of 1.77 Gy and an extrapolation number of 1.7, similar to that found with HeLa cells studied in the same laboratory. WEININGER et al. (1978) studied three cell lines derived from three different patients, two from lymph node metastases, one from a primary nodular melanoma. Survival curves were established for cells in exponential and in plateau growth phases. There was very little difference in radiosensitivity between growth phases. The survival curves did not differ much between patients: All were very similar to those of HeLa cells. One did have a somewhat higher extrapolation number (of 7.8), which, however, was due to only one unusually low survival point after 11 Gy (surviving fraction less than 0.001); all other survival data were similar to those of the other melanomas.

Thus, the two studies which followed the original experiments of Dewey and Barranco et al. failed to confirm the observation of a wide shoulder as a characteristic feature of melanoma cell survival

curves. With standard cell culture techniques, however, it is notoriously difficult to define the shoulder region of a cell survival curve. Dr. Malaise gave me one of his melanoma cell lines for which he published a D_0 of 1.2 Gy and an extrapolation number of 7.8. In our laboratory, we determined a D_0 of 0.9 Gy and an extrapolation number of 100

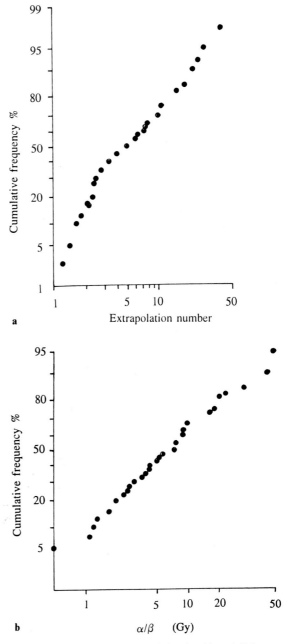

Fig. 7.2a,b. The heterogeneity of the shoulder of 40 human melanoma cell lines (data from ROFSTAD 1986). **a** The cumulative frequency distribution of extrapolation numbers. **b** The cumulative frequency distribution of α/β values

for the same cell line (TROTT et al. 1981a). There were no significant differences in cell survival between the two experiments up to about 7 Gy but with even higher doses surviving fractions were lower in our laboratory than in the laboratory of Dr. Malaise. The differences affected the estimated survival curve parameters very much, which should warn against overinterpreting the biological significance of D_0 and n.

A few more survival curves for melanoma cells derived from rodents have been published, e.g. for the hamster melanoma Amel 3, which is a popular animal model for studies on the biology of melanomas. The D_0 was 1.5, the extrapolation number, 10 (TROTT et al. 1981a). Yet a large number of human melanoma lines have been studied in vitro, especially in the laboratory of Dr. Rofstad in Oslo. In his review of human melanoma cell survival curves (ROFSTAD 1986), 24 of the reported 43 lines came from his laboratory. He compared survival curve parameters of established melanoma cell lines, of cells isolated from melanoma xenografts and of cells directly isolated from surgical specimens but did not find any influence of the source of melanoma cells on the survival curve parameters. Yet within each group there was a wide range of values, with D_0 values ranging from 0.57 Gy to 2.11 Gy and extrapolation numbers ranging from 1 to 78. In this review, the new and old data were also analysed using the linear-quadratic model and values of α, β and α/β were determined. The distribution of extrapolation numbers and α/β values for the 40 human melanoma cell lines for which both values are available is plotted in Fig. 7.2. Both show a wide variation; the median extrapolation number is 5 but 30% are below 3 or above 10. The median α/β value is 7 Gy; 30% are below 3 Gy and 30% above 10 Gy. For no other cell type do we have such a large number of independent assessments of survival curve parameters but it is obvious that the heterogeneity of values of melanoma cell lines is particularly large.

7.3 Repair in Melanoma Cells In Vitro

The wide shoulder of the survival curves displayed by some melanoma cell lines suggests a pronounced repair capacity of melanomas, yet few experiments have been performed that address the repair capacity of melanoma cells in vitro directly. BARRANCO et al. (1971) found a fourfold increase in

the surviving fraction if a dose of 7 Gy was split into two fractions separated by 3 h. TROTT et al. (1981a) observed an eightfold increase using a higher dose of twice 6 Gy separated by 3–4 h. COURDI et al. (1992) compared the survival curve parameters of ten human cancer cell lines, among them three melanomas, to their split-dose recovery after two fractions of 2 Gy. The melanomas were not in any way outside the normal range; their α/β values ranged from less than 1 to 31 Gy and their recovery factor from 1.9 to 4.3, which was in the central range of the ten tumour cell lines.

WEICHSELBAUM et al. (1982) suggested that the radioresistance of some human tumours might be due to more effective repair of potentially lethal radiation damage in those tumour cells. This hypothesis was supported by delayed plating experiments after irradiation of plateau phase cultures. The two melanoma cell lines were among those most proficient at repair of potentially lethal damage. This pronounced repair was also observed after repeated daily doses of 1.75 Gy in the two melanoma cell lines (WEICHSELBAUM et al. 1984). Similar studies by MARCHESE et al. (1985), however, failed to demonstrate any repair of potentially lethal damage in other melanoma cell lines.

7.4 Intrinsic Radiosensitivity and Fractionation Sensitivity of Melanoma Cells In Vitro

The intrinsic radiosensitivity of tumour cells is presently regarded to be a major factor determining the outcome of cancer radiotherapy. The most relevant and most commonly used parameter to describe inherent radiosensitivity is the surviving fraction after 2 Gy (SF_2) (PETERS et al. 1989), i.e. the dose which typically is given daily in 25–35 fractions. DEACON et al. (1984) related the clinical response of different human tumour types to the SF_2 values determined for cells isolated from those tumours. The class of the most radioresistant tumours contained some glioblastomas and osteosarcomas but mostly melanomas (18/25); the SF_2 values of the latter ranged from 0.20 to 0.82 with a mean value of 0.52, which was higher than for any other group of tumours.

High SF_2 values are not necessarily associated with low α/β values, which is the most relevant parameter to describe the shoulder of the survival curve and thus the fractionation sensitivity. From the data compiled by ROFSTAD (1986) on 40 human melanoma cell lines in vitro, the SF_2 values were

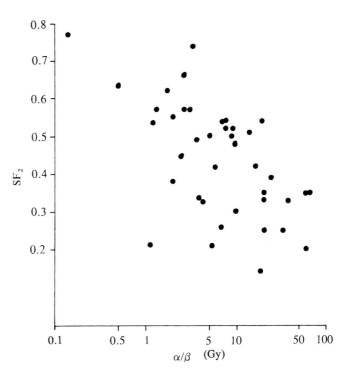

Fig. 7.3. The relationship of intrinsic radio-sensitivity (SF$_2$) to fractionation sensitivity (α/β) in 40 human melanoma cell lines (derived from data of ROFSTAD 1986)

calculated and plotted in relation to the α/β value of the individual melanoma cell lines (Fig. 7.3). Although there is wide scatter of the data points there appears to be some correlation between intrinsic radiosensitivity as expressed by SF$_2$ and fractionation sensitivity as expressed by α/β: the more radioresistant a cell line to 2 Gy, the lower the α/β value. All cell lines with an SF$_2$ exceeding 0.55 have an α/β value of less than 4 Gy; however, this relationship is very sensitive to the chosen boundaries: for an SF$_2$ of more than 0.5, α/β values range from 0 to 20 Gy.

If the survival curve parameters determined in vitro are representative of the response of the tumour to fractionated radiotherapy, one might conclude that it is especially the most radioresistant melanomas (with a high SF$_2$) which should be treated with hypofractionated radiotherapy as they have a fractionation sensitivity similar to that found with chronic reactions of normal tissues which usually limit radiotherapy. But these melanomas may comprise less than one-quarter of all human melanoma cell lines reviewed by ROFSTAD (1986).

The observed relationship of intrinsic radio-resistance to a wide shoulder of the survival curve in the presence of the most pronounced heterogeneity of cellular radiation sensitivity of melanoma cells makes any conclusions as to the most appropriate

radiotherapeutic schedule a very complex under-taking.

7.5 The Radiation Response of Melanoma Spheroids In Vitro

Multicellular spheroids have several biological features in common with tumours, such as hypoxic and necrotic regions, and time-dependent changes in these cellular compartments after cytotoxic insults, such as reoxygenation. This makes them an interesting in vitro model for studies of human tumour radiobiology in which different endpoints can be studied, i.e. those commonly used in cell cultures like clonogenic survival and those commonly used in vivo like regrowth delay or local control. POURREAU-SCHNEIDER and MALAISE (1981) demonstrated close agreement between these different response criteria in spheroids established from a human melanoma cell line. Moreover, ROFSTAD et al. (1986) found a high degree of conformity in the results on cellular radiosensitivity, regrowth delay etc. between the spheroids grown in vitro and the original xenografted human tumour in vivo. However, although spheroids would be a good experimental system to study the fractiona-tion sensitivity of the different cell lines under semi-physiological conditions, no such experiments have been reported to date.

7.6 The Radiation Response of Human Melanoma Xenografts

Human melanomas have been transplanted into immunosuppressed or immunoincompetent mice with particular success. Their radiation response has been assessed either by in situ criteria like regrowth delay or local control or by determining clonogenic cell survival after removal of the tumour and preparation of a single-cell suspension.

The cell survival curves determined from xeno-transplanted human melanomas irradiated in situ and assayed in vitro were not different from those obtained from melanoma cells in vitro. CHAVAUDRA et al. (1981) found very similar dose-response curves in two xenografted human melanoma lines, but also uncommonly high hypoxic fractions (of 40% and 62%) and some repair of potentially lethal damage. Six xenografts reviewed by ROFSTAD (1986) displayed the same wide range of survival curve parameters as the large sample of melanoma cell lines in vitro, with α/β values between 1.2 Gy and 66 Gy. The correlation of the α/β values determined for the same melanoma line in vitro and in the xenograft is, however, very poor (ROFSTAD 1986). This is probably due to the great influence experimental procedures have on the shape of the survival curve, which might be even greater in xenografts than in established cell lines in vitro. These factors, which greatly affect the α/β value derived from single-dose experiments, could be reduced by determining the fractionation sensitivity in the xenografted tumour directly by giving different fractionation schedules but in such a way as to exclude the influence of reoxygenation and repopulation. Unfortunately no results of such experiments have been reported although experiments of this nature are presently being performed on a number of xenografted human melanomas in Oslo (ROFSTAD, personal communication, July 1992). Only GUICHARD and MALAISE (1982) reported on some fractionation experiments in one xenografted human melanoma. After two fractions of 10 Gy they observed very little split-dose recovery in the melanoma, with an α/β value of 9 Gy. The interpretation of these data is complicated by the fact that the first dose was given under ambient conditions. This way only the split-dose recovery of hypoxic cells can be studied, which

might not be representative of the fractionation response of the total melanoma cell population.

Human melanoma xenografts have also been studied for their intrinsic radiosensitivity, as defined by SF_2. ROFSTAD and BRUSTAD (1987) found a close correlation between the SF_2 value determined in vitro (i.e. in the cell line grown, irradiated and assayed in vitro) and the specific regrowth delay after 12–30 fractions of 2 Gy each given in an accelerated schedule to reduce the influence of repopulation. Still, the melanomas were more radioresistant in vivo than in vitro. This was entirely due to extensive repopulation between radiation fractions. Inadequate reoxygenation or significant potentially lethal damage repair, however, did not have any major effect on the response of the five malignant melanomas treated with multiple doses of 2 Gy (ROFSTAD 1992).

HINKELBEIN (personal communication, May 1992) determined SF_2 values from 16 human melanoma xenografts and found a wide spread of values ranging from 0.10 to 0.89 with a median of 0.48. This compares well with the data of ROFSTAD (1986) in vitro (cf. Fig. 7.3) and in vivo.

7.7 Fractionation Sensitivity of Rodent Melanomas

The direct method to determine the fractionation sensitivity (i.e. the α/β value) of a tumour in situ is by a suitable fractionation experiment and by determining iso-effective total doses for different doses per fraction. A number of experiments have been performed on various rodent carcinomas and sarcomas following a rigid protocol which eliminates as much as possible the influence of other complicating factors such as reoxygenation, redistribution and repopulation (e.g. GUTTENBERGER et al. 1990). WILLIAMS et al. (1985) have reviewed a large number of experiments, including those not specifically designed to quantitate the fractionation sensitivity of the tumour, and found that except in a very few cases the α/β value of tumours was close to or higher than that observed for acute reactions of normal tissues ($\alpha/\beta > 10$ Gy). However, no data on rodent melanomas were included in this review. In an unpublished MD thesis from Munich, HAIDER (1987) determined α/β ratios of the Harding-Passey and the B-16 melanomas in vivo using the TCD_{50} assay and the regrowth delay assay after fractionated irradiation with two, four or eight fractions given in an overall time of less than 36 h to clamped tumours. The derived α/β ratios varied between experiments, assays and melanoma types; the mean of five separate experiments was 12 Gy.

The only published study on the fractionation sensitivity of the B-16 melanoma (TAKAI et al. 1992) unfortunately is flawed by several insufficiencies in the experimental design and analysis of the results so that the reported α/β value of 10.5 Gy may or may not be correct. Up to ten daily fractions were given under ambient conditions to the transplanted melanoma and the period from the start of treatment to reach five times treatment size was determined. The true fractionation sensitivity of the melanomas could have been significantly obscured by time-dependent processes occurring in the fractionation intervals: repopulation during the intervals could have reduced the apparent α/β value, while reoxygenation could have increased the apparent α/β value. One observation from the published growth curves might indicate that the true α/β value is indeed lower than the reported 10 Gy: the B-16 melanoma displays a pronounced tumour bed effect which does not change at a defined regrowth delay level with increasing fractionation. This suggests that the α/β value for the melanoma is similar to that of the tumour stroma. In other tumour systems, the fractionation sensitivity of the tissue responsible for the tumour bed effect is equivalent to an α/β value of 5–7 Gy (BEGG and TERRY 1984; TROTT and KUMMERMEHR 1982).

An as yet unpublished reanalysis of the above-mentioned study of Haider which avoided most of the cited pitfalls was performed by KUMMERMEHR in 1993. The results are given in Table 7.1.

7.8 Retrospective Studies on the Fractionation Sensitivity of Human Melanomas Treated by Radiotherapy Alone

Although radiotherapy does not play any significant role in the primary treatment of cutaneous malignant melanomas today, extensive experience on the effect of palliative radiotherapy of metastatic melanomas has been published. A prominent question in the discussion of these data has been the optimal radiation dose per fraction in the treatment of malignant melanomas. However, certain features common to all studies render them of only limited value for this purpose. Since until recently melanomas were not considered suitable for radiotherapy, radiotherapists only saw very

Table 7.1. α/β ratios of murine malignant melanomas, determined in vivo by giving different fractionation schedules to clamped tumours. Values corrected by an OER of 2.7. (From KUMMERMEHR, unpublished)

Melanoma	Assay	Experiment	α/β (Gy)
Harding-Passey	Growth delay	1	12.1
		2	13.7
		3	8.1
B-16	Growth delay		6.2
	Local control		6.1

advanced cases, often with multiple metastases at different sites, for palliative radiotherapy which usually was prescribed on a very individualised basis taking into account the general condition of the patient, life expectancy, lesion size and expected side-effects. In practically all reports patient numbers were small, the size and site of metastases varied, follow-up was short owing to the limited survival of the advanced stage of disease and response criteria were more related to palliation than to objective response.

The first retrospective studies to emphasise the importance of the dose per fraction as suggested by ELLIS (1974) were by HABERMALZ and FISHER (1976), HORNSEY (1978) and OVERGAARD (1980). HABERMALZ (1981) summarised the results of these studies. There was a 38% (85/221) complete response rate of cutaneous, subcutaneous and lymph node melanoma metastases. Response rate was not related to total dose but to dose per fraction (Gy/f). The complete response rate was 32% (35/110) if the dose per fraction was less than 4 Gy/f but 45% (50/110) with a dose per fraction of 4 Gy or more ($P < 0.05$). The difference became even larger if partial responses were included: overall response rates were 54% (59/110) with less than 4 Gy/f, rising to 83% (92/111) with fractional doses of more than 4 Gy/f.

These results were taken as evidence that malignant melanomas were special in that they respond better to large fractional doses than to conventional dose fractionation. Yet each of these and subsequent studies are flawed by a very heterogeneous distribution of tumour sizes (large tumours were more often treated with lower doses per fraction) and of total doses (most tumours were clearly underdosed with conventional fractionation, the maximum usually being 20×2.5 Gy), by a short follow-up and by small numbers of comparable cases.

Not all retrospective studies, however, demonstrated the superiority of large-fraction-size radiotherapy. We analysed 44 lymph node or skin metastases of malignant melanomas treated with megavoltage radiotherapy and with curative intent. Doses per fraction ranged from 2 to 9 Gy. Of the 44, 20 (45%) were locally controlled after 2 years. There was no indication of an improved local control rate with higher fractional doses: it was 33% (3/9) with more than 4.5 Gy/f and 47% (16/34) with less than 4.5 Gy/f. This study did, however, suggest an influence of overall treatment time. Among 22 patients who received the same dose of 54 Gy in 20–24 fractions, local control rate decreased from 75% (6/8) if treatment lasted less than 30 days to 40% (4/10) if treatment lasted 30–39 days and further to 25% (1/4) if treatment lasted more than 40 days (TROTT et al. 1981b).

Other studies which did not find any influence of dose per fraction on the response of melanomas have been published, e.g. by KONEFAL et al. (1988), who studied mainly palliation of bone and brain metastases (which was 68% and 39% respectively) and failed to observe any differential effect of fractional doses ranging from 2 Gy to 6 Gy. ZIEGLER and COOPER (1986) confirmed these results. In 72 patients with brain metastases, results were similar with ten times 3 Gy or six times 5 Gy. In 59 patients with brain metastases, CHOI et al. (1985) found a better response with ten fractions of 3–3.7 Gy in 1 week than with 20 fractions of 1.9–2.4 Gy in 2 weeks, but it is impossible to separate the effects of time and dose per fraction in this study. In bone metastases, KATZ (1981) did not see any better response with six fractions of 6 Gy than with ten fractions of 3 Gy whereas there was some indication of better response of lymph nodes or skin metastases to 6 Gy/f.

The largest retrospective study was performed by OVERGAARD and co-workers (OVERGAAD 1980; OVERGAARD et al. 1986) and BENTZEN et al. (1989) on more than 100 patients with skin or lymph node metastases. It was further elaborated by combining the study results with other published cases by OVERGAARD (1986). Forty-nine percent (83/171) of the lesions achieved a complete response, which was persistent in 43% (74/171) (OVERGAARD et al. 1986). The complete response rate was independent of total dose (ranging from 30 to more than 60 Gy) or dose per fraction except for those 38 lesions which received less than 3 Gy per fraction. Yet with low doses per fraction the majority of patients received doses which would be regarded as too low for the control of any carcinoma. In the group of patients treated with 2.5 Gy/per fraction, 52% (12/23) received less than 50 Gy and all of these failed. But of the nine patients who received 55–60 Gy, five achieved a complete response. Overall the data of OVERGAARD et al. (1986) demonstrated a greater than 50% local control rate with 55–60 Gy given with 2.5 Gy/f or with about 40 Gy given in eight fractions of 5 Gy or with 27 Gy given in three fractions of 9 Gy.

Submitting these values to the FE plot of DOUGLAS and FOWLER (1976) an α/β value of 2.5 Gy is found. This is, however, a very rough estimate since in the group of 61 patients who received 5-Gy fractions, no dose response was apparent between 25 Gy and 60 Gy. Moreover, with 9 Gy per fraction all patients received the same total dose. Therefore, except for the 2.5 Gy per fraction group, no reasonable TCD_{50} value could be derived. BENTZEN et al. (1989) demonstrated that the absence of a dose-response relationship in the group of patients treated with 5 Gy per fraction (the latter sample contained 85 patients) was due to the marked heterogeneity of tumour size. Only after corrections had been made for tumour size could all cases (239 lesions) be subjected to a single direct analysis which yielded an even lower value for α/β than before, i.e. 0.6 Gy with 95% confidence limits of − 1 Gy and + 2.5 Gy.

This low α/β value depends critically on the procedure for correcting the radiosensitivity of melanomas for differences in tumor volume. Small nodules of less than 1 cm diameter were readily controlled [88% (7/8)], but with comparable doses the control rate dropped to 67% (36/54) for 1 to 4.9-cm tumours and to 47% (7/15) for 5 to 9.9-cm tumours. An empirical correction factor of (tumour diameter)$^{0.33}$ was developed which, if built into the

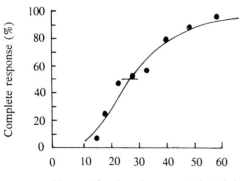

Fig. 7.4. The dependence of complete response of 618 human melanomas on radiation dose, corrected for a tumour diameter of 1 cm and a fraction size of 5 Gy (data from OVERGAARD 1986)

linear-quadratic equation, led to a smooth sigmoid dose-response curve. Although the principles of this procedure are convincing, some scepticism remains regarding the influence of the normalisation process on the derived α/β value, especially as the calculated value of 0.6 Gy is well below any value ever produced in any of the experimental studies mentioned above.

The formula developed by OVERGAARD et al. (1986) on their own melanoma cases with the graphically derived α/β value of 2.5 Gy and the volume correction factor was checked on a large sample of 618 published melanoma lesions from the literature by OVERGAARD (1986) and found to fit very well (Fig. 7.4).

The most important conclusion from the careful work of OVERGAARD et al. (1986) and OVERGAARD (1986) is that malignant melanoma is a highly radioresponsive tumour. Moreover, patients with complete response have a high probability of longterm local control and significantly improved survival. Therefore radiotherapy with curative intent is the treatment of choice in melanoma metastases to skin or lymph nodes. The optimal irradiation schedule was suggested to be with a few high-dose fractions in a short overall time, which differs from recommendations for curative radiotherapy to all other cancers. Since this conclusion was entirely based on retrospective analysis, a prospective randomized clinical trial was set up to resolve the question of the optimal dose per fraction in radiotherapy of malignant melanomas.

7.9 Prospective Study on the Fractionation Sensitivity of Human Melanomas Treated by Radiotherapy Alone

In 1983, the Radiotherapy Oncology Group started a prospective randomised trial on patients with measurable melanoma lesions, who received either four fractions of 8 Gy in 21 days or 20 fractions of 2.5 Gy in 4 weeks. Lesions were stratified by location and according to size greater or smaller than 5 cm. Between 1983 and 1988, 123 patients were treated; the results were published in 1991 (SAUSE et al. 1991). Both treatment groups were very similar with regard to all selection criteria. Normal tissue toxicity was greater in the four times 8 Gy arm (three grade IV and three grade III) than in the 20 times 2.5 Gy arm (four grade III). The response rates were strikingly similar for both arms of the study (Table 7.2). No statistical difference exists between any arms of the study but the overall response to irradiation was good and much better than for any chemotherapeutic regimen, refuting the concept that melanoma is a radioresistant tumour.

The problem with this clinical trial lies in the choice of doses to be compared. Whereas the one arm with 20 times 2.5 Gy gives a commonly used conventional treatment of proven effectiveness which yields response rates of about 50%, the high-fractional-dose schedule of four times 8 Gy is consistent with an intermediate level of fractionation sensitivity, i.e. an α/β ratio of 7 Gy. This is higher than proposed by OVERGAARD et al. (1986) or BENTZEN et al. (1989) but lower than for most other human cancers (THAMES et al. 1989). If an α/β ratio of 2.5 Gy were correct, the isoeffective dose should have been four times 6.8 Gy; if, however, the α/β were 15 Gy, the isoeffective dose should have been four times 9 Gy. Given the shallow slope of the dose-response curve for malignant melanomas (Fig. 7.4) with a change in the complete response rate of 10% if the dose changes by 20%, an increase or decrease of the given intermediate dose of four times 8 Gy by 12%–16% would go unrecognised in any trial. Therefore, an α/β ratio for melanomas of 7 Gy or considerably less cannot be ruled out by the results of this study—nor can there be an α/β

Table 7.2. Results of the randomised clinical trial on the effect of dose per fraction on melanomas (SAUSE et al. 1991)

Best response	Diameter of nodule < 5 cm		Diameter of nodule ≥ 5 cm		All sizes		
	4×8 Gy	20×2.5 Gy	4×8 Gy	20×2.5 Gy	4×8 Gy	20×2.5 Gy	Total
Complete	33.3%	28.6%	17.1%	19.4%	24.2%	23.4%	23.8%
Partial	18.0%	28.6%	48.6%	38.9%	35.5%	34.4%	34.9%
No change	33.3%	39.3%	34.3%	38.9%	33.9%	39.1%	36.5%
Progression	14.8%	3.6%		2.8%	6.5%	3.1%	4.8%
Total no.	27	28	35	36	62	64	126
CR + PR rate	0.52	0.57	0.66	0.58	0.60	0.58	

CR, complete remission; PR, partial remission

ratio of 15 Gy, as has been estimated for squamous cell carcinomas. Yet it may look rather unlikely that four times 5.9 Gy (which would be isoeffective to 20 times 2.5 Gy with an α/β ratio of 0.6 Gy) could be expected to produce the same response rates as four times 8 Gy (TROTT 1991).

7.10 Conclusion

The experimental and clinical data discussed here demonstrate clearly that there is no evidence for the claim that malignant melanomas in general are radioresistant tumours. There may, however, be greater heterogeneity in the biology and the radiation response of melanomas compared to some other more common tumours like squamous cell carcinomas. Clinical studies including a prospective randomised trial have clearly demonstrated that moderate radiation doses which produce little risk of normal tissue complications produce a high rate of response including complete responses in one-third of the patients or more.

The question of the optimal treatment schedule, which was raised more than 20 years ago when experimental studies suggested that malignant melanomas may differ from other tumours by having a much higher fractionation sensitivity, has not been completely resolved. As more experimental data have accumulated, the case for the special fractionation sensitivity of melanomas in general has been weakened but, for reasons difficult to understand, the definitive experiment to answer that question has not yet been performed, i.e. direct determination of the α/β value (i.e. of the fractionation sensitivity) in a range of human melanoma xenografts by a suitable fractionation experiment (TROTT 1991).

The retrospective analyses of response rates of melanomas to different fractionation protocols have produced conflicting results, and there is even reason to assume that melanoma lesions in lymph nodes may respond differently to those in brain or bone. The randomised clinical trial, however, failed to demonstrate any significant advantage of high-dose-fraction radiotherapy for melanomas. Whereas the clinical message is obvious, i.e. that conventional fractionation to doses also given to squamous cell carcinomas may produce a good local control rate, it is also clear that clinical data are just too heterogeneous to allow any stringent analysis of the fractionation sensitivity of malignant melanomas. This has to be done in the laboratory.

References

Barranco SC, Romsdahl MM, Humphrey RM (1971) The radiation response of human malignant melanoma cells grown in vitro. Cancer Res 31: 830–833
Begg AC, Terry NMA (1984) The sensitivity of normal stroma to fractionated radiotherapy measured by a tumour growth rate assay. Radiother Oncol 11: 337–347
Bentzen SM, Overgaard J, Thames HD, Overgaard M, Vejby Hansen P, von der Maase H, Meder J (1989) Clinical radiobiology of malignant melanoma. Radiother Oncol 16: 169–182
Chavaudra N, Guichard M, Malaise EP (1981) Hypoxic fraction and repair of potentially lethal radiation damage in two human melanomas transplanted into nude mice. Radiat Res 88: 56–61
Choi KN, Withers HR, Rotman M (1985) Metastatic melanoma in brain, rapid treatment or large dose fractions. Cancer 56: 10–15
Courdi A, Bensadaun R-J, Gioanni J, Caldani C (1992) Inherent radiosensitivity and split-dose recovery in plateau-phase cultures of 10 human tumour cell lines. Radiother Oncol 24: 102–107
Deacon J, Peckham MJ, Steel GG (1984) The radio-responsiveness of human tumours and the initial slope of the cell survival curve. Radiother Oncol 2: 317–323
del Regato JA, Spjut MJ (1977) Ackerman's and del Regato's cancer, diagnosis, treatment and prognosis, 5th edn. Mosby, St Louis
Dewey DL (1971) The radiosensitivity of melanoma cells in culture. Br J Radiol 44: 816–817
Douglas BG, Fowler JF (1976) The effect of multiple small doses of x-rays on skin reactions in the mouse and a basic interpretation. Radiat Res 66: 401–426
Ellis F (1974) The NSD concept and radioresistant tumours. Br J Radiol 47: 909
Elsmann HJ, Ernst K, Suter L (1991) Radiotherapy of primary human melanomas—experiences and suggestions. Strahlenther Onkol 167: 387–391
Guichard M, Malaise EP (1982) Radiosensitivity of Na 11 human melanoma transplanted into nude mice. Repair, reoxygenation and dose fractionation. Int J Radiat Oncol Biol Phys 8: 1005–1009
Guttenberger R, Kummermehr J, Chmelewsky D (1990) Kinetics of recovery from sublethal radiation damage in four murine tumours. Radiother Oncol 18: 79–88
Habermalz HJ (1981) Irradiation of malignant melanoma: experience in the past and present. Int J Radiat Oncol Biol Phys 7: 131–133
Habermalz HJ, Fischer JJ (1976) Radiation therapy of malignant melanoma, experience with high individual treatment doses. Cancer 38: 2258–2262
Hornsey S (1972) The radiosensitivity of melanoma cells in culture. Br J Radiol 45: 158
Hornsey S (1978) The relationship between total dose, number of fractions and fraction size in the response of malignant melanoma in patients. Br J Radiol 51: 905–909
Katz HR (1981) The results of different fractionation schemes in the palliative irradiation of metastatic melanoma. Int J Radiat Oncol Biol Phys 7: 901–911
Konefal JB, Emami B, Pilepich MV (1988) Analysis of dose fractionation in the palliation of metastases from malignant melanoma. Cancer 61: 243–246
Kummermehr J (1978) Kurabilität des Harding-Passey-Melanoms durch Einzeitbestrahlung. Strahlentherapie 154: 578–581

Marchese MJ, Minarik L, Hall EJ, Zaider M (1985) Potentially lethal damage repair in cell lines of radio-resistant human tumours and normal skin fibroblasts. Int J Radiat Biol 48: 431–436

Miescher G (1926) Zur Frage der Strahlenresistenz der Melanome. Schweiz Med Wochenschr 788–812

Overgaard J (1980) Radiation treatment of malignant melanoma. Int J Radiat Oncol Biol Phys 6: 41–44

Overgaard J (1986) The role of radiotherapy in recurrent and metastatic malignant melanoma: a clinical radiobiological study. Int J Radiat Oncol Biol Phys 12: 867–872

Overgaard J, Overgaard M, Vejby Hansen P, von der Maase H (1986) Some factors of importance in the radiation treatment of malignant melanoma. Radiother Oncol 5: 183–192

Peters LJ, Tofilon PJ, Goepfert H, Brock WA (1989) Radiosensitivity of primary tumour cultures as a determinant of curability of human head and neck cancers. In: BIR Report 19: The scientific basis of modern radiotherapy. British Institute of Radiology

Pourreau-Schneider N, Malaise EP (1981) Relationship between surviving fractions using the colony method, the CD_{50}, and the growth delay after irradiation of human melanoma cells grown as multicellular spheroids. Radiat Res 85: 321–332

Rofstad EK (1986) Radiation biology of malignant melanoma. Review article. Acta Radiol Oncol 25: 1–10

Rofstad EK (1992) Are human melanoma cells more radioresistant in vivo than in vitro? In: Dewey WC, Edington M, Fry RJM, Hall EJ, Whitmore GF (eds) Radiation research, a twentieth century perspective. Academic, New York, pp 739–744

Rofstad EK, Brustad T (1987) Radioresponsiveness of human melanoma xenografts given fractionated irradiation in vivo—relationship to the initial slope of the cell survival curves in vitro. Radiother Oncol 9: 45–56

Rofstad EK, Wahl A, Brustad T (1986) Radiation response of human melanoma multicellular spheroids measured as single cell survival, growth delay and spheroid cure: comparisons with the parent tumour xenograft. Int J Radiat Oncol Biol Phys 12: 975–982

Rohde B, Wiskemann A (1964) Über das Wachstum röntgenbestrahlter Melanomalignome in der Gewebekultur und im Tierversuch. Strahlentherapie 123: 534–544

Sause WT, Cooper JS, Rush S et al. (1991) Fraction size in external beam radiation therapy in the treatment of melanoma. Int J Radiat Oncol Biol Phys 20: 429–432

Storck H, Ott F, Schwarz K (1972) Maligne Melanoma. In: Zuppinger A, Krokowski E (eds) Encyclopedia of medical radiology, vol XIX/1. Springer, Heidelberg Berlin New York, pp 161–257

Takai V, Goodman GB, Chaplin DJ, Grulkey W, Lam GKY (1992) The response of murine B-16 melanoma to fractionated doses of pions. Int J Radiat Oncol Biol Phys 23: 573–578

Thames HD, Bentzen SM, Turesson I, Overgaard M, van den Bogaert W (1989) Fractionation parameters for human tissues and tumours. In: Steel G (ed) The radiobiology of human cells and tissues. Taylor and Francis, London, pp 701–710

Trott KR (1991) The optimal radiation dose per fraction for the treatment of malignant melanomas. Int J Radiat Oncol Biol Phys 20: 905–907

Trott KR, Kummermehr J (1982) Split dose recovery of a mouse tumour and its stroma during fractionated irradiation. Br J Radiol 55: 841–846

Trott KR, von Lieven H, Kummermehr J, Skopal D, Lukacs S, Braun-Falco O (1981a) The radiosensitivity of malignant melanomas part I: experimental studies. Int J Radiat Oncol Biol Phys 7: 9–13

Trott KR, von Lieven H, Kummermehr J, Skopal D, Lukacs S, Braun-Falco O, Kellerer AM (1981b) The radiosensitivity of malignant melanomas part II: clinical studies. Int J Radiat Oncol Biol Phys 7: 15–20

von Lieven H, Skopal D (1976) Zur Strahlenempfindlichkeit des malignen Melanoms. Strahlentherapie 152: 1–4

Weichselbaum RR, Schmit A, Little JB (1982) Cellular repair factors influencing radiocurability of human malignant tumours. Br J Cancer 45: 10–16

Weichselbaum RR, Little JB, Tomkinson K, Evans S, Yuhas J (1984) Repair of fractionated radiation in plateau phase cultures of human tumor cells and human multicellular tumor spheroids. Radiother Oncol 2: 41–47

Weininger J, Guichard M, Joly AM, Malaise EP, Lachet B (1978) Radiosensitivity and growth parameters in vitro of three human melanoma cell strains. Int J Radiat Biol 34: 285–290

Wheldon TE (1979) Optimal fractionation for the radiotherapy of tumour cells possessing wide-shouldered survival curves. Br J Radiol 52: 417–418

Williams MV, Denekamp J, Fowler JF (1985) A review of α/β ratios for experimental tumors. Implications for clinical studies of altered fractionation. Int J Radiat Oncol Biol Phys 11: 87–96

Zeitz L, McDonald JM (1978) Pitfalls in the use of in vitro survival curves for the determination of tumour cell survival with fractionated doses. Br J Radiol 51: 637–639

Zeitz L, Silagi S (1977) Radiosensitivity of melanoma cells in culture: implications for the radiotherapy of malignant melanoma. Br J Radiol 50: 604–608

Ziegler JC, Cooper JS (1986) Brain metastases from malignant melanoma: conventional vs. high-dose-per-fraction radiotherapy. Int J Radiat Oncol Biol Phys 12: 1839–1842

8 Radiosensivity of Tumor Cells: The Predictive Value of SF2

M. Baumann, A. Taghian, and W. Budach

CONTENTS

8.1 Introduction

Early the history of radiation therapy, clinicians recognized that some tumor entities can be controlled considerably more easily by radiation therapy than others (WETTERER 1913–1914; HOLTHUSEN 1936; PATERSON 1948.) Table 8.1 summarizes the ranking of the radiosensitivities of selected tumor histologies. The judgment of the responsiveness of different tumors has changed little from Paterson's textbook, published in 1948, to recent reviwes such as Wang's textbook from 1988. Today, knowledge of the relative radiosensitivities of tumors of given histologies and grades, together with careful assessment of tumor size, stage, location, and patient characteristics such as sex, age, hemoglobin level, and Karnofsky score, forms the basis of prediction of the outcome of radiation therapy in individual patients (PETERS et al. 1986, 1988; SUIT and WALKER 1988; BENTZEN et al. 1991). Typical examples of radiosensitive tumors are seminomas

M. BAUMANN, MD, Department of Radiation Therapy, University of Hamburg, University Hospital Eppendorf, Martinistraße 52, 20246 Hamburg 20, Germany
A. TAGHIAN, MD, Department of Radiation Oncology, Massachusetts General Hospital, Harvard Medical School, Fruit Street, Boston, MA 02114, USA
W. BUDACH, MD, Department of Radiation Therapy, University of Essen, Hufelandstraße 55, 45147 Essen, Germany

and lymphomas, with total doses of 30–45 Gy being highly effective in achieving local tumor control (RUBIN et al. 1974; PEREZ and BRADY 1992). Adenocarcinomas and squamous cell carcinomas are generally considered moderately radiosensitive: if not too large, these tumors are radiocurable by doses between 50 and 75 Gy (RUBIN et al. 1974; PEREZ and BRADY 1992). A uniquely radioresistant tumor is glioblastoma multiforme: This entity is almost never controlled permanently by radiation doses between 60 and 80 Gy (DAVIS 1989), and in-field recurrences have been reported even after doses as high as 115 Gy (LOEFFLER et al. 1990a,b).

In addition to this heterogeneity of radiation response between tumor entities, clinicians have suspected for a long time that the response of individual tumors of the same histology also varies considerably. This suspicion is mainly based on the experience that even if all available predictive parameters (vide supra) are thoroughly applied, local recurrence after state-of-the-art radiation therapy develops in a considerable proportion of patients in whom local tumor control was expected. Vice versa, every clinician oversees patients in whom local tumor control is achieved against all

Table 8.1. Radiosensitivity of different tumor entities

Radiosensitivity	PATERSON (1948)	WANG (1988)
Sensitive	Lymphomas, leukemia, embryonal tumors (e.g., Wilms), neuroblastoma	Lymphomas, leukemia, seminoma, dysgerminoma
Limited sensitivity	Squamous cell carcinoma, bladder carcinoma, retinal glioma	Squamous cell carcinoma, adenocarcinoma
Resistant	Osteosarcoma, soft tissue sarcoma, melanoma	Osteosarcoma, soft tissue sarcoma glioma, melanoma

expectations based on the prognostic factors cited above. This clinical experience of heterogeneous radiation responses within the same tumor entity has recently been substantiated by quantitative evaluation of slopes of dose-response curves for local control of human tumors showing that even in stratified data the increase in percentage local control per unit dose is less steep than would be expected from theoretical considerations (THAMES et al. 1980; PETERS et al. 1982; BRAHME 1984; WILLIAMS et al. 1984; DUTREIX et al. 1988; SUIT and WALKER 1988; THAMES et al. 1992; SUIT et al. 1993). The clinical observations are strongly supported by results of studies performed in the laboratory on mouse tumors, and on human tumor xenografts in nude mice: even under well-defined experimental conditions, the radiation dose necessary to obtain local control shows significant heterogeneity in different tumor lines of the same histology (HILL and MILAS 1989; ROFSTAD 1989; SUIT et al. 1990; ROFSTAD 1991; BAUMANN et al. 1992a).

At present, important efforts are being made to develop assays that quantitate factors which contribute to the heterogeneous response of individual tumors to radiation therapy. Such *predictive assays* could aid clinicians to tailor-fit treatment strategies to individual patients and would thereby improve the outlook of patients suffering from cancer. This chapter addresses the potential of determinations of tumor cell radiosensitivity at 2 Gy as a predictor of the outcome of treatment.

8.2 The Concept of SF2

The low-dose "shoulder" region of radiation cell survival curves was the subject of intense investigation following the publication of the first in vitro survival curve of mammalian cells (PUCK and MARCUS 1956; ELKIND and SUTTON 1959). Nevertheless, most of the classic work on intrinsic radiosensitivity concentrated on the terminal slope of cell survival curves at high doses, that is D_0. Since this terminal slope was found to be very similar in many different tumor cell lines, the general opinion emerged that differences in cellular radiosensitivity are of only minor importance for explaining the diversity of response of tumors to clinical radiation therapy (BERRY 1974).

This picture changed with the sixth L.H. Gray Conference (ALPER 1975), and with the work of FERTIL and MALAISE (1981) and DEACON et al. (1984), who focused interest on examination of

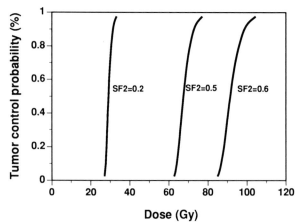

Fig. 8.1. Tumor control probability as a function of total dose applied as 2 Gy per fraction for hypothetical tumors composed of 10^{10} clonogenic cells with SF2 values of 0.2, 0.5, and 0.6

cellular radiation sensitivity at radiation doses that are actually applied in clinical practice, e.g., the surviving fraction of clonogenic cells at 2 Gy (SF2). Since clinical radiation therapy is given as a course of, for example, 30 fractions over 6 weeks, small differences in SF2 are expected to potentiate and should result in important differences in the dose necessary for local tumor control.

This is illustrated in Fig. 8.1 for a hypothetical tumor composed of 10^{10} clonogenic cells with SF2 values of 0.2, 0.5, and 0.6. Assuming that (a) only the number of clonogenic tumor cells and their radiosensitivity determine treatment outcome, (b) the SF2 is constant during treatment, and (c) every clonogenic cell surviving radiation eventually will proliferate and produce a recurrent tumor, the doses necessary to control 50% of the tumors according to Poisson's statistics would be 29, 68, and 92 Gy.

8.3 SF2 of Cells of Tumor Entities with Different Clinical Radioresponsiveness

SF2 values for different classes of tumors with known differences in clinical radioresponsiveness are listed in Table 8.2: the data were reevaluated by FERTIL and MALAISE (1981, 1985) and DEACON et al. (1984) from a variety of published cell survival curves using the linear-quadratic model. Two principal conclusions can be drawn from these studies:

1. *SF2 values vary considerably between tumor lines of different histologies.* Tumor classes which

are known to be resistant to radiation therapy are on average characterized by higher SF2 values than radiosensitive entities. This observation suggests an important impact of cellular radiation sensitivity on local tumor control.

2. *SF2 values also vary substantially between tumor lines of the same histology.* Thus, the variable radiation response clinically observed for tumors of the same class might be explained by different cellular radiosensitivities. If this is the case, determinations of SF2 in tumors of individual patients may be expected to be a powerful predictor of the outcome of radiation therapy.

However, certain problems have to be considered in interpreting the results of SF2 measurements. For example, clinical experience clearly shows that the radiation sensitivity of malignant lymphoma, squamous cell carcinoma, and malignant glioma is significantly different. In fact, no or only very little overlapping is expected between the clinical dose-response relationships of these three entities. This is in sharp contrast to the cumulative distribution of SF2 values shown in Fig. 8.2. The data for this comparison were taken from publications of several laboratory groups which used colony formation assays on early- or late-passage cell lines (ALLALUNIS-TURNER et al. 1992a; BELLAMY et al. 1984; DREWINKO et al. 1972; FERTIL et al. 1980; GERWECK et al. 1977; INADA et al. 1977; KELLAND and STEEL 1988; LEHNERT et al. 1986; LEITH et al. 1982; MASUDA et al. 1983; NILSSON et al. 1980; RAAPHORST et al. 1989; SCHULTZ and GEARD 1990; SESHADRI et al. 1985; SZEKELY and LOBREAU 1985; TAGHIAN et al.

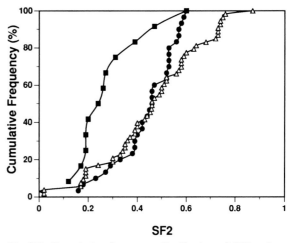

Fig. 8.2. Cumulative frequency distribution of SF2 values for malignant lymphomas/lymphocytic leukemias (*squares*), squamous cell carcinomas (*circles*), and malignant gliomas (*triangles*) given in the literature. All assays were performed on early- or late- passage established cell lines using colony formation as an endpoint. Where SF2 values were not given by the authors, the cell survival curves were reevaluated as described by DEACON et al. (1984). When different SF2 values were reported for the same cell line by different authors, the mean value was chosen

1993; WEICHSELBAUM et al. 1976, 1981, 1990; YANG et al. 1990). Whereas the distribution of SF2 values of malignant lymphoma is almost separated from the SF2 distributions of squamous cell carcinomas and malignant gliomas, the curves for the two latter entities almost superimpose. In addition, at "tumoricidal" doses for malignant lymphoma, say tumor control probability = 80%–90%, local control rates

Table 8.2. SF2 values for human tumor cell lines of different origin

FERTIL and MALAISE (1981, 1985), MALAISE et al. (1986)		DEACON et al. (1984)	
Tumor type	SF2	Tumor type	SF2
Oat cell carcinomas (6)[a]	0.22 (0.42)[b]	Burkitt (1), neuroblastoma (3), myelom (2)	0.19 (0.56)[c]
Lymphomas (7) ·	0.34 (0.27)	Small cell (6), medulloblastoma(2)	0.22 (0.40)
Adenocarcinomas (6)	0.48 (0.37)	Breast (1), bladder (1), cervix (2)	0.46 (0.26)
Squamous cell ca. (6)	0.49 (0.18)	Pancreas (1), colon (5), rectum (1), lung SCC (1)	0.43 (0.52)
Melanomas (6)	0.51 (0.28)	Glioblastoma (4), melanoma (18), osteosarcoma (2), renal ca. (1)	0.52 (0.34)
Gliobastoma (5)	0.58 (0.34)		

SCC, squamous cell carcinoma
[a] Number of cell lines studied
[b] Coefficient of variation
[c] Coefficient of variation recalculated from the data given in the publication

Table 8.3. Differences in SF2 values for five human glioblastoma cell lines studied by three different investigators in two different laboratories (TAGHIAN et al., unpublished data)

Cell line	SF2		
	Investigator 1/Lab 1	Investigator 2/Lab 2	Investigator 3/Lab 2
D54MG	0.52	0.49	0.37
U251MG	0.35	0.40	0.42
A7	0.58[a]	0.59	0.55
MMC1	0.40	0.52	0.56
HGL4	0.24	0.39	0.54

[a] For the same cell line an SF2 value of 0.86 can be calculated from the data of GERWECK et al. (1977)

of 20%–50% for squamous cell carcinoma and malignant glioma would be expected from simple extrapolation of the SF2 distributions. Similar unrealistic results are obtained when SF2 distributions of other tumor entities such as melanoma (ROFSTAD 1986), colorectal adenocarcinoma (LEITH et al. 1991a, b), ovarian carcinoma (ROFSTAD and SUTHERLAND 1988; WEICHSELBAUM et al. 1989), and sarcoma (WEICHSELBAUM et al. 1989, 1990) are included in this evaluation. Further limitations arise from the observation that absolute SF2 values appear to be poorly related to tumor control doses in patients and that the steepness of SF2 distributions does not correspond well to the steepness of clinical dose-control curves (SUIT et al. 1989, 1993; BENTZEN et al. 1990; BENTZEN 1992).

Tumor heterogeneity may account for some of these problems. BROCK and colleagues (1989, 1990a) have found in head and neck squamous cell carcinoma that the intratumoral coefficient of variation for determination of SF2 values was 23%. In three human malignant gliomas, ALLAM et al. (Department of Radiation Oncology, Massachusetts General Hospital, Boston, USA, unpublished data) found coefficients of variation for intratumoral variability of SF2 between 27% and 48%. In this ongoing study some of the SF2 values obtained from different parts of the same tumor were significantly different. In contrast, DAVIDSON et al. (1990) did not find significant variability between intratumor SF2 values in cervical carcinoma.

Technical factors also contribute to the difficulties in the interpretation of SF2 distributions cumulated from different laboratory groups that are outlined above. This is illustrated in Table 8.3 showing that the SF2 values of five human malignant glioma lines varied substantially between three different

investigators from two different laboratories who used the same assay technique for determination of SF2. Such variability is expected to be even more pronounced when different assay techniques are used, e.g., primary cultures vs established cell lines, colony formation assays vs cell prolifertion techniques, and plastic surface vs soft agar assays (FERTIL and MALAISE 1981; DEACON et al. 1984; SUIT et al. 1989; MALAISE et al. 1989).

Therefore, it may be more appropriate to restrict comparisons of SF2 distributions to data that have been obtained by the same laboratory group using a constant technique. However, Table 8.4 indicates that this kind of analysis, too, does not provide completely unequivocal results:

1. ROFSTAD et al. (1987) studied tumor biopsies using a colony formation assay in soft agar (COURTENAY and MILLS 1978). Analysis of variance showed no significant differences. However, corresponding to clinical experience, melanoma tended to be more resistant and seminoma to be more sensitive than carcinoma of the breast, cervix, head and neck, and ovary.

2. BROCK et al. (1989) studied primary cultures of five different tumor histologies using population growth as an endpoint (BAKER et al. 1986). Analysis of variance of their data revealed significant differences: lung adenocarcinoma and melanoma were more resistant than breast carcinoma, head and neck squamous cell carcinoma, and Ewing's sarcoma. Although tumor control doses for melanoma and lung adenocarcinoma are not well defined, the results of this group agree with clinical practice.

3. WEICHSELBAUM et al. (1989, 1990) studied SF2 in sarcomas, ovarian carcinomas and head and neck squamous cell carcinomas by colony formation of early-passage cell lines. In contrast to the judgment of most clinicians, sarcomas were significantly more sensitive than the epithelial tumors.

4. ALLALUNIS-TURNER (1991, 1992a), using early-passage cell lines and a colony formation assay on plastic, demonstrated a tendency for higher SF2 values in malignant gliomas compared to cervical and endometrial carcinomas. Nevertheless, this difference was not significant, and similar to the pooled data from several laboratories shown in Fig. 8.2, the wide overlapping of the SF2 distributions does not track clinical experience.

5. RUKA et al. (Department of Radiation Oncology, Massachusetts General Hospital, Boston, USA, unpublished data) used established cell lines and a colony formation assay on plastic. They

Table 8.4. SF2 values for tumors of different clinical responsiveness obtained by the same group of investigators using the same culture technique. The original data were read from figures or tables given in the publications and analysis of variance was performed to test for significant differences

Investigator and assay technique	Tumor[a]	SF2[b]	ANOVA[c]
ROFSTAD et al. 1987 (primary culture, colony formation in soft agar)	Bladder (6) Breast (9) Cervix (8) H + N SCC (7) Melanoma (19) Ovarian (14) Seminoma (3)	0.28(0.44) 0.30(0.37) 0.31(0.45) 0.30(0.37) 0.40(0.45) 0.30(0.35) 0.24(0.62)	$P = 0.26$
BROCK et al. 1989 (primary culture, population growth)	H + N SCC (72) Breast (14) Ewing's sarcoma (4) Lung adenoca. (8) Melanoma (15)	0.33(0.43) 0.34(0.49) 0.31(0.34) 0.53(0.22) 0.65(0.27)	$P < 0.0001$ (breast vs lung adenoca., breast vs melanoma, Ewing's vs melanoma, H + N SCC vs lung adenoca., H + N SCC vs melanoma
WEICHSELBAUM et al. 1989, 1990 (early-passage cell lines, colony formation on plastic)	Sarcoma (13) H + N SCC (20) Ovarian (15)	0.27(0.46) 0.45(0.26) 0.46(0.33)	$P < 0.001$ (sarcoma vs H + N SCC, sarcoma vs ovarian)
ALLALUNIS-TURNER et al. 1991, 1992a, b (early-passage cell lines, colony formation on plastic)	Cervix (26) Endometrium (18) Malignant glioma (20)	0.29(0.41) 0.30(0.50) 0.36(0.62)	$P = 0.29$
RUKA et al., unpublished data (early- and late-passage cell lines, colony formation on plastic)	GBM (21) Sarcoma (7) Breast (8)	0.51(0.27) 0.39(0.24) 0.38(0.25)	$P < 0.01$ (breast and sarcoma vs GBM)

H + N SCC, head and neck squamous cell carcinoma; GBM, glioblastoma multiforme
[a] Figures in parentheses are the number of cell lines
[b] Mean values. Coefficients of variation are given within parentheses
[c] ANOVA, analysis of variance. Tumour entities that exhibit significantly different SF2 values in the Bonferroni-Dunn test are cited within parentheses

found that the mean SF2 values of glioblastoma multiforme was significantly higher than the mean values of breast carcinomas and sarcomas. This difference in the average SF2 values clearly reflects clinical observations; however, the SF2 distribution of glioblastoma and sarcoma/breast carcinoma overlap widely, which does not accord with the much better clinical outcome of the latter entities.

In summary, measurements of SF2 on tumor cells of varying origin have provided a promising possibility to explain some of the clinically well-documented variation in radiation response between tumors of different histologies. The wide coefficient of variation of SF2 values within the same histology is a necessary basis to pursue studies on the predictive value of cellular radiosensitivity on the outcome of radiation therapy. However, the wide overlapping of SF2 distributions of tumor entities that do not overlap in their clinical radioresponsiveness indicates that determination of SF2 alone is not sufficient to predict accurately the outcome of treatment in individual patients.

8.4 Comparison of SF2 and Response to Fractionated Radiation Therapy in Tumor Models

Several research groups have compared SF2 values to the outcome of fractionated radiation therapy in tumor models. This experimental approach is straightforward and has, in contrast to studies performed on clinical samples, the important advantage that dose-response relationships can be determined for each tumor model under investigation. Figure 8.3 summarizes the results published to data. Since a variety of models and endpoints were used, SF2 values and treatment outcome were ranked for each individual study. Increasing ranks indicate increasing radioresistance.

ROFSTAD and BRUSTAD (1987) studied five human melanoma xenografts in nude mice and compared specific growth delay, that is absolute growth delay over the growth rate of untreated control tumors, after fractionated radiation therapy to survival parameters of the tumors assayed in soft agar. Figure 8.3a shows a correlation approaching signif-

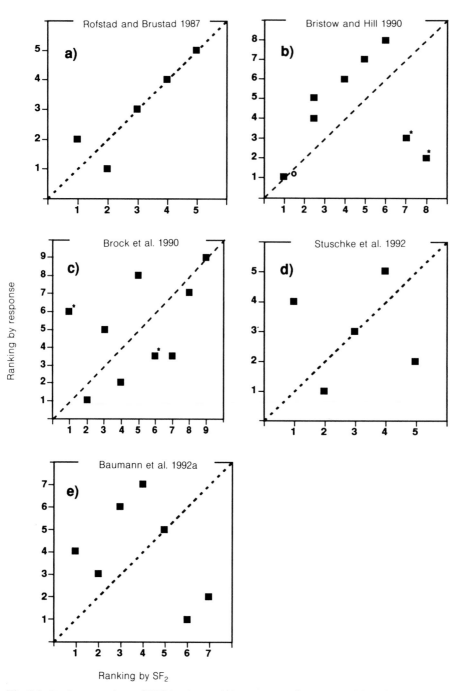

Fig. 8.3. Rank comparison of SF2 in vitro and the response of tumor models to fractionated irradiation. Increasing ranks indicate incrasing radioresistance. Under the assumption that the SF2 in vitro directly determines the radiation response of the tumor models, all data points are expected to lie on the *dotted line*. Tumors proven or suspected by the authors to be immunogenic are marked by an *asterisk*, tumors excluded for other reasons by *a circle*

icance (Spearman's rank $P = 0.07$) between specific growth delay after $10 \times 2\,\mathrm{Gy}$ given as three fractions per day and SF2. This correlation was later extended to local tumor control as the experimental endpoint for three of the five melanomas, which were *not immunogenic* in nude mice (ROFSTAD 1989,

1991). The lack of a demonstrable immune response reaction in these models in important insofar as such reactions may impact the results of therapy studies, and variable degrees of immune reactivity have been demonstrated for different xenotransplanted human tumor lines (ZIETMAN et al. 1988;

ROFSTAD 1989; SUIT et al. 1990; BAUMANN et al. 1990, 1992b). It should be noted, however, that immune response reactions may affect not only studies using xenografts but also studies using murine tumor models.

In a comprehensive study, BRISTOW and HILL (1990) compared the specific growth delay of eight murine tumor lines after 10×2 Gy to the SF2 values of the same cell lines assayed by colony formation in vitro (BRISTOW et al. 1990) (Fig. 8.3b). They found a significant correlation between the in vivo and in vitro parameters when three of the eight tumors, two of which were likely to be immunogenic, were excluded from analysis. (In Fig. 8.3b the immunogenic tumors are marked by an asterisk, the third excluded tumor by a circle).

BROCK and colleagues (1990) determined specific growth delay after 10×2 Gy in nine murine tumors and compared the results to SF2s obtained from a population growth assay (Fig. 8.3c). When two immunogenic tumors were excluded from the analysis, the correlation between cellular radiosensitivity and in vivo response approached significance. (The excluded tumors are marked by an asterisk.)

A different technique was used by STUSCHKE and colleagues (1992), who compared the SF2 of five human soft tissue sarcoma cell lines assayed in soft agar to the dose necessary to control the same cell lines grown as multicellular spheroids. Compared to tumors in vivo, multicellular spheroids in vitro are a less complex three-dimensional tumor model, because several parameters which may impact tumor response in vivo (e.g., immune response) will not affect spheroid control doses. Nevertheless, no correlation between SF2 and spheroid control dose fractionated irradiation was observed in this study (Fig. 8.3d).

BAUMANN et al. (1992a) investigated growth delay and tumor control after radiation therapy with 30 fractions in five human gliomas and two human squamous cell carcinomas in nude mice. The results were compared to SF2 values obtained for the same cell lines by a colony formation assay in vitro. Using local tumor control as the experimental endpoint, four of the five gliomas were more resistant than the squamous cell carcinomas, suggesting that the unique radioresistance of malignant gliomas observed in patients is at least in part reflected in human tumor xenografts. No correlation was observed between SF2 values in vitro and tumor control doses in vivo (Fig. 8.3e). It appears unlikely that the residual immune reactivity of nude mice against human tumor xenografts has significantly influenced this study since the results were confirmed in subsequent experiments using experimental endpoints that are not at all or only very slightly dependent on immune reactions (DuBois et al. 1991, and unpublished data).

Summing up, from a total of five studies, three show a correlation between SF2 in vitro and tumor response. Out of these, two studies were performed using specific growth delay as the only experimental endpoint. In theory, growth delay does not depend on the number of tumor stem cells (BEGG 1987; DENEKAMP 1980). Thus, studies that compare SF2 and growth delay might overlook influences of the number of tumor stem cells on the dose necessary to obtain local tumor control. That such an influence exists has been demonstrated for murine tumors in vivo, as well as for multicellular spheroids in vitro (HILL and MILAS 1989; STUSCHKE et al. 1992). However, differences between in vitro assay techniques, the overall treatment time, and undetected immune responses may also have contributed to the different results of the five studies reported to date.

8.5 Comparison of SF2 and Tumor Response in Patients Undergoing Radiation Therapy

Despite the many problems involved in clinical studies, comparison to the outcome of radiation therapy in patients is the most relevant endpoint for assessment of the predictive value of SF2. Most studies designed to test this correlation are still ongoing, and only preliminary results can be summarized here (Table 8.5).

Indirect evidence that intrinsically radioresistant cells determine local control rates of tumors was reported by WEICHSELBAUM et al. (1988). The SF2 values of 14 head and neck carcinoma cell lines derived from tumors that had failed radiation therapy were on average higher than the SF2 values of eight-head and neck tumor lines obtained prior to irradiation. The study was later extended to follow patients whose biopsies were obtained prior to radiotherapy for treatment outcome (WEICHSELBAUM et al. 1990; SCHWARTZ et al. 1992). Intrinsic radiation sensitivity in this study was not determined as SF2 but as mean inactivation dose (KELLERER and HUG 1972); however, for the purpose of the present chapter interpretation of mean inactivation dose values corresponds to the interpretation of SF2 (FERTIL et al. 1984; TUCKER 1986). In contrast to the earlier

Table 8.5. Preliminary results of prospective clinical studies evaluating the predictive value of SF2 in respect of the outcome of radiation therapy

Investigator	Assay technique	Tumors	Results
WEICHSELBAUM et al. (1990) SCHWARZ et al. (1992)	Early-passage cell lines, colony formation on plastic	H + N SCC (34)[a]	No difference in cellular radiosensitivity between patients with LC and LF
BROCK et al. (1990)	Primary culture, population growth	H + N SCC (72)	Average SF2 slightly but not significantly higher in patients with LF
WEST et al. (1989, 1992)	Primary culture, colony formation in soft agar	Cervix ca. (51)	Mean SF2 significantly lower in patients with LC
ALLALUNIS-TURNER et al. (1992a,b)	Early-passage cell lines, colony formation on plastic	Endometr. ca. (22) Cervix ca. (36) GBM/AA (17)	No difference in SF2 between patients with LC and LF
GIRINSKY et al. (1992)	Primary culture, population growth	H + N ca. cervix ca. (56)	Tendency ($P = 0.13$) for decreased LC rate of tumors with SF2 > 0.36. Significant differences when linear component of LQ model is used
TAGHIAN et al. (1993)	Early- and late-passage cell limes, colony formation on plastic	GBM/AA (46)	No correlation between SF2 and survival

H + N SCC, head and neck squamous cell carcinoma; LC, local tumor control; LF, failure to control the tumor locally; GBM, glioblastoma multiforme; AA, anaplatic astrocytoma
[a] Figures in parentheses are the number of patients reported to date

results, intrinsic radiation sensitivity in the prospective study was similar in 13 patients who suffered in-field recurrences and in 21 patients with local tumor control.

BROCK and colleagues (1990) compared SF2 measurements to the outcome of radiation therapy in patients with head and neck squamous cell carcinomas. All patients in this study were treated with postoperative radiotherapy, the surgical margins were negative, and patients who received chemotherapy were excluded. The average SF2 (= 0.4) of cultures derived from 12 patients who developed recurrences was slightly, but not significantly higher than the average SF2 (= 0.3) of cultures from 60 patients in whom local tumor control was achieved. In a further analysis the authors selected a subset of 29 patients with high risk of local failure as predicted from clinical and pathological parameters (BROCK et al. 1992). In this stratified group increased radioresistance was associated with a lower probability of cure; however, this association was not statistically significant.

The group of WEST et al. (1989, 1992) studied SF2 in primary specimens of cervical carcinoma obtained prior to treatment and compared the results to local tumor control. The mean SF2 value of 0.41 for 32 patients who were disease free was significantly lower than the mean SF2 of 0.62 in ten patients with local recurrence ± metastatic disease ($P = 0.02$). The average SF2 of 0.44 for nine patients who developed metastases was almost identical to the SF2 of patients with local tumor control. In order to discriminate radioresistant and radiosensitive tumors, a cut-off point of SF2 (= 0.55) was chosen. The probability of local recurrence was 5% in patients with SF2 values < 0.55 vs 57% in patients with SF2 > 0.55, this difference being highly significant ($P < 0.001$).

ALLALUNIS-TURNER and colleagues (1992a, b) compared SF2 values obtained from colony formation assays on early-passage cell lines with treatment outcome in endometrical and cervical carcinomas, and in gliomas. Only one out of 22 patients with endometrial carcinoma developed a local recurrence. The SF2 value measured for this patient's tumor was 0.67, which was the highest value determined for endometrial carcinoma in this study. Twenty-five of 36 patients with carcinoma of the cervix were free of disease at > 1 year after therapy, eight patients had local failure, and three patients developed distant metastases. No differences in radiosensitivity were observed; the mean SF2 values were 0.31 for patients with local control and 0.27 for patients with local failure. Also no evident correlation of SF2 and clinical outcome was found in 17 patients irradiated for malignant gliomas.

GIRINSKY et al. (1992) used the same technique as Brock's group and reported SF2 values for 56 patients with head and neck cancers and cervical carcinomas who were treated with radiation alone or combined with surgery. The local control rate was 93% in 16 patients with SF2 values < 0.36 compared at 67% for 40 patients with SF2 > 0.36. This difference was not significant ($P = 0.13$); however, a significant separation was found when the linear component of the linear-quadratic model was used instead of SF2.

In a collaborative study involving three centers, TAGHIAN et al. (1993) compared SF2 and clinical outcome in 46 patients suffering from glioblastoma multiforme and anaplastic astrocytoma. All patients were treated by some form of surgery and postoperative irradiation ± chemotherapy. The mean SF2 value of anaplastic astrocytoma (0.36) was lower than the mean SF2 of glioblastoma multiforme (0.45), this difference being of borderline significance. No evident correlation was found between SF2 and survival of individual patients.

Thus, from a total of six clinical reports only the study of WEST et al. (1989, 1992) shows a significant correlation between SF2 in vitro and tumor response in patients. Two of the remaining five studies show a trend for tumors with high SF2 values also to be more resistant in vivo, and three studies do not reveal a correlation between SF2 and tumor response. Even if differences in the assay techniques, particularities of the histologies studied, small numbers of patients, unstratified patient groups, and variable treatment strategies may all have obscured to some degree correlations between SF2 and treatment outcome, currently available clinical data indicate that determinations of SF2 in vitro do not simplistically reflect tumor response in vivo.

8.6 Summary and Outlook

Experimental and clinical results reported to date clearly demonstrate that the radiation response of tumors cannot be predicted from SF2 values with sufficient accuracy to base therapeutic decisions for *individual* patients solely upon such measurements. However, the observation that *mean SF2 values* of tumor classes correspond to the ranking of their clinical responsiveness and the fact that correlations between intrinsic radiosensitivity and outcome of

treatment were found in some studies indicate that cellular radiation sensitivity is *one important parameter among others* that impact tumor response. This is supported by single-dose studies under clamp hypoxia demonstrating that under such highly standarized experimental conditions tumor control doses can be predicted from the number of tumor stem cells and their radiosensitivity (SUIT et al. 1965; BAUMANN et al. 1990). For the much more complex situation during fractionated radiation therapy, additional influences will result from repopulation of clonogenic tumor cells, hypoxic cell fraction, reoxygenation, cell age distribution, and others (WITHERS 1975). It is therefore expected that a *combination of SF2 values with determinations of other radiobiologically important parameters* will eventually improve the accuracy of predictive assays of tumor response. Animal tumor models appear to be especially useful for developing such panels of predictive assays since the relative impact of a variety of variables on local tumor control can be concurrently evaluated.

Another promising approach employing measurements of intrinsic radiosensitivity for radiation treatment planning that should briefly be mentioned here is the determination of the radiation sensitivity of normal cells. Several hereditary disorders such as *ataxia telangiectasia* are associated with increased cellular radiosensitivity (TAYLOR et al. 1975; ABADIR and HAKAMI 1983; DESCHAVANNE et al. 1986; HART et al. 1987). These genetic disorders are extremely rare in their homozygote forms, but heterozygotes, who constitute a considerable proportion of cancer patients, e.g., 8% of breast cancer patients (SWIFT et al. 1987, 1991), also may exhibit increased radiosensitivities (ARLETT and PRIESTLEY 1985; DESCHAVANNE et al. 1986). Determinations of the intrinsic radiosensitivity of normal cells might be used to detect this subpopulation of radiosensitive patients and would thereby improve the therapeutic ratio of radiation therapy (NORMAN et al. 1988; SUIT et al. 1989; BUDACH et al. 1993).

References

Abadir R, Hakami N (1983) Ataxia telangiectasia with cancer. An indication for reduced radiotherapy and chemotherapy doses. Br J Radiol 56: 343–345

Allalunis-Turner MJ, Pearcey RG, Barron GM, Buryn DA, Babiak JC, Honore LH (1991) Inherent radiosensitivity testing of tumor biopsies obtained from patients with carcinoma of the cervix or endometrium. Radiother Oncol 22: 201–205

Allalunis-Turner MJ, Barron MG, Day RS, Fulton DS, Urtasun RC (1992a) Radiosensitivity testing of human primary brain tumor specimens. Int J Radiat Oncol Biol Phys 23: 339–343

Allalunis-Turner MJ, Day RS, Pearcey RG, Urtasun RC (1992b) Radiosensitivity testing in gynecological tumors and malignant gliomas. In: Dewey WC, Edington M, Fry RJM, Hall EJ, Whitmore GF (eds) Radiation research, a twentieth-century perspective. Academic, San Diego, pp 712–715

Alper T (ed) (1975) Cell survival after low doses of radiation. John Wiley, London

Arlett CF, Priestley A (1985) An assessment of the radiosensitivity of ataxic telangiectasia heterozygotes. In: Gatti RA, Swift M (eds) Ataxic telangiectaxic genetics: neuropathology and immunology of a degenerative disease of childhood. Alan R. Liss, New York, pp 101–109

Baker FL, Spitzer G, Ajani JA et al. (1986) Drug and radiation sensitivity measurements of successful primary monolayer culturing of human tumor cells using cell adhesive matrix and supplemented medium. Cancer Res 46: 1263–1274

Baumann M, duBois W, Suit HD (1990) Response of a human squamous cell carcinoma xenograft to irradiation at different sizes: relationship of clonogenic cells, cellular radiation sensitivity in vivo, and tumor rescuing units. Radiat Res 123: 325–330

Baumann M, duBois W, Pu A, Freeman J, Suit HD (1992a) Response of xenografts of human malignant gliomas and squamous cell carcinomas to fractionated irradiation. Int J Radiat Oncol Biol Phys 23: 803–809

Baumann M, Pu A, duBois W, Suit HD (1992b) Quantitative evaluation of the effects of cotransplantation of heavily irradiated tumor cells and of different immunosuppressive measures on the xenotransplantability of a human squamous cell carcinoma into athymic nude mice. In: Fiebig HH, Berger D (eds) Immunodeficient mice in oncology. Karger, Basel (Contributions to Oncology, vol 42, pp 89–107)

Begg A (1987) Principles and practices of the tumor growth delay assay. In: Kallman RF (ed) Rodent tumor models in experimental cancer therapy. Pergamon, New York, pp 114–121

Bellamy AS, Whelan RDH, Hill BT (1984) Studies of variation in inherent sensitivities to radiation, 5-fluorouracil and methotrexate in a series of human and murine tumor cell lines in vitro. Int J Radiat Oncol Biol Phys 10: 87–93

Bentzen SM, (1992) Steepness of the clinical dose-control curve and variation in the in vitro radiosensitivity of head and neck squamous cell carcinoma. Int J Radiat Biol 61: 417–423

Bentzen SM, Thames HD, Overgaard J (1980) Does variation in the in vitro cellular radiosensitivity explain the shallow clinical dose-control curve for malignant melanoma. Int J Radiat Biol 57: 117–126

Bentzen SM, Johansen L, Overgaard J, Thames HD (1991) Clinical radiobiology of squamous cell carcinoma of the oropharynx. Int J Radiat Oncol Biol Phys 20: 1197–1206

Berry RJ (1974) Population distribution in tumors and normal tissues: a guide to tissue radiosensitivity. In: Friedmann M (ed) The biological and clinical basis of radiosensitivity. Charles C. Thomas, Cicago, Ill, pp 141–155

Brahme A (1984) Dosimetric precision requirements in radiation therapy. Acta Radio Oncol 23: 379–391

Bristow RG, Hill RP (1990) Comparison between in vitro radiosensitivity and in vivo radioresponse in murine tumor cell lines. II: In vivo radioresponse following fractionated treatment and in vitro/in vivo correlations. Int J Radiat Oncol Biol Phys 18: 331–345

Bristow RG, Hardy PA, Hill RP (1990) Comparison between in vitro radiosensitivity and in vivo radioresponse of murine tumor cell lines. I. Parameters of in vitro radiosensitivity and endogenous cellular glutathione levels. Int J Radiat Oncol Biol Phys 18: 133–145

Brock WA, Baker F, Peters LJ (1989) Radiosensitivity of human head and neck squamous cell carcinomas in primary culture and its potential as a predictive assay of tumor radiocurability. Int J Radiat Biol 56: 751–760

Brock WA, Baker FL, Wike JL, Sivon SL, Peters LJ (1990a) Cellular radiosensitivity of primary head and neck squamous cell carcinomas and local tumor control. Int J Radiat Oncol Biol Phys 18: 1283–1286

Brock WA, Wike JL, Hunter NR, Milas L (1990b) Radiosensitivity of murine tumor cells in primary culture and tumor response to single and fractionated doses of irradiation. Poster. 38 Annual Meeting of the Radiation Research Society, New Orleans

Brock WA, Brown BW, Goepfert, Peters LJ (1992) In vitro radiosensitivity of tumor cells and local control by radiotherapy. In: Dewey WC, Edington M, Fry RJM, Hall EJ, Whitmore GF (eds) Radiation research, a twentieth-century perspective. Academic, San Diego, pp 696–699

Budach W, Hartford A, Gioioso D, Freeman J, Taghian A, Suit HD (1992) Radiation response of normal tissue as a predictor of tumor response in a murine model. Cancer Res 52: 6292–6296

Courtenay VD, Mills J (1978) An in-vitro colony assay for human tumours growth in immune-suppressed mice and treated in vivo with cytotoxic agents. Br J Cancer 37: 261–268

Davidson SE, West CML, Roberst SA, Hendry JH, Hunter RD (1990) Radiosensitivity testing of primary cervical carcinoma: evaluation of intra- and inter-tumour heterogeneity. Radiother Oncol 18: 349–356

Davis LW (1989) Presidential address: malignant glioma—a nemesis which requires clinical and basic investigation in radiation oncology. Int J Radiat Oncol Biol Phys 16: 1355–1365

Deacon J, Peckham MJ, Steel GG (1984) The radioresponsiveness of human tumours and the initial slope of the cell survival curve. Radiother Oncol 2: 317–323

Denekamp J (1980) Is any single in situ assay of tumor response adequate? Br J Cancer [Suppl IV]: 56–63

Deschavanne PJ, Debieu S, Fertil B, Malaise EP (1986) Reevaluation of in-vitro radiosensitivity of human fibroblasts of different genetic origins. Int J Radiat Biol 50: 279–293

Drewinko B, Humphrey RM, Trujillo JM (1972) The radiation response of a long-term culture of human lymphoid cells. Int J Radiat Biol 21: 361–373

duBois W, Suit HD, Baumann M, Taghian A, Gerweck L (1991) Factors influencing the radiation response of human tumor xenografts in nude mice. Int J Radiat Oncol Biol Phys 21 [Suppl 1]: 150

Dutreix J, Tubiana M, Dutreix A (1988) An approach to the interpretation of clinical data on the tumor control probability-dose relationship. Radiother Oncol 11: 239–248

Elkind MM, Sutton HA (1959) X-ray damage and recovery in mammalian cells in culture. Nature 184: 1293–1295

Fertil B, Malaise EP (1981) Inherent cellular radiosensitivity as a basic concept for human tumor radiotherapy. Int J Radiat Oncol Biol Phys 7: 621–629

Fertil B, Malaise EP (1985) Intrinsic radiosensitivity of human cell lines is correlated with radioresponsiveness of human tumors: analysis of 101 published survival curves. Int J Radiat Oncol Biol Phys 11: 1699–1707

Fertil B, Deschavanne PJ, Lachet B, Malaise EP (1980) In vitro radiosensitivity of six human cell lines. Radiat Res 82: 297–309

Fertil B, Dertinger H, Courdi A, Malaise EP (1984) Mean inactivation dose: a useful concept for intercomparison of human cell survival curves. Radiat Res 99: 73–84

Gerweck LE, Kornblith PL, Burlett P, Wang J, Sweigert S (1977) Radiation sensitivity of cultured human glioblastoma cells. Radiology 125: 231–234

Girinsky T, Lubin R, Chavaudra N, et al. (1992) In vitro radiosensitivity and calculated cell growth fraction in primary cultures from head and neck cancers and cervical carcinomas: preliminary correlations with treatment outcome. In: Dewey WC, Edington M, Fry RJM, Hall EJ, Whitmore GF (eds) Radiation research, a twentieth-century perspective. Academic, San Diego, pp 700–705

Hart RM, Kimler BF, Evans RG, Park CH 91987) Radiotherapeutic management of medulloblastoma in a pediatric patient with ataxia telangiectasia. Int J Radiat Oncol Biol Phys 13: 1237–1240

Hill RP, Milas L (1989) The proportion of stem cells in murine tumors. Int J Radiat Oncol Biol Phys 16: 513–528

Holthusen H (1936) Erfahrungen über die Verträglichkeitsgrenze für Röntgenstrahlen und deren Nutzanwendung zur Verhütung von Schäden. Strahlentherapie 57: 254–269

Inada T, Kasuga T, Nojiri I, Hiraoka T, Furuse T (1977) Comparative study on radiosensitivities of cultured cell lines derived from several human tumours under hypoxic conditions. Gann 68: 357–362

Kelland LR, Steel GG (1988) Differences in radiation response among human cervix carcinoma cell lines. Radiother Oncol 13: 225–232

Kellerer AM, Hug O (1972) Theory of dose-effect relations. In: Encyclopedia of medical radiology, vol 2. Springer, Berlin Heidelberg New York, pp 1–42

Lehnert S, Rybka WB, Suissa S, Giambattisto D (1986) Radiation response of haematopoietic cell lines of human origin. Int J Radiat Biol 49: 423–431

Leith JT, Dexter DL, DeWyngaert JK, Zeman EM, Chu MY, Calabresi P, Glicksman AS (1982) Differential responses to x-irradiation of subpopulations of two heterogeneous human carcinomas in vitro. Cancer Res 42: 2556–2561

Leith JT, Padfield G, Faulkner LE, Quinn P, Michelson S (1991a) Effects of feeder cells on the x-ray sensitivity of human colon cancer cells. Radiother Oncol 21: 53–59

Leith JT, Faulkner LA, Papa G, Quinn P, Michelson S (1991b) In vitro radiation survival parameters of human colon tumor cells. Int J Radiat Oncol Biol Phys 20: 203–206

Loeffler JS, Alexander E, Hochberg FH, et al. (1990a) Clinical patterns of failure following stereotactic interstitial irradiation for malignant gliomas. Int J Radiat Oncol Biol Phys 19: 1455–1462

Loeffler JS, Alexander E, Wen PY, et al. (1990b) Results of stereotactic brachytherapy used in the initial management of patients with glioblastoma. J Natl Cancer Inst 82: 1918–1921

Malaise EP, Fertil B, Chavaudra N, Guichard M (1986) Distribution of radiation sensitivities for tumor cells of specific histological types: comparison of in vitro to in vivo data. Int J Radiat Oncol Biol Phys 12: 617–624

Malaise EP, Fertil B, Chavaudra N, Brock WA, Rofstad EK, Weichselbaum RR (1989) The influence of technical factors of the in vitro measurement of intrinsic radiosensitivity of cells derived from human tumors. In: Paliwal BR, Fowler JF, Herbert DE, Kinsella TJ, Orton CG (eds) Prediction of response in radiation therapy: the physical, biological and analytical basis. American Institute of Physics, New York, pp 61–78

Masuda K, Aramaki R, Takaki T, Wakisaka S (1983) Possible explanation of radioresistance of glioblastoma in situ. Int J Radiat Oncol Biol Phys 9: 255–258

Nilsson S, Carlson J, Larson B (1980) Survival of irradiated glia and glioma cells studied with a new cloning technique. Int J Radiat Biol 37: 267–279

Norman A, Kagan Ar, Chan SL (1988) The importance of genetics for the optimization of radiation therapy. Am J Clin Oncol 11: 84–88

Paterson R (1948) The treatment of malignant disease by radium and x-rays. Edward Arnold, London

Perez CA, Brady LW (1992) Overview. In: Perez CA, Brady LW (ed) Principles and practice of radiation oncology. J.B. Lippincott, Philadelphia, p 6

Peters LJ, Withers HR, Thames HD, Fletcher GH (1982) Keynote address—the problem: tumor radioresistance in clinical radiotherapy. Int J Radiat Oncol Biol Phys 8: 101–108

Peters LJ, Brock WA, Johnson T, Meyn RE, Tofilon PJ, Milas L (1986) Potential methods for predicting tumor radiocurability. Int J Radiat Oncol Biol Phys 12: 459–467

Peters LJ, Brock WA, Chapman JD, Wilson G (1988) Predictive assays of tumor radiocurability. Am J Clin Oncol 11: 275–287

Puck TT, Marcus PI (1956) Action of x-rays on mammalian cells. J Exp Med 103: 653–666

Raaphorst GP, Feeley MM, DaSilva VF, Danjoux CE, Gerig LH (1989) A comparison of heat and radiation sensitivity of three human glioma cell lines. Int J Radiat Oncol Biol Phys 17: 615–622

Rofstad Ek (1986) Radiation biology of malignant melanoma. Acta radio Oncol 25: 1–10

Rofstad EK (1989) Local tumor control following single dose irradiation of human melanoma xenograft: relationship to cellular radiosensitivity and influence of an immune response by the athymic mouse. Cancer Res 49: 3163–3167

Rofstad EK (1991) Influence of cellular radiation sensitivity on local tumor control of human melanoma xenografts given fractionated radiation treatment. Cancer Res 51: 4609–4612

Rofstad EK, Brustad TB (1987) Radioresponsiveness of human melanoma xenografts given fractionated irradiation in vivo—relationship to the initial slope of the cell survival curve. Radiother Oncol 9: 45–56

Rofstad EK, Sutherland RM (1988) Radiation sensitivity of human ovarian carcinoma cell lines in vitro: effects of growth factors and hormones, basement membrane, and intercellular contact. Int J Radiat Oncol Biol Phys 15: 921–929

Rofstad EK, Wahl A, Brustad T (1987) Radiation sensitivity in vitro of cells isolated from human tumor surgical specimens. Cancer Res 47: 106–110

Rubin P, Keller B, Quick R (1974) The range of prescribed tumor lethal doses in the treatment of different human tumors. In: Friedman M (ed) The biological and clinical basis of radiosensitivity. Charles C. Thomas, Springfield, Ill., pp 435–484

Schultz CJ, Geard CR (1990) Radioresponse of human astrocytic tumors across grade as a function of acute and chronic irradiation. Int J Radiat Oncol Biol Phys 19: 1397–1403

Schwartz JL, Beckett MA, Mustafi R, Vaughan ATM, Weichselbaum RR (1992) Evaluation of different in vitro assays of inherent sensitivity as predictors of radiotherapy response. In: Dewey WC, Edington M, Fry RJM, Hall EJ, Whitmore GF (eds) Radiation research, a twentieth-century perspective. Academic, San Diego, pp 716–721

Seshadri R, Matthews C, Morley AA (1985) Radiation sensitivity of human malignant lymphocytes. Acta Radiol Oncol 24: 411–414

Stuschke M, Budach V, Klaes W, Sack H (1992) Radiosensitivity, repair capacity, and stem cell fraction in human soft tissue tumors: an in vitro study using multicellular spheroids and the colony assay. Int J Radiat Oncol Biol Phys 23: 69–80

Suit HD, Walker Am (1988) Predictors of radiation response in use today: criteria for new assays and methods of verification. In: Chapman JD, Peters LJ, Withers HR (eds) Prediction of tumor treatment response. Pergamon, New York, pp 3–19

Suit HD, Shalek RJ, Wette R (1965) Radiation response of mouse mammary carcinoma evaluated in terms of cellular radiation sensitivity. In: The University of Texas HD Anderson Hospital (Ed) Cellular radiation biology. Williams and Wilkins, Baltimore, pp 514–530

Suit HD, Baumann M, Skates S, Convery K (1989) Clinical interest in determinations of cellular radiation sensitivity. Int J Radiat Biol 5: 725–737

Suit HD, Zietman A, Tomkinson K, Ramsay J, Gerweck L, Sedlacek R (1990) Radiation response of xenografts of a human squamous cell carcinoma and a gliobolastoma multiforme: a progress report: Int J Radiat Oncol Biol Phys 18: 365–373

Suit HD, Skates S, Taghian A, Okunieff P, Efird JT (1992) Clinical implications of heterogeneity of tumor response to radiation therapy. Radiother Oncol 25: 251–260

Swift M, Reitnauer PJ, Morrell D, Chase CL (1987) Breast and other cancers in families with ataxia telangiectasia. N Engl J Med 316: 1289–1294

Swift M, Morrell D, Massey RB, Chase CL (1991) Incidence of cancer in 161 families affected by ataxia telangiectasia. N Engl J Med 325: 1831–1836

Szekely JG, Lobreau AU (1985) High radiosensitivity of the MOLT-4 leukaemic cell line. Int J Radiat Biol 48: 277–284

Taghian A, Suit HD, Pardo A, Gioioso D, Tomkinson K, duBois W, Gerweck L (1992) In vitro intrinsic radiation sensitivity of gioblastoma multiforme. Int J Radiat Oncol Biol Phys 23: 55–62

Taghian A, Ramsay J, Allalunis-Turner J et al. (1993) Intrinsic radiation sensitivity may not be the major determinant of the poor clinical outcome of glioblastoma multiforme. Int J Radiat Oncol Biol Phys 25: 243–249

Taylor AMR, Harnden DG, Arlett CF, Harcourt SA, Lehmann AR, Stevens S, Bridges BA (1975) Atexia telangiec-tasia: a human mutation with abnormal radiation sensitivity. Nature 258: 427–429

Thames HD, Peters LJ, Spanos W, Fletcher GH (1980) Dose-response curves for squamous cell carcinomas of the upper respiratory and digestive tracts. Br J Cancer 41: 35–38

Thames HD, Schultheiss TE, Hendry JH, Tucker SL, Dubray BM, Brock WA (1992) Can modest escalations of dose be detected as increased tumor control? Int J Radiat Oncol Biol Phys 22: 241–246

Tucker SL (1986) Is the mean inactivation dose a good measured of cell radiosensitivity? Radiat Res 105: 18–26

Wang CC (1988) Clinical radiation oncology. Indications, techniques, and results. PSG, Littleton

Weichselbaum RE, Epstein J, Little JB, Kornblith P (1976) Inherent cellular radiosensitivity of tumours of varying clinical curability. Am J Roentgenol 127: 1027–1032

Weichselbaum RR, Greenberger JS, Schmidt A, Karpas A, Moloney WC, Little JB (1981) In vitro radiosensitivity of human leukemia cell lines. Radiology 139: 485–487

Weichselbaum RR, Beckett MA, Schwartz JL, Dritschilo A (1988) Radioresistant cells are present in head and neck carcinomas that recur after radiotherapy. Int J Radiat Oncol Biol Phys 15: 575–579

Weichselbaum RR, Rotmensch J, Ahmed-Swan S, Beckett MA (1989) Radiobiological characterization of 53 human tumor cell lines. Int J Radiat Biol 56: 553–560

Weichselbaum RR, Beckett MA, Vijayakumar S et al. (1990) Radiobilogical characterization of head and neck and sarcoma cells derived from patients prior to radiotherapy. Int J Radiat Oncol Biol Phys 19: 313–319

West CML, Davidson SE, Hunters RD (1989) Evaluation of surviving fraction at 2 Gy as a potential prognostic factor for the radiotherapy of carcinoma of the cervix. Int J Radiat Biol 56: 761–765

West CML, Davidson SE, Hunter RD (1992) Surviving fraction at 2 Gy versus control of human cervical carcinoma—update of the Manchester study. In: Dewey WC, Edington M, Fry RJM, Hall EJ, Whitmore GF (eds) Radiation research, a twentieth-centuary perspective. Academic, San Diego, pp 706–711

Wetterer J (1913–1914) Handbuch der Röntgentherapie, 2nd edn, vol I. Otto Neminch, Leipzig

Williams MV, Denkamp J, Fowler F (1984) Dose-response relationships for human tumors: implications for clinical trials of dose modifying agents. Int J Radiat Oncol Biol Phys 10: 1703–1707

Withers HR (1975) The four R's of radiotherapy. In: Lett JT, Alder H (eds) Advances in radiation biology, vol 5. Academic, New York, p 241

Yang X, Darling JL, McMillan TJ, Peacock JH, Steel GG (1990) Radiosensitivity, recovery and dose-rate effect in three human glioma cell lines. Radiother Oncol 19: 49–56

Zietman AL, Suit HD, Ramsay JR, Silobrcic V, Sedlaek RS (1988) Quantitative studies on the transplantability of murine and human tumors into brain and subcutaneous tissues of NCr/Sed nude mice. Cancer Res 48: 6510–6516

9 Hypoxia in Tumours: Its Relevance, Identification, and Modification

M.R. Horsman

CONTENTS

9.1 Introduction

It is well known that cells irradiated under conditions of oxygen deprivation are more resistant to sparsely ionizing radiation than well-oxygenated cells (HALL 1988). Additional studies have now shown that oxygen-deficient cells exist in most animal solid tumours (GUICHARD et al. 1980; MOULDER and ROCKWELL 1984). There is strong evidence to suggest that hypoxic cells can also be found in human tumours and that they are probably one of the major reasons for failure to locally control certain tumor types with conventional radiation therapy (DISCHE 1989; OVERGAARD 1989).

Perhaps the best illustration for the presence of hypoxic cells in human tumours comes from a recent study by OVERGAARD (1993), in which he performed a meta-analysis using the results from all clinical trials that addressed the question of hypoxic modification in solid tumours undergoing primary radiotherapy. He identified some 9315 patients in 72 trials. The treatments included hyperbaric oxygen, radiation sensitizers, oxygen or

carbogen breathing, and blood transfusion, with the tumour sites being bladder, uterine cervix, CNS, head and neck, and lung (two of the trials contained a variety of mixed tumours). None of the treatments resulted in any significant improvement on the incidence of distant metastasis or radiation complications. Overall survival did show a significant improvement, but probably the most impressive results were seen with the 44 trials looking at local tumour control and these are summarized in Fig. 9.1. It is obvious that while eight of the trials showed no benefit of the hypoxic treatment over radiation alone, the remaining 36 gave an improved response; for seven of these 36 trials, primarily concerning squamous cell carcinoma of the head and neck, this improvement was statistically significant.

Tumour hypoxia is therefore clearly an important problem in radiation therapy and overcoming hypoxia continues to be a major interest in radia-

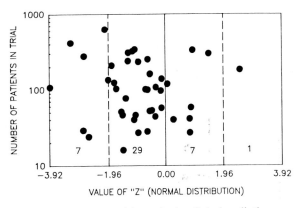

Fig. 9.1. Importance of hypoxia in clinical radiotherapy. These results show a meta-analysis of 44 trials with patients undergoing primary radiotherapy combined with a treatment to modify tumour hypoxia, in which the endpoint was local-regional control. The value of "Z" represents the observed minus expected control rates divided by a measure of the uncertainty of this difference. Negative values denote results that favour the treatment arm, while positive values favour radiation alone. Results falling between 0 and ± 1.96 indicate non-significant trends, while from ± 1.96 to ± 3.92 the differences become significant. (OVERGAARD, unpublished observations)

M.R. HORSMAN, PhD, Danish Cancer Society, Department of Experimental Clinical Oncology, Nørrebrogade 44, DK-8000 Aarhus C, Denmark

tion biology and oncology (see *Radiotherapy and Oncology*, supplement 20, 1991). In the current chapter the hypoxia problem is reviewed with specific reference to (a) the different ways in which hypoxia can arise in animal and human tumours, (b) the methods currently available for its detection in both qualitative and quantitative terms and (c) the various clinically applicable techniques that can be used to modify hypoxia and thereby improve tumour response to subsequent therapy.

9.2 Types of Tumour Hypoxia

9.2.1 Diffusion-Limited Chronic Hypoxia

For solid tumours to grow beyond a size of 1 mm^3 it is necessary for the tumour cells to develop a blood supply, a process which is referred to as angiogenesis (FOLKMAN 1976). These new blood vessels, which are formed following angiogenic stimulus, differ in many ways from the normal tissue blood vessels from which they are derived (WARREN 1979; VAUPEL et al. 1989a). Structurally these differences

include a lack of smooth muscle, incomplete or missing endothelial lining, interrupted or absent basement membranes, lack of nervous innervation, tortuosity, lack of a collateral supply, existence of arteriovenous shunts, abnormal vessel branching patterns and elongated vessels (WARREN 1979; VAUPEL et al. 1989a). Furthermore, many solid tumours lack a lymphatic system for interstitial fluid drainage, which can lead to abnormally high interstitial fluid pressures within the tumour (WIIG and GADEHOLT 1985). These factors coupled with the rapid proliferation of the tumour cells often result in a blood supply which is actually inadequate for meeting the needs of all the tumour cells. Regions within the tumours can therefore develop which are nutrient deprived, highly acidic and low in oxygen (VAUPEL 1979; WIKE-HOOLEY et al. 1984), yet the hypoxic cells which exist in these areas can still be viable.

The first real indication that hypoxia could be present in tumours came in 1955 from observations on histological sections of fresh specimens from human carcinoma of the bronchus (THOMLINSON and GRAY 1955). These authors found that the

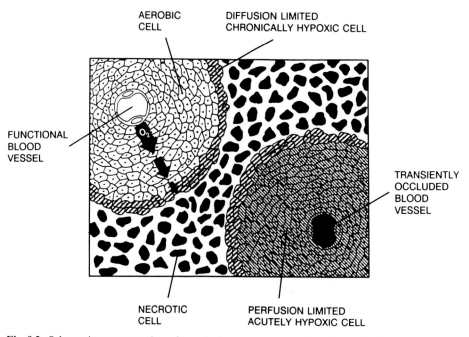

Fig. 9.2. Schematic representation of a typical tumour cross-section illustrating how hypoxia can develop. Viable aerobic tumour cells growing around a functional blood vessel consume the oxygen that diffuses from the vessel. Beyond the diffusion distance of oxygen, typically around 150 μm, the cells become necrotic, but immediately prior to the necrotic zone is a layer of cells which are oxygen deprived yet viable. These cells remain hypoxic until they become either reoxygenated or die and hence are often referred to as chronically hypoxic cells. If blood flow through a vessel is transiently stopped then all the normally aerobic cells downstream of the occlusion are suddenly made hypoxic. These cells are considered acutely hypoxic because they only remain hypoxic as long as the occlusion continues, becoming oxygenated again when blood flow resumes. (Redrawn for HORSMAN 1992c)

tumours grew as solid rods surrounded by vascular stroma from which the tumour cells obtained their nutrient and oxygen requirements. As the tumours grew, areas of necrosis appeared in the tumour centre. Since the radii of the resulting tumour cords were found to be equivalent to the calculated diffusion distance of oxygen in respiring tissues, it was suggested that as oxygen diffused from the stroma it was consumed by the cells, and while those cells beyond the diffusion distance were unable to survive, those cells immediately prior to the necrosis were viable yet existing in areas of low oxygenation. The "corded" structure of tumours described by Thomlinson and Gray is more typically seen as cords of viable tumour tissue growing around individual blood vessels, as illustrated in Fig. 9.2.

9.2.2 Perfusion-Limited Acute Hypoxia

Recently it was suggested that hypoxia in tumours could also be acute (BROWN 1979; SUTHERLAND and FRANKO 1980). Using recently developed fluorescent staining techniques which not only allow for selection and analysis of cells in tumours as a function of their distance from the blood supply but also enables observations of blood flow at the microregional level, the presence of acutely hypoxic cells in tumours was confirmed and found to result from transient fluctuations in tumour blood flow (CHAPLIN et al. 1986, 1987). This is also shown in Fig. 9.2.

These cessations in blood flow have been shown to involve around 4% of vessels in a FaDu human head and neck squamous cell carcinoma xenograft

and up to 7% in a Nall malignant melanoma xenograft, both grown in nude mice (CHAPLIN and TROTTER 1991). Values of about 8% have also been reported in a murine SCCVII carcinoma (CHAPLIN and TROTTER 1991), a C3H mouse mammary carcinoma (HORSMAN et al. 1990a), and an SMT-2A rat tumour (JIRTLE 1988). Interestingly, intermittent flow has been found to be higher in the tumour centre than in the periphery (CHAPLIN and TROTTER 1991). In addition, for SCCVII tumours transient fluctuations in flow were seen to increase with increasing tumour size (TROTTER et al. 1991a), an efffect that correlates with the finding that acute hypoxia is more pronounced in larger tumours (CHAPLIN et al. 1986, 1987). The mechanisms responsible for this intermittent blood flow in tumours is not entirely clear. Suggestions for the causative factors include vessel plugging by white blood cells, red blood cell rouleaux or circulating tumour cells (JAIN 1988); collapse of vessels in regions of high tumour interstitial pressure (SEVICK and JAIN 1989); and spontaneous vasomotion in incorporated host arterioles affecting flow in downstream capillaries (INTAGLIETTA et al. 1977; REINHOLD et al. 1977).

9.3 Identifying and Estimating Hypoxia in Tumours

9.3.1 Animal Tumour Studies

Not only is it relatively easy to identify hypoxia in experimental animal tumours, one can also quantitatively estimate the percentage of cells which are

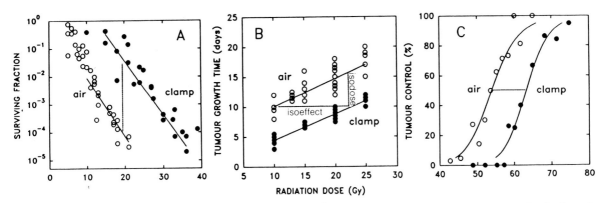

Fig. 9.3A–C. In vivo procedures used to estimate hypoxic fractions in tumours. All tumours were grown in the feet of mice and treated when they had reached 200 mm³ in volume. Irradiations were given locally to tumours under either normal air breathing or clamped conditions. **A** Survival of SCCVII tumour cells measured by an excision assay performed 24 h after irradiation. Individual tumour results are shown. **B** Time taken for C3H/Tif tumours to regrow to three times their treatment volume. *Points* represent separate animals. **C** Percentage of mice showing local control of C3H/Tif tumours 90 days after treatment. (GRAU, unpublished observations)

hypoxic. Three major assay techniques are routinely used and these are illustrated in Fig. 9.3. All of them involve a comparison of the response of tumours when irradiated in animals either under normal air breathing conditions or when the tumours are artificially made fully hypoxic.

The first procedure is often referred to as the paired survival curve assay, since one uses an in vivo/in vitro excision assay to determine the survival of the tumour cells following irradiation and then compares the survival dose-response curves obtained under the two conditions (Fig. 9.3A). Hypoxia can be achieved either by killing the mice or by clamping the tumours immediately prior to irradiation. The hypoxic fraction can then be calculated from the vertical distance between the two parallel curves (VAN PUTTEN and KALLMAN 1968), and in this example the hypoxic fraction is $\sim 1\%$.

Tumour hypoxia can also be determined using the so-called clamped tumour growth delay assay (Fig. 9.3B). Basically, this requires irradiation of tumours under either normal or clamped conditions and then measuring the time taken for tumours to reach a specific size (tumour growth time). From the dose-response curves the hypoxic fraction can then be estimated either by the isodose method, which involves comparing the differences in tumour growth time at a particular radiation dose, or by the isoeffect method, which uses the differences in radiation dose at the same tumour growth time (MOULDER and ROCKWELL 1984). From the data of Fig. 9.3B the isodose method gives a hypoxic fraction of $\sim 40\%$, while with the isoeffect procedure a value of only $\sim 2\%$ was obtained.

The third technique used to calculate hypoxic fractions is the clamped tumour control assay (Fig. 9.3C). This involves determining the percent local tumour control following irradiation under normal or clamped conditions and estimating, from the dose-response curves, the radiation dose necessary to control 50% of the tumours (TCD_{50} dose). Hypoxic fractions can then be obtained from these values by direct analysis (BENTZEN and GRAU 1991), and in this example was found to be $\sim 12\%$.

Several studies have used these different assay procedures to calculate hypoxic fractions in the same tumour models and found that the assay procedures gave different results (McNALLY and SHELDON 1977; SIEMANN 1980; MOULDER and MARTIN 1984). Why this should be is not entirely clear. It may be due to differences in the underlying assumptions upon which each method is based, or it may

simply reflect differences in the fate of cells analysed by in situ and excision assays. It is also dependent on the endpoint of the assay, and this is seen from the data of Fig. 9.3B in which the hypoxic fractions calculated by the isodose and isoeffect methods were different. Nevertheless, using these procedures hypoxia has been directly identified in most animal solid tumours, with the values ranging from $< 1\%$ to well over 50% (GUICHARD et al. 1980; MOULDER and ROCKWELL 1984). Unfortunately, none of these procedures can be applied to the clinical situation. One therefore has to rely on techniques which indirectly indicate the presence of hypoxia.

9.3.2 Techniques Applicable to Human Tumours

There are a number of ways that this problem has been approached clinically. Since the degree of hypoxia in tumours is strongly dependent on the vascular supply, several studies have focused their attention on tumour vascularization. The endpoints have included measurements of intercapillary distance (KOLSTAD 1968; AWWAD et al. 1986), vascular density (DELIDES et al. 1988; RÉVÉSZ et al. 1989; STREFFER et al. 1989) and the distance from tumour cells to the nearest vessel (LAUK et al. 1989). By far the most extensive studies have involved carcinoma of the cervix (KOLSTAD 1968; AWWAD et al. 1986; RÉVÉSZ et al. 1989) and in all of these a clear correlation was seen between tumour vascularity and response to radiotherapy. In the Kolstad and Awwad studies it was reported that poor treatment outcome was actually associated with those tumours which had an intercapillary distance greater than $300-350\,\mu m$, which is consistent with the presence of hypoxia if one assumes a diffusion distance of oxygen of around $150\,\mu m$. Similar positive correlations between vascularization and treatment outcome were seen for nasopharyngeal tumours (DELIDES et al. 1988) and rectal carcinomas (STREFFER et al. 1989). But the study by LAUK et al. (1989) using oral squamous cell cancers surprisingly showed that those tumours which had the poorest treatment outcome were actually better vascularized. Whatever the explanation for this apparent anomaly, the results strongly suggest that using estimates of tumour vasculature alone may not be a reliable prognostic indicator of hypoxia in all situations.

Cryospectrophotometric measurements of intercapillary haemoglobin oxygen (HbO_2) saturations may also be a potentially useful method for characterizing the oxygenation status of tumours. VAUPEL and colleagues (1978, 1979) have shown that tumour HbO$_2$ values agree well with oxygen partial pressure measurements obtained with microelectrodes. Other studies have shown that for certain tumour cell lines, as the radiobiological hypoxic fraction changes with tumour volume, there is a concomitant change in HbO$_2$ distributions (FENTON et al. 1988; ROFSTAD et al. 1989). However, when the HbO$_2$ values and hypoxic fraction between different tumour cell lines are compared, now such changes are seen (ROFSTAD et al. 1989).

Tumour metabolic activity has also been suggested as a possible prognostic indicator of hypoxia, since the metabolism of hypoxic cells is likely to be different from that of cells which are well oxygenated. There are several ways in which tumour metabolism can be studied. From tumour extracts one can perform either biochemical (TAMULEVICIUS et al. 1987) or high performance liquid chromatographic (GERWECK et al. 1989) analysis. A refinement of these techniques and one that allows for the regional distribution of substrates and metabolites in tumours to be determined is the method based on the measurement of luminescence produced when tumour cryosections are brought into contact with a frozen bioluminescent enzyme cocktail and then thawed (MÜLLER-KLIESER et al. 1991). Alternatively, tumour metabolism can be determined non-invasively when intact tumours are imaged using nuclear magnetic resonance (NMR) spectroscopy (OKUNIEFF 1990) or positron emission tomography (PET) (McEWAN 1989).

Using either invasive or non-invasive procedures, investigators have shown significant changes in tumour metabolic status after treatment with a variety of agents which can substantially decrease tumour blood flow and subsequently increase tumour hypoxia, such as hyperthermia (STREFFER et al. 1992), hydralazine (OKUNIEFF 1990) and flavone acetic acid (EVELHOCH et al. 1990). Other workers have reported that tumour metabolism changes with tumour volume and thus presumably with hypoxic fraction (ROFSTAD et al. 1989; VAUPEL et al. 1989b; KOUTCHER et al. 1990). In addition, a recent study comparing the adenosine triphosphate (ATP) measured by bioluminescence in biopsies from cervical cancer patients with direct measurements of tumour oxygenation made using a microelectrode reported that as ATP concentration increased, so did modal pO$_2$, although there was no significant correlation (VAUPEL and MÜLLER-KLIESER 1992). However, the relationship between

tumour metabolic state and radiation response is somewhat controversial, in that no studies have yet shown any direct correlation between metabolic activity and response to radiation. In fact, one study using two types of human melanoma xenografts with different radiobiologically hypoxic cell fractions reported that the differences in ATP and lactate levels measured by bioluminescence did not reflect the differences in tumour radiosensitivity (MÜLLER-KLIESER et al. 1991). Furthermore, no significant differences were seen in metabolism, measured by NMR, of two small cell lung cancer xenografts which had dissimilar radiosensitivities (KRISTJANSEN et al. 1990). Nor were any clear correlations seen between the NMR results from two rodent tumours and two human xenografts with differing radiobiological hypoxic fractions (ROFSTAD et al. 1989).

Another approach which has been made to directly identify hypoxia in human tumours has been the use of radioactive or fluorescent labelled compounds. The observation that the nitroimidazole compound misonidazole was preferentially metabolized in hypoxic cells and then covalently bound to the macromolecules in these cells for substantial periods led to the proposal that such agents might be used as hypoxic markers (CHAPMAN et al. 1979). This was later demonstrated in tumours using misonidazole labelled with carbon-14 or hydrogen-3, an effect that was shown to be not only dependent on oxygen level but also correlated with hypoxia fraction (for review see FRANKO 1986). Efforts to use this procedure to identify hypoxia in human tumours have been undertaken. In a recent study URTASUN (1992) looked at the binding of ^{3}H-misonidazole in 27 tumours in 26 patients. Following total resection of the metastatic lesion the tumours were analysed by liquid scintillography and autoradiography to determine whether they contained significant areas of heavy labelling indicative of hypoxia. The results showed areas of dense labelling in 0% (0/2) of squamous cell carcinomas of the head and neck, 10% (1/10) of sarcomas, 67% (8/12) of small cell lung cancers and 100% (3/3) of melanomas. Currently work is being undertaken to find more rapid, non-invasive labelling techniques for identifying hypoxia. Iodoazamycin arabinoside is an agent which has been shown to undergo hypoxia-dependent binding in EMT-6 tumours and when labelled with iodine-131 has the potential to be used to detect tumour hypoxia using single-photon emission computed tomography techniques (URTASUN 1992). Preliminary studies have shown binding in

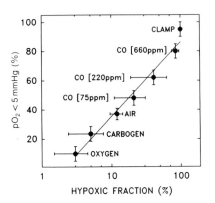

Fig. 9.4. Relationship between tumour oxygen partial pressure (pO_2) measurements and radiobiological hypoxic fraction. Experiments were performed on a C3H/Tif mammary carcinoma grown in the feet of CDF1 mice and treated at 200 mm³. The pO_2 values were obtained using an Eppendorf microelectrode and hypoxic fractions calculated from full radiation dose-response curves as shown in Fig. 9.3C. Mice were allowed to breath oxygen or carbogen for 5 min and carbon monoxide (CO) for 35 min prior to treatment. Gassing continued throughout the pO_2 measurement or irradiation period. Tumour clamping was also for 5 min prior to and during treatment. Results show mean values ± 95% confidence intervals. (HORSMAN, unpublished observations)

one of three patients with sarcomas, none of five with glioblastomas, and five of ten with small cell lung cancers (URTASUN 1992). Fluoromisonidazole is another agent being considered to identify hypoxic cells. Labelling experiments in murine tumours showed that the binding of ³H-fluoromisonidazole was consistent with the presence of tumour hypoxia (RASEY et al. 1989). The compound can also be labelled with the positron emitter fluorine-18,

allowing it to be imaged with PET (RASEY and EVANS 1991), and early clinical studies with ¹⁸F-fluoromisonidazole showed that five of six head and neck malignancies and one of three non-head and neck tumours contained significant numbers of hypoxic cells (RASEY and EVANS 1991).

Perhaps the most direct method for identifying hypoxia in human tumours is to determine oxygen partial pressure (pO_2) distributions using microelectrodes. This technique involves insertion of a microelectrode probe into the tissue and then oxygen measurements are made after each stepwise movement through the tissue. A frequency distribution of intratumour pO_2 is then obtained. The use of this procedure to measure oxygenation in tumours has recently been reviewed (VAUPEL et al. 1989a). Several studies have shown a decrease in median pO_2 values in animal tumours with increasing tumour size (VAUPEL 1979; VAUPEL et al. 1987, 1989b; KALLINOWSKI et al. 1990). Tumour pO_2 measurements can also be related to radiation response and this is shown in Fig. 9.4. In these experiments a C3H mammary carcinoma was locally irradiated in mice under a variety of treatment conditions. From the local tumour control results similar to those shown in Fig. 9.3C the various hypoxic fractions were calculated by direct analysis (BENTZEN and GRAU 1991), and then compared to the percentage of tumour pO_2 values less than or equal to 5 mmHg, determined using an Eppendorf microelectrode in similarly treated mice. Clearly there is an excellent correlation in this tumour between the level of oxygenation estimated from the pO_2 measurements and radiobiological hypoxia.

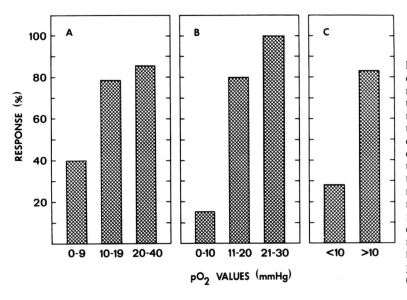

Fig. 9.5A–C. Influence of tumour pO_2 on clinical outcome in response to radiation therapy. **A** Absence of local tumour recurrence 5 years after radiation treatment as a function of the lowest pO_2 values measured in 31 cases of stage I and II cancers of the cervix (KOLSTAD 1968). **B** Complete tumour response 90 days after radiation treatment as a function of mean pO_2 in 31 fixed lymph node metastases from squamous cell carcinoma of the head and neck (GATENBY et al. 1988). **C** Patient survival 22 months after radiation treatment as a function of median pO_2 values in 31 patients with uterine cervix carcinoma (HÖCKEL et al. 1992)

The pO_2 histograph has also been used to measure tumour oxygenation in human tumours and the results correlated with response to radiation therapy (KOLSTAD 1968; GATENBY et al. 1988; HÖCKEL et al. 1993). These results are summarized in Fig. 9.5. There is a clear indication that the level of oxygenation in both cervical cancers and head and neck tumours will influence the tumour response to radiation, with the less well oxygenated tumours showing the poorest response. Although this microelectrode technique appears to be an excellent way to identify hypoxia in tumours, it does have the disadvantage that it is invasive and can only be used on tumours which are readily accessible to the electrodes. In addition, care must be taken in interpreting the data since not only is intratumour variability sometimes seen but also tumour-to-tumour differences often occur even if tumours of the same pathological stage and histological grade are compared (VAUPEL et al. 1991; VAUPEL and MÜLLER-KLIESER 1992).

9.4 Modifying Tumour Hypoxia

9.4.1 Overcoming Hypoxic Cell Resistance

Numerous attempts have been made to try and eliminate radiation-resistant hypoxic cells in tumours. Approaches to the problem of diffusion-limited chronic hypoxia have involved improving the diffusion distance of oxygen, directly sensitizing hypoxic cells to radiation or preferentially killing these cells. One of the more popular methods that has been used to improve tumour oxygenation has involved the use of agents which can increase tumour blood flow. Improved blood flow to tumours has been reported to occur with angiotensin II (SUZUKI et al. 1981; BURTON et al. 1985), noradrenaline (HAFSTRÖM et al. 1980), calcium antagonists (KAELIN et al. 1982; WOOD and HIRST 1989), anaesthetics (ZANELLI et al. 1975; MENKE and VAUPEL 1988), hyperthermia (SONG 1984) and nicotinamide (HORSMAN et al. 1988a, 1989a). Unfortunately, many of these agents can, under certain conditions, also decrease tumour blood flow. This is true for angiotensin II (JIRTLE et al. 1978), noradrenaline (JIRTLE et al. 1978; MATTSON et al. 1978), calcium antagonists (KNAPP et al. 1985; WOOD and HIRST 1989), anaesthetics (KALLMAN et al. 1972; MENKE and VAUPEL 1988) and hyperthermia (SONG 1984). No studies as yet

have reported that nicotinamide can decrease tumour blood flow.

Tumour oxygenation can also be improved by increasing the oxygen-carrying capacity of blood. This can occur following oxygen or carbogen breathing under normobaric or hyperbaric conditions (SUIT et al. 1972; ROJAS 1991), or using perfluorochemical emulsions (ROCKWELL 1985; ROCKWELL et al. 1991). To this list can be added haemoglobin-oxygen affinity modifiers, which, although they do not increase the amount of oxygen in the blood, do increase the ease with which haemoglobin releases oxygen (HIRST and WOOD 1989; SIEMANN et al. 1989).

A final approach that has been extensively used to combat chronic hypoxia is the use of agents such as bioreductive/radiosensitizing drugs or hyperthermia. These agents can both directly sensitize hypoxic cells to radiation and specifically kill them (ADAMS 1984; OVERGAARD et al. 1987), although in the case of hyperthermia, cytotoxicity is not a consequence of hypoxia per se but rather is due to cellular metabolic changes—especially an increase in acidity, which is the result of prolonged oxygen deprivation (OVERGAARD and NIELSEN 1980).

Although the above-listed procedures work extremely well against diffusion-limited chronic hypoxia, most of them have little or no influence on hypoxia that is acute and results from a perfusion limitation. Increasing blood flow or oxygenation, for example, will be of little benefit if flow is inhibited. Similarly acutely hypoxic cells are probably not sensitive to hyperthermia because it is unlikely that these cells are hypoxic for a period sufficient to induce the necessary metabolic changes. Acutely hypoxic cells, however, can be attacked by bioreductive or radiosensitizing drugs since these agents can kill or radiosensitize any hypoxic cell (ADAMS 1984; COLEMAN 1988). The ability of such drugs to influence acute hypoxia is also illustrated in experiments in which tumours are treated with radiation and heat, a combination which can effectively kill the aerobic and chronically hypoxic populations, but not those that are acutely hypoxic. However, if the radiosensitizers misonidazole or nimorazole, or the bioreductive drug SR-4233, are introduced into this treatment protocol, then a substantial improvement in tumour response is observed (OVERGAARD 1980; TIMOTHY and OVERGAARD 1984; HERMAN et al. 1990).

An alternative approach to the acute hypoxia problem would be to make these cells chronically hypoxic and then attack them with a treatment that specifically kills such cells, for example hyperthermia. The antihypertensive drug hydralazine is one agent capable of decreasing blood flow to tumours and thereby making them fully radiobiologically hypoxic for several hours (HORSMAN et al. 1989b). Although giving hydralazine prior to irradiation will protect the tumour, it will enhance the tumour response to heat (HORSMAN et al. 1989b). Now if mice are injected with hydralazine several hours after local tumour irradiation, a sequence which has no influence on radiation response alone, and the tumours are subsequently heated, then the resulting response of the tumour is greater than that seen with the combination of radiation and heat (HORSMAN 1992a), an effect which is entirely consistent with acutely hypoxic cells being made chronically hypoxic before the heat treatment.

Probably the best method for overcoming acute hypoxia would be to actually prevent it from occurring in the first place. Several years ago it was demonstrated that the vitamin B_3 analogue, nicotinamide, could enhance radiation damage in a variety of murine tumour models and did so in preference to its effects in normal tissues (HORSMAN et al. 1989c). Mechanistic studies have since shown that nicotinamide can decrease ^{14}C-misonidazole binding in tumours (HORSMAN et al. 1988a, 1989a) and increase metabolic activity as measured by both biochemical analysis (HORSMAN et al. 1992) and ^{31}P-NMR (WOOD et al. 1991), all of these findings being consistent with an improvement in tumour oxygenation. Additional data have now indicated that the nicotinamide effect is primarily the result of the drug preventing the transient fluctuations in tumour blood flow (CHAPLIN et al. 1990b; HORSMAN et al. 1990a) which normally lead to the development of acute hypoxia (CHAPLIN et al. 1986, 1987). Similar results have also been reported with angiotensin II (TROTTER et al. 1991b) and flunarizine (JIRTLE 1988). How these agents prevent acute hypoxia from occurring is not clear. Angiotensin II increases arterial blood pressure (TROTTER et al. 1991b), which could decrease the likelihood of vessel collapse due to high interstitial pressure in tumours. On the other hand, flunarizine can increase red blood cell deformability (DECREE et al. 1979) and thus may reduce vessel plugging. While the mechanism for the nicotinamide effect is unknown, it is unlikely to be the same as for angiotensin II because at high doses nicotinamide actually decreases arterial blood pressure in mice (HORSMAN et al. 1992). It is also possible that the ability of nicotinamide to prevent the transient fluctuations in blood

flow may fully explain the reported increases in tumour blood flow alluded to earlier (HORSMAN et al. 1988a, 1989a), and, if so, it is unlikely that nicotinamide will have any large effect on diffusion-limited chronic hypoxia.

It was recently suggested that if one were to take a treatment like nicotinamide which primarily eliminates radiation-resistant acute hypoxia and combine it with an agent which specifically overcomes chronic hypoxia, then a better tumour response to radiation might be achievable (HORSMAN et al. 1990b). This has now been done. Originally it was shown that nicotinamide could substantially enhance the tumour response to heat (HORSMAN et al. 1990a) or fluosol DA + carbogen (CHAPLIN et al. 1990a) when combined with single-dose radiation treatments. More recent studies have demonstrated that nicotinamide can also influence radiosensitization by oxygen or carbogen breathing when given with fractionated radiation schedules (KJELLEN et al. 1991). Limited normal tissue studies suggest that although combination therapy of this type does enhance normal tissue damage, the enhancement ratios are smaller than those seen in tumours, thus resulting in a therapeutic gain (HORSMAN et al. 1990a; KJELLEN et al. 1991).

9.4.2 Exploiting Tumour Hypoxia

Although hypoxic cells are resistant to certain therapies, there is evidence that these same cells are sensitive to other modalities. Now, rather than trying to reduce hypoxia in tumours, some studies are suggesting that it might be beneficial to actually increase the level of tumour hypoxia before subsequent exposure to agents that specifically kill hypoxic cells. There are a number of ways in which tumour hypoxia can be increased experimentally. One can alter the oxygen-carrying capacity of the blood either by allowing mice to breath carbon monoxide, which has a greater affinity for haemoglobin than oxygen (GRAU et al. 1992), or by using a drug like BW12C, which modifies haemoglobin–oxygen binding in such a way as to increase the affinity of haemoglobin for oxygen and thereby makes the haemoglobin less likely to release oxygen (BEDDALL et al. 1984).

Alternatively, one can decrease oxygen availability by simply decreasing blood flow to the tumour. As we have already discussed, there are certain physiological modifiers of tumour blood flow which not only increase flow but under certain conditions also decrease it. Other agents which physiologically decrease tumour blood flow include hydralazine (CHAPLIN and ACKER 1987; HORSMAN et al. 1989b), 5-hydroxytryptamine (KNAPP et al. 1985; SHRIVASTAR et al. 1985) and glucose (WIKE-HOOLEY et al. 1984; HIRAOKA and HAHN 1990). Tumour blood flow can also be reduced by the use of agents which directly damage tumour vasculature. These include flavone acetic acid (EVELHOCH et al. 1988; HORSMAN et al. 1991), tumour necrosis factor (KALLINOWSKI et al. 1989a, b), photodynamic therapy (STAR et al. 1986; HORSMAN and WINTHER 1989) and even hyperthermia (SONG 1984). Typically the physiological modifiers of tumour blood flow produce effects lasting anywhere from a few minutes to several hours, whereas with the vascular damaging agents blood flow can be reduced for up to several days.

A number of these blood flow modifiers have now been combined with hypoxic cell cytotoxins. The antitumour effects of bioreductive drugs have been enhanced by hydralazine (CHAPLIN and ACKER 1987; BREMNER et al. 1990), 5-hydroxytryptamine (CHAPLIN 1986), flavone acetic acid (SUN and BROWN 1989), photodynamic therapy (ADAMS et al. 1992) and heat (HORSMAN et al. 1988b; HERMAN et al. 1990). An improvement of the in vivo cytotoxic action of heat has also been observed after treatment with hydralazine (HORSMAN et al. 1989b; KALMUS et al. 1990), glucose (URANO et al. 1983; HIRAOKA and HAHN 1990), anaesthetics (URANO et al. 1980), flavone acetic acid (HORSMAN et al. 1991), tumour necrosis factor (KALLINOWSKI et al. 1989a) and photodynamic therapy (WALDOW and DOUGHERTY 1984; HENDERSON et al. 1985). As has already been mentioned, this increased sensitivity to heat is the result of a decrease in pH occurring after the metabolic changes resulting from long-term hypoxia (OVERGAARD and NIELSEN 1980). A reduction in tumour blood flow should therefore enhance the anti-tumour activity of other agents for which cytotoxicity is dependent on low pH and not hypoxia per se. One such agent is melphalan (CHAPLIN et al. 1989), and indeed a significant enhancement of melphalan toxicity in tumours has been observed after hydralazine treatment (CHAPLIN et al. 1989; ADAMS et al. 1989).

9.5 Conclusions

It is clear that hypoxia exists in human tumours and that it can influence the response to therapy in some situations (DISCHE 1989; OVERGAARD 1989).

What is now needed is a reliable, reproducible and non-invasive procedure for accurately identifying which human tumours contain hypoxic cells. None of the currently available techniques fit these criteria, and until one is developed it might be prudent to actually use as many different techniques as possible on each tumour. What is also required is a clinically acceptable method for identifying acute hypoxia in human tumours. The fluorescent staining techniques now used for this purpose in animal models are in fact too toxic for clinical use (CHAPLIN, personal communication).

Although several of the procedures which have been used in patients to combat radiation resistance due to hypoxic cells have met with some success, the results are far from satisfactory. One explanation for this is that most of the procedures used clinically have little or no influence on acute hypoxia. The best approach to the hypoxia problem in human tumours is probably therefore to combine treatments which separately attack chronic and acute hypoxia. Of the treatments which experimentally have been shown to work against acute hypoxia, nicotinamide probably has the greatest clinical potential, since it shows low toxicity in humans (ZACKHEIM et al. 1981), with an oral dose of 6 g being considered acceptable for prolonged administration and perhaps even higher doses possible with shorter treatment times. Recent pharmacokinetic studies have shown that 6 g in humans is equivalent to 100–200 mg/kg in mice, and such doses in mice will enhance radiation damage in tumours (HORSMAN 1992b). But, with which treatment should nicotinamide be combined? Experimentally, the drug has been shown to improve tumour radiosensitization induced by hyperthermia (HORSMAN et al. 1990a), a perfluorochemical emulsion (CHAPLIN et al. 1990a) and normobaric carbogen or oxygen breathing (KJELLEN et al. 1991). In fact, preliminary clinical testing is now being undertaken with nicotinamide in combination with carbogen (DENEKAMP 1991), although whether or not this is the best combination remains to be seen.

Overcoming acute hypoxia in human tumours may actually be more important than eliminating chronic hypoxia. Figure 9.6 shows the results of an experiment in which tumours were made totally hypoxic for up to 6 h at different temperatures. Clamping tumours for 6 h at room temperature has no effect on tumour growth. However, if tumours are heated to 37°C, which is the normal intratumour temperature expected for deep-seated tumours, then tumour growth changes substantially even after

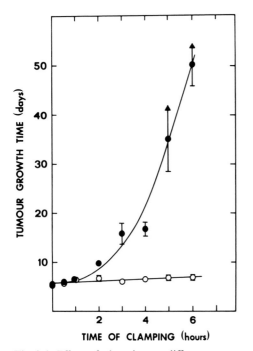

Fig. 9.6. Effect of clamping at different temperatures on tumour growth. C3H/Tif mammary carcinomas grown in the feet of CDF1 mice were clamped for up to 6 h either at room temperature (*open circles*) or when tumours were heated to 37°C (*closed circles*) by immersion of the tumour-bearing foot in a water bath. The time taken for tumours to regrow to five times their treatment volume of 200 mm³ was recorded. Results show means ($\pm$ 1 SE). *Arrows* on errors indicate those groups in which some tumours were controlled, and in such cases the tumour growth time was assigned an arbitrary value of 60 days. (HORSMAN and CHAPLIN, unpublished observations)

being made hypoxic for only 1–2 h, and by 6 h the tumour growth time is so long that some tumours never recover and local control occurs. Of course, what we have here is technically anoxia and not chronic hypoxia; nevertheless, it strongly suggests that the adverse physiological conditions in tumours at normal temperatures make the lifetime of hypoxic cells relatively short and it is possible that the presence of acutely hypoxic cells may be a more important reason for failure to control tumours after radiation treatment.

Increasing hypoxia in tumours prior to treatment is currently under a great deal of investigation, and while this is a novel approach to try and kill tumour cells, it is one that must be carefully controlled because if some of the "new" hypoxic cells survive treatment with the hypoxic cell cytotoxin, they may become a problem. If they remain hypoxic, they could reduce the effect of subsequent conventional therapy used against the aerobic population. They may also be a problem if they reoxygenate, since it

has been shown that prolonged exposure of tumour cells to hypoxia can increase their metastatic potential when they are subsequently incubated in normal aerobic conditions (YOUNG and HILL 1988, 1990).

Finally, now may be a good time to actually change our terminology of hypoxia, since the distinction between chronic and acute hypoxia may not be as clear as it at first seems. If, for example, blood flow through a vessel is stopped and remains so for a long period, the "long-term" acute hypoxia could be identified as chronic. In such situations an agent like nicotinamide, which prevents fluctuations in flow, could appear to affect both acute and chronic hypoxia. This may in fact explain why nicotinamide appears to affect chronic hypoxia in some tumours (HORSMAN et al. 1990b) and not in others (HORSMAN et al. 1990a). Acute and chronic hypoxia are therefore somewhat obsolete phrases and it might be better in the future if we simply referred to hypoxia as diffusion or perfusion limited.

Acknowledgements. This work was supported by a grant from the Danish Cancer Society.

References

Adams GE (1984) Radiosensitizers: a conference preview. Int J Radiat Oncol Biol Phys 10: 1181–1184

Adams GE, Stratford IJ, Godden J, Howells N (1989) Enhancement of the anti-tumor effect of melphalan in experimental mice by some vaso-active agents. Int J Radiat Oncol Biol Phys 16: 1137–1139

Adams GE, Bremner J, Edwards HS, Fielden EM, Naylor M, Stratford IJ, Wood P (1992) Bioreductive drugs—dual function agents and related compounds. In: Dewey WC, Edington M, Fry RJM, Hall EJ, Whitmore GF (eds) Radiation research: a twentieth-century perspective, vol II. Academic, San Diego, p 802

Awwad HK, Nagger M, Mocktar N, Barsoum M (1986) Intercapillary distance measurement as an indicator of hypoxia in carcinoma of the cervix uteri. Int J Radiat Oncol Biol Phys 12: 1329–1333

Beddell CR, Goodford PJ, Kneen G, White RD, Wilkinson S, Wootton R (1984) Substituted benzaldehydes designed to increase the oxygen affinity of human haemoglobin and inhibit the sickling of sickle erythrocytes. Br J Pharmacol 82: 397–407

Bentzen SM, Grau C (1991) Direct estimation of the fraction of hypoxic cells from tumour-control data obtained under aerobic and clamped conditions. Int J Radiat Biol 59: 1435–1440

Bremner JCM, Stratford IJ, Bowler J, Adams GE (1990) Bioreductive drugs and the selective induction of tumour hypoxia. Br J Cancer 61: 717–721

Brown JM (1979) Evidence for acutely hypoxic cells in mouse tumours and a possible mechanism of reoxygenation. Br J Radiol 52: 650–656

Burton MA, Gray BN, Self GW, Heggie JC, Townsend PS (1985) Manipulation of experimental rat and rabbit liver tumor blood flow with angiotensin II. Cancer Res 45: 5390–5393

Chaplin DJ (1986) Potentiation of RSU-1069 tumour cytotoxicity by 5-hydroxytryptamine. Br J Cancer 54: 727–731

Chaplin DJ, Acker B (1987) The effect of hydralazine on the tumor cytotoxicity of the hypoxic cell cytotoxin RSU-1069: evidence of therapeutic gain. Int J Radiat Oncol Biol Phys 13: 579–585

Chaplin DJ, Trotter MJ (1991) Chemical modifiers of tumour blood flow. In: Vaupel P, Jain RK (eds) Tumour blood supply and metabolic microenvironment. Gustav Fischer, Stuttgart, p 65

Chaplin DJ, Durand RE, Olive PL (1986) Acute hypoxia in tumors: implication for modifiers of radiation effects. Int J Radiat Oncol Biol Phys 12: 1279–1282

Chaplin DJ, Olive PL, Durand RE (1987) Intermittent blood flow in a murine tumor: radiobiological effects. Cancer Res 47: 597–601

Chaplin DJ, Acker B, Olive PL (1989) Potentiation of the tumor cytotoxicity of melphalan by vasodilating drugs. Int J Radiat Oncol Biol Phys 16: 1131–1135

Chaplin DJ, Horsman MR, Aoki D (1990a) Nicotinamide, fluosol DA and carbogen: a strategy to reoxygenate acutely and chronically hypoxic cells in vivo. Br J Cancer 63: 109–113

Chaplin DJ, Horsman MR, Trotter MJ (1990b) Effect of nicotinamide on the microregional heterogeneity of oxygen delivery within a murine tumour. J Natl Cancer Inst 82: 672–676

Chapman JD, Raleigh JA, Pedersen JE, Ngan J, Shum FY, Meeker BE, Urtasun RC (1979) Potentially three distinct roles for hypoxic cell sensitizers in the clinic. In: Okada S, Imamura M, Terashima T, Yamaguchi H (eds) Radiation research. Proceedings of the sixth international congress of radiation research. Tokyo, p 885

Coleman CN (1988) Hypoxia in tumours: a paradigm for the approach to biochemical and physiological heterogeneity. J Natl Cancer Inst 80: 310–317

DeCree J, DeCock W, Guckens H, DeClerck F, Beerens M, Verhaegen H (1979) The rheological effects of cinnarizine and flunarizine in normal and pathological conditions. Angiology 30: 505–515

Delides GS, Venizelos J, Révész L (1988) Vascularization and curability of stage III and IV nasopharyngeal tumours. J Cancer Res Clin Oncol 114: 321–323

Denekamp J (1991) ARCON: accelerated radiotherapy with carbogen and nicotinamide. Eur Cancer News 4: 3–5

Dische S (1989) The clinical consequences of the oxygen effect. In: Steel GG, Adams GE, Horwich A (eds) The biological basis of radiotherapy, 2nd edn. Elsevier Science, Amsterdam, p 135

Evelhoch JL, Bissery MC, Chabot GG, Simpson NE, McCoy CL, Heilbrun LK, Corbett TH (1988) Flavone acetic acid (NSC 34512)-induced modulation of murine tumor physiology monitored by in vivo nuclear magnetic resonance spectroscopy. Cancer Res 48: 4749–4755

Evelhoch JL, Simpson NE, Valeriote FA, Corbett TH (1990) 31-P and 2-H MRS studies of flavone acetic acid and analogues. In: Evelhoch JL, Negendank W, Valeriote FA, Baker LH (eds) Magnetic resonance in experimental and clinical oncology. Kluwer Academic, Boston, p 121

Fenton BM, Rofstad EK, Degnar FL, Sutherland RM (1988) Cryospectrophotometric determination of tumour intravascular oxyhemoglobin saturations: dependence on vascular geometry and tumour growth. J Natl Cancer Inst 80: 1612–1619

Folkman J (1976) The vascularization of tumours. Sci Am 234: 58–73

Franko AJ (1986) Misonidazole and other hypoxic markers: metabolism and applications. Int J Radiat Oncol Biol Phys 12: 1195–1202

Gatenby RA, Kessler HB, Rosenblaum JS, Coia LR, Moldofsky PJ, Hartz WH, Broder GJ (1988) Oxygen distribution in squamous cell carcinoma metastases and its relationship to outcome of radiation therapy. Int J Radiat Oncol Biol Phys 14: 831–838

Gerweck LE, Urano M, Koutcher J, Fellenz MP, Kahn J (1989) Relationship between energy status, hypoxic cell fraction, and hyperthermic sensitivity in a murine fibrosarcoma. Radiat Res 117: 448–458

Grau C, Horsman MR, Overgaard J (1992) Influences of carboxyhemoglobin level on tumour growth, blood flow and radiation response in an experimental model. Int J Radiat Oncol Biol Phys 22: 421–424

Guichard M, Courdi A, Malaise EP (1980) Experimental data on the radiobiology of solid tumours. Eur J Radiother 1: 171–191

Hafström L, Nobin A, Persson B, Sundqvist K (1980) Effects of catecholamines on cardiovascular response and blood flow distribution to normal tissue and liver tumours in rats. Cancer Res 40: 481–485

Hall EJ (1988) Radiobiology for the radiologist. Harper and Row, Philadelphia

Henderson BW, Waldow SM, Potter WR, Dougherty TJ (1985) Interaction of photodynamic therapy and hyperthermia: tumor response and cell survival studies after treatment of mice in vivo. Cancer Res 45: 6071–6077

Herman TS, Teicher BA, Coleman CN (1990) Interaction of SR-4233 with hyperthermia and radiation in the FSaIIC murine fibrosarcoma tumour system in vitro and in vivo. Cancer Res 50: 5055–5059

Hiraoka M, Hahn GM (1990) Changes in pH and blood flow induced by glucose, and their effects on hyperthermia with or without BCNU in RIF-1 tumours. Int J Hyperthermia 6: 97–103

Hirst DG, Wood PJ (1989) Chlorophenoxyacetic acid derivatives as hemoglobin modifiers and tumour radiosensitizers. Int J Radiat Oncol Biol Phys 16: 1183–1186

Höckel M, Knoop C, Schlenger K, Vorndran B, Mitz M, Knapstein PG, Vaupel P (1993) Intratumoral pO_2 predicts survival in advanced cancer of the uterine cervix. Radiother Oncol (to be publ.)

Horsman MR (1992) Modifiers of tumor blood supply. In: Urano M, Double EB (eds) Hyperthermia and oncology. VSP, Netherlands

Horsman MR (1992b) Carbogen and nicotinamide: expectations too high? Radiother Oncol 24: 121–122

Horsman MR (1992c) Overcoming tumour radiation resistance resulting from acute hypoxia. Eur J Cancer 28A: 717–718

Horsman MR, Winther J (1989) Vascular effects of photodynamic therapy in an intraocular retinoblastoma-like tumour. Acta Oncol 28: 693–697

Horsman MR, Brown JM, Hirst VK, Lemmon MJ, Wood PJ, Dunphy EP, Overgaard J (1988a) Mechanism of action of the selective tumor radiosensitizer nicotinamide. Int J Radiat Oncol Biol Phys 15: 685–690

Horsman MR, Overgaard J, Chaplin DJ (1988b) The interaction between RSU-1069, Hydralazine and hyperthermia in a C3H mammary carcinoma as assessed by tumour growth delay. Acta Oncol 27: 861–862

Horsman MR, Chaplin DJ, Brown JM (1989a) Tumor radiosensitization by nicotinamide: a result of improved blood perfusion and oxygenation. Radiat Res 118: 139–150

Horsman MR, Christensen KL, Overgaard J (1989b) Hydralazine-induced enhancement of hyperthermic damage in a C3H mammary carcinoma in vivo. Int J Hyperthermia 5: 123–136

Horsman MR, Hansen PV, Overgaard J (1989c) Radiosensitization by nicotinamide in tumors and normal tissues: the importance of tissue oxygenation status. Int J Radiat Oncol Biol Phys 16: 1273–1276

Horsman MR, Chaplin DJ, Overgaard J (1990a) Combination of nicotinamide and hyperthermia to eliminate radioresistant chronically and acutely hypoxic tumor cells. Cancer Res 50: 7430–7436

Horsman MR, Wood PJ, Chaplin DJ, Brown JM, Overgaard J (1990b) The potentiation of radiation damage by nicotinamide in the SCCVII tumour in vivo. Radiother Oncol 18: 49–57

Horsman MR, Chaplin DJ, Overgaard J (1991) The effect of combining flavone acetic acid and hyperthermia on the growth of a C3H mammary carcinoma in vivo. Int J Radiat Biol 60: 385–388

Horsman MR, Kristjansen PEG, Mizuno M, Christensen K, Chaplin DJ, Quistorff B, Overgaard J (1992) Biochemical and physiological changes induced by nicotinamide in a C3H mouse mammary carcinoma and CDF1 mice. Int J Radiat Oncol Biol Phys 22: 451–454

Intaglietta M, Myers RR, Gross JF, Reinhold HS (1977) Dynamics of microvascular flow in implanted mouse mammary tumours. Bibl Anat 15: 237–276

Jain RK (1988) Determinants of tumor blood flow: a review. Cancer Res 48: 2641–2658

Jirtle RL (1988) Chemical modification of tumour blood flow. Int J Hyperthermia 4: 355–371

Jirtle R, Clifton KH, Rankin JHG (1978) Effects of several vasoactive drugs on the vascular resistance of MT-W9B tumors in W/Fu rats. Cancer Res 38: 2385–2390

Kaelin WG, Shrivastava S, Shand DG, Jirtle RL (1982) Effect of verapamil on malignant tissue blood flow in SMT-2A tumor-bearing rats. Cancer Res 42: 3944–3949

Kallinowski F, Moehle R, Vaupel P (1989a) Substantial enhancement of tumor hyperthermic response by tumor necrosis factor. In: Sugahara T, Saito M (eds) Hyperthermic oncology, vol 1. Summary papers. Taylor & Francis, London, p 258

Kallinowski F, Schaefer C, Tyler G, Vaupel P (1989b) In vivo targets of recombinant human tumour necrosis factor—alpha: blood flow, oxygen consumption and growth of isotransplanted rat tumours. Br J Cancer 60: 555–560

Kallinowski F, Zander R, Höckel M, Vaupel P (1990) Tumor tissue oxygenation as evaluated by computerised—pO2—histography. Int J Radiat Oncol Biol Phys 19: 953–961

Kallman RF, Denardo GL, Stasch MJ (1972) Blood flow in irradiated mouse sarcoma as determined by the clearance of xenon–133. Cancer Res 32: 483–490

Kalmus J, Okunieff P, Vaupel P (1990) Dose-dependent effects of hydralazine on microcirculatory function and hyperthermic response of murine FSaII tumors. Cancer Res 50: 15–19

Kjellen E, Joiner MC, Collier JM, Johns H, Rojas A (1991) A therapeutic benefit from combining normobaric carbogen or oxygen with nicotinamide in fractionated x-ray treatments. Radiother Oncol 22; 81–91

Knapp WH, Debatin J, Layer K, Helus F, Altmann A, Sinn HJ, Ostertag H (1985) Selective drug-induced reduction of blood flow in tumour transplants. Int J Radiat Oncol Biol Phys 11: 1357–1366

Kolstad P (1968) Intercapillary distance, oxygen tension and local recurrence in cervix cancer. Scand J Clin Lab Invest 106: 145–157

Koutcher JA, Barnett D, Kornblith AB, Cowburn D, Brady TJ, Gerweck LE (1990) Relationship of changes in pH and energy status to hypoxic cell fraction and hyperthermia sensitivity. Int J Radiat Oncol Biol Phys 18: 1429–1435

Kristjansen PEG, Pederson EJ, Quistorff B, Elling F, Spang-Thomsen M (1990) Early effects of radiotherapy in small cell lung cancer xenografts monitored by 31-P-magnetic resonance spectroscopy and biochemical analysis. Cancer Res 50: 4880–4884

Lauk S, Skates S, Goodman M, Suit HD (1989) Morphometric study of the vascularity of oral squamous cell carcinomas and its relation to outcome of radiation therapy. Eur J Cancer Clin Oncol 25: 1431–1440

Mattson J, Appelgren L, Karlsson L, Peterson HI (1978) Influence of vasoactive drugs and ischaemia on intratumour blood flow distribution. Eur J Cancer 14: 761–764

McEwan AJB 91989) Positron-emission tomography and predicting tumor treatment response. In: Chapman JD, Peters LJ, Withers HR (eds) Prediction of tumor treatment response. Pergamon, New York, p 277

McNally NJ, Sheldon PW (1977) The effect of radiation on tumour growth delay, cell survival, and cure of the animal using a single tumour system. Br J Radiol 50: 321–328

Menke H, Vaupel P (1988) Effect of injectable or inhalational anaesthetics and of neuroleptic, neuroleptanalgesic, and sedative agents on tumour blood flow. Radiat Res 114: 64–76

Moulder JE, Martin DF (1984) Hypoxic fraction determinations in the BA1112 rat sarcoma: variations within and among assay techniques. Radiat Res 98: 536–548

Moulder JE, Rockwell S (1984) Hypoxic fractions of solid tumors. Int J Radiat Oncol Biol Phys 10: 695–712

Müller-Klieser W, Kröger M, Wallenta S, Rofstad EK (1991) Comparative imaging of structure and metabolites in tumours. Int J Radiat Biol 60: 147–159

Okunieff P (1990) Relationship of 31-P NMR measurements to tumor biology. In: Evelhoch JL, Negendank W, Valeriote FA, Baker LH (eds) Magnetic resonance in experimental and clinical oncology. Kluwer Academic, Boston, p 23

Overgaard J (1980) Effect of misonidazole and hyperthermia on the radiosensitivity of a C3H mammary carcinoma and its surrounding normal tissue. Br J Cancer 41: 10–21

Overgaard J (1989) Sensitization of hypoxic tumour cells—clinical experience. Int J Radiat Biol 56: 801–811

Overgaard J (1993) Modification of tumour hypoxia. A meta-analysis of controlled clinical trials. Br J Radiol (to be publ.)

Overgaard J, Nielsen OS (1980) The role of tissue environmental factors on the kinetics and morphology of tumor cells exposed to hyperthermia. Ann NY Acad Sci 335: 254–280

Overgaard J, Nielsen OS, Lindegaard JC (1987) Biological basis for rational design of clinical treatment with combined hyperthermia and radiation. In: Field SB, Franconi C (eds) Physics and technology of hyperthermia. Martinus Nijhoff, Amsterdam, p 54

Rasey JS, Evans ML (1991) Detecting hypoxia in human tumors. In: Vaupel P, Jain RK (eds) Tumor blood supply and metabolic microenvironment. Gustav Fischer, Stuttgart, p 187

Rasey JS, Koh W-J, Grierson JR, Grunbaum Z, Krohn KA (1989) Radiolabelled fluoromisonidazole as an imaging agent for tumor hypoxia. Int J Radiat Oncol Biol Phys 17: 985–991

Reinhold HS, Blackiewicz B, Block A (1977) Oxygenation and reoxygenation in "sandwich" tumours. Bibl Anat 15: 270–272

Révész L, Siracka E, Siracky J, Delides G, Pavlaki K (1989) Variation of vascular density within and between tumors of the uterine cervix and its predictive value for radiotherapy. Int J Radiat Oncol Biol Phys 16: 1161–1163

Rockwell S (1985) Use of a perfluorochemical emulsion to improve oxygenation in a solid tumour. Int J Radiat Oncol Biol Phys 11: 97–103

Rockwell S, Kelley M, Irvin CG, Hughes CS, Porter E, Yabuki H, Fisher JJ (1991) Modulation of tumor oxygenation and radiosensitivity by a perfluorooctylbromide emulsion. Radiother Oncol 22: 92–98

Rofstad EK, DeMuth P, Fenton BM, Ceckler TL, Sutherland· RM (1989) 32-P NMR spectroscopy and HbO_2 cryospectrophotometry in prediction of tumor radioresistance caused by hypoxia. Int J Radiat Oncol Biol Phys 16: 919–923

Rojas A (1991) Radiosensitization with normobaric oxygen and carbogen. Radiother Oncol [Suppl] 20: 65–70

Sevick EM, Jain RK (1989) Geometric resistance to blood flow in solid tumors perfused ex vivo: effects of tumor size and perfusion pressure. Cancer Res 49: 3506–3512

Shrivastava S, Joines WT, Jirtle RL (1985) Effect of 5-hydroxytryptamine on tissue blood flow and microwave heating of rat tumors. Cancer Res 45: 3203–3208

Siemann DW (1990) Tumour size: a factor influencing the isoeffect analysis of tumour response to combined modalities. Br J Cancer 41 [Suppl IV] : 294–298

Siemann DW, Alliet KL, Macler LM (1989) Manipulations in the oxygen transport capacity of blood as a means of sensitizing tumors to radiation therapy. Int J Radiat Oncol Biol Phys 16: 1169–1172

Song CW (1984) Effect of local hyperthermia on blood flow and microenvironment: a review. Cancer Res 44 [Suppl]: 4721s–4730s

Star WM, Marijnissen HPA, van den Berg-Blok AE, Versteeg JAC, Franken KAP, Reinhold HS (1986) Destruction of rat mammary tumor and normal tissue microcirculation by hematoporphyrin derivative photoradiation observed in vivo in sandwich observation chambers. Cancer Res 46: 2532–2540

Streffer C, van Beuningen D, Gross E, Eigler FW, Pelzer T (1989) Determination of DNA, micronuclei and vascular density in human rectum carcinomas. In: Chapman JD, Peters LJ, Withers HR (eds) Prediction of tumour treatment response. Pergamon, London, p 217

Streffer C, Zölzer F, Tamulevicius P (1992) Studies on combined treatment with X-rays, hyperthermia and hypoxic cell sensitizers on tumors. In: Dewey WC, Edington M, Fry RJM, Hall EJ, Whitmore GF (eds) Radiation research: a twentieth-century perspective, vol II. Academic, San Diego, p 1021

Suit HD, Marshall N, Woerner D (1972) Oxygen, oxygen plus carbon dioxide, and radiation therapy of a mouse mammary carcinoma. Cancer 30: 1154–1158

Sun JR, Brown JM (1989) Enhancement of the antitumor effect of flavone acetic acid by the bioreductive cytotoxic drug SR 4233 in a murine carcinoma. Cancer Res 49: 5664–5670

Sutherland RM, Franko AJ (1980) On the nature of the radiobiologically hypoxic fraction in tumors. Int J Radiat Oncol Biol Phys 6: 117–120

Suzuki M, Hori K, Abe I, Saito S, Sato H (1981) A new approach to cancer chemotherapy: selective enhancement of tumor blood flow with angiotensin II. J Natl Cancer Inst 67: 663–669

Tamulevicius P, Luscher G, Streffer C (1987) Effects on intermediary metabolism in mouse tissues by Ro-03-8799. Br J Cancer 56: 315–320

Thomlinson RH, Gray LH (1955) The histological structure of some human lung cancers and the possible implications for radiotherapy. Br J Cancer 9: 539–549

Timothy AR, Overgaard J (1984) In vivo radiosensitization by nimorazole and hyperthermia. In: Overgaard J (ed) Hyperthermic oncology, vol 1. Summary Papers. Taylor & Francis, London, p 309

Trotter MJ, Chaplin DJ, Olive PL (1991a) Possible mechanisms for intermittent blood flow in the murine SCCVII carcinoma. Int J Radiat Biol 60: 139–146

Trotter MJ, Chaplin DJ, Olive PL (1991b) Effect of angiotensin II on intermittent tumour blood flow and acute hypoxia in the murine SCCVII carcinoma. Eur J Cancer 27: 887–893

Urano M, Cunningham M, Rice L (1980) Effect of general anaesthetics on the thermal response of normal and malignant murine tissues. Int J Radiat Biol 38: 667–671

Urano M, Montoya V, Booth A (1983) Effect of hyperglycemia on the thermal response of murine normal and tumor tissue. Cancer Res 43: 453–455

Urtasun RC (1992) Tumor hypoxia, its clinical detection and relevance. In: Dewey WC, Edington M, Fry RJM, Hall EJ, Whitmore GF (eds) Radiation research: a twentieth-century perspective, vol II. Academic, San Diego, p 725

Van Putten LM, Kallman RF (1968) Oxygenation status of a transplantable tumour during fractionated radiation therapy. J Natl Cancer Inst 40: 441–451

Vaupel P (1979) Oxygen supply to malignant tumors. In: Peterson HI (ed) Tumor blood circulation: angiogenesis, vascular morphology and blood flow of experimental and human tumors. CRC Press, Boca Raton, Fl., p 143

Vaupel P, Müller-Klieser W (1992) Oxygenation and bioenergetic status of human tumors. In: Dewey WC, Edington M, Fry RJM, Hall EJ, Whitmore GF (eds) Radiation research: a twentieth-century perspective, vol II. Academic, San Diego, p 772

Vaupel P, Grunewald WA, Manz R, Sowa W (1978) Intracapillary HbO_2 saturation in tumor tissue of DS-carcinosarcoma during normoxia. Adv Exp Med Biol 94: 367–375

Vaupel P, Manz R, Müller-Klieser W, Grunewald WA (1979) Intracapillary HbO_2 saturation in malignant tumors during normoxia and hyperoxia. Microvasc Res 17: 181–191

Vaupel P, Fortmeyer HP, Runkel S, Kallinowski F (1987) Blood flow, oxygen consumption and tissue oxygenation of human breast cancer xenografts in nude mice. Cancer Res 47: 3496–3503

Vaupel P, Kallinowski F, Okunieff P (1989a) Blood flow, oxygen and nutrient supply, and metabolic microenvironment of human tumors: a review. Cancer Res 49: 6449–6465

Vaupel P, Okunieff P, Kallinowski F, Neuringer LJ (1989b) Correlations between ^{31}P-NMR spectroscopy and tissue O_2 tension measurements in a murine fibrosarcoma. Radiat Res 120: 477–493

Vaupel P, Schlenger K, Höckel M (1991) Blood flow and oxygenation of human tumors. In: Vaupel P, Jain RK (eds) Tumor blood supply and metabolic microenvironment. Gustav Fischer, Stuttgart, p 165

Waldow SM, Dougherty TJ (1984) Interaction of hyperthermia and photoradiation therapy. Radiat Res 97: 380–385

Warren BA (1979) The vascular morphology of tumors. In: Peterson H-I (ed) Tumor blood circulation: angiogenesis, vascular morphology and blood flow of experimental tumors. CRC Press, Boca Raton, Fl., p 1

Wiig H, Gadeholt G (1985) Interstitial fluid pressure and hemodynamics in a sarcoma implanted in the rat tail. Microvasc Res 29: 176–189

Wike-Hooley JL, Haveman J, Reinhold HS (1984) The relevance of tumor pH to the treatment of malignant disease. Radiother Oncol 2: 343–366

Wood PJ, Hirst DG (1989) Calcium antagonists as radiation modifiers: site specificity in relation to tumor response. Int J Radiat Oncol Biol Phys 16: 1141–1144

Wood PJ, Counsell CJR, Bremner JCM, Horsman MR, Adams GE (1991) The measurement of radiosensitizer-induced changes in mouse tumour metabolism by 31-P magnetic resonance spectroscopy. Int J Radiat Oncol Biol Phys 20: 291–294

Young SD, Hill RP (1988) Hypoxia induces DNA over-replication and enhances metastatic potential of murine tumour cells. Proc Natl Acad Sci USA 85: 9533–9537

Young SD, Hill RP (1990) Effects of reoxygenation on cells from hypoxic regions of solid tumours: anticancer drug sensitivity and metastatic potential. J Natl Cancer Inst 82: 371–380

Zackheim HS, Vasily DB, Westphal ML, Hastings CW (1981) Reactions to niacinamide. J Am Acad Dermatol 4: 736–737

Zanelli GD, Lucas PB, Fowler JF (1975) The effect of anaesthetics on blood perfusion I. Br J Cancer 32: 380–390

10 The Impact of Local Tumor Control on the Outcome in Human Cancer

S.A. LEIBEL and Z. FUKS

CONTENTS

10.1 Introduction

The impact of local tumor control on the outcome in human cancer has been an issue of debate in the recent literature. Obviously, this question is primarily relevant in patients receiving treatment for tumors still confined to their original local or local-regional sites. While it is obvious that eradication of the primary tumor is essential for the achievement of cure, several investigators have argued that the presence of incurable micrometastases from spread before initial diagnosis is the most important determinant of the ultimate fate in early-stage patients (DeVITA et al. 1986; SUIT 1982). Concerns have, therefore, been raised that efforts to improve local control will be offset by the eventual development of metastatic disease and will thus represent a futile endeavor in many types of tumors. However, while relapse due to early micrometastatic dissemination is a relevant pattern of failure in a fraction of.locally controlled patients, recent retrospective studies have demonstrated that local recurrence at the primary tumor site is associated with a significant increase in metastatic disease in nearly every

S.A. LEIBEL, MD, Department of Radiation Oncology, Memorial Sloan-Kettering Cancer Center, New York, NY 10021, USA
Z. FUKS, MD, Department of Radiation Oncology, Memorial Sloan-Kettering Cancer Center, New York, NY 10021, USA

type of tumor tested (FUKS et al. 1991a; LEIBEL et al. 1991b). Some investigators have interpreted these data as indicating that local failure represents a "marker" for tumors with a high propensity for metastatic dissemination, and therefore, improvements in local control are unlikely to affect the outcome in a major way (FISHER et al. 1991; WALSH 1987). On the other hand, recent studies on the temporal relationship between local recurrence and the first detection of metastatic disease in the same patients are most consistent with the hypothesis that distant metastases in such patients are derived from residual tumor clonogens which acquire a metastatic potential after the failure to eradicate the primary tumor (FUKS et al. 1991a; LEIBEL et al. 1991b). These observations indicate a possible causative relationship between local relapse and metastatic spread and highlight the relative importance of local control as a biological determinant that impacts on the metastatic outcome and the likelihood of survival. This review discusses some of these issues in the context of the need to develop new therapeutic methods for improving local control in human tumors.

10.2 The Curative Potential of Localized Modes of Cancer Therapy

While chemotherapy has occasionally been used to eradicate localized tumors, especially in the case of malignant lymphomas, surgey and/or radiation therapy have been the mainstays of localized treatment aimed at attaining a local cure in the great majority of human tumors. Data from the National Cancer Institute Surveillance, Epidemiology, and End Results (SEER) program (U.S. Department of Health and Human Services 1988) and the National Cancer Data Base (NCDB) (MENICK et al. 1991) indicate that approximately 65% of invasive cancer patients initially present with tumors still confined to their original local or local-regional sites and without clinical evidence of distant spread. Only two-thirds of such patients attain a permanent local control with the current modes of radiation and/or surgey (MYERS and RIES 1989). An accurate assessment of the patterns of failure in those who relapse are not available, but published estimates suggest that approximately one-third of the patients fail at the primary tumor sites alone, one-third recur at primary sites with concurrent or subsequent failures at distant sites, and one-third relapse at distant metastatic sites only (DEVITA 1983; SUIT 1982; PEREZ and BRADY 1992). Obviously, patients who recur at local sites alone are those who would be the primary candidates for gains from improved local tumor control. However, some of the patients who relapse at both local and distant sites may also benfit from treatments that improve local control since, as discussed later in this review, clinical and experimental studies suggest that metastatic disease in patients who fail local-regional therapy frequently occurs significantly later than the local recurrence and probably second-ary to the regrowth process of the residual primary tumor (FUKS et al. 1991a; LEIBEL et al. 1991b). Based on these considerations, it is estimated that if local relapses were to be completely eliminated, an incre-ment of up to one-third of the cancer patients who currently succumb to metastatic disease could perhaps be rescued by the prevention of metastatic dissemination due to the spread of clonogenic tumor cells with freshly acquired metastatic poten-tial, arising from locally relapsing tumors.

10.3 Causes of Local Failure in Clinical Radiation Therapy

Analysis of the causes of local failure in radiation therapy requires consideration of multiple biological and treatment-related factors. There is good evi-dence that the radiosensitivity of human tumors varies from one tumor type of another (FERTIL and MALAISE 1981, 1985; DEACON et al. 1984; WEICHSELBAUM et al. 1989). This heterogeneity is a function of inherent factors, such as the tumor cell radiosensitivity, the size of the clonogenic stem cell pool, tumor cell kinetics during the course of radiation therapy, and the prevalence of various microenvironmental factors. These factors determine the potential and proficiency of radiation damage repair, which have been shown to correlate with the relative response of tumors to ionizing irradiation (MCMILLAN 1992). Unfortunately, at the present time it is not possible to effectively modu-late these parameters and, hence, affect the local outcome in clinical radiation therapy. However, because of the random nature in which lethal radiation lesions are produced, the inactivation of tumor clonogens by ionizing irradiation is dose dependent, mathematically described as an expo-nential function (ALPER 1980). Hence, dose-related factors, including the size of the dose per fraction, the overall treatment duration, and the total dose, as well as the homogeneity of the dose distribution within the tumor (in particular the presence of geo-graphical volumes of tumor underdosage), strongly affect the therapeutic outcome. If optimized, these treatment-related factors may serve to partially or completely overcome the relative radiation resis-tance in some types of human tumors.

In animal experiments, where all variables can be carefully controlled, there is a distinctive rela-tionship between dose and tumor control that is best described by Poisson distributions (MUNRO and GILBERT 1961; HENDRY and MOORE 1984). Accordingly, at low radiation dose levels, tumor control probabilities are small, but at higher doses there is a sigmoid shape to the curve relating tumor control to dose, with a steep increase in control from 10% to 90% over a relatively narrow dose range until a plateau is reached (PORTER 1980). A similar dose-response pattern has been observed for radiation-induced damage in normal tissues. Dose-response studies in human tumors have been rare, but available clinical data confirm the sigmoidal nature of dose-tumor control curves (FISHER and MOULDER 1975; THAMES et al. 1980; METZ et al. 1982; PETERS and FLETCHER 1983; ZAGARS et al. 1987). The steepness of published curves varies sig-nificantly between reported series, suggesting the existence of significant variations in the sensitivity of the clonogenic cell populations within human tumors, but treatment-related inaccuracies have also contributed to the flattening of dose-response curves in human tumors (DUTREIX et al. 1988; PETERS et al. 1981). In early-stage tumors where the accuracy of target coverage is more certain, dose-response curves have been relatively steep. For example, FOWLER (1986) reported on dose-response relationships in T1–2 head and neck tumors and found that in the steep segments of the curves a 10% increase in dose led to an 8%–20% increase (full range 5%–50%) in local control. On the other hand, THAMES et al. (1980) showed that in T3 and T4 pharyngeal wall tumors, in which the technical aspects of treatment are more challenging, a 30% dose increment was required to increase local control from 37% to 50% (i.e., a 13% increase). Because the curves flattened at the 50% control level, a further increase in local control could not be achieved without exceeding unacceptably toxic dose levels. Similarly, METZ et al. (1982) found a steep dose-response curve for T1–T2 nasopharyngeal lesions, but a flatter dose-response relationship in T3 and T4 lesions.

While the number of patient series which have analyzed dose-response relationships are too small to provide detailed definitions of tumor control probabilities and curve steepness, existing data suggest that the range of doses necessary to increase tumor control by about 1% varies from 10 cGy to 60 cGy (TAYLOR and WITHERS 1992; THAMES et al. 1992). The slope of the dose-response curve is defined by the γ factor, which describes the percentage increase in tumor control for a 1% increase in dose (BRAHME 1984). Representative clinical series suggest that the median value for γ is approximately 1.8 (TAYLOR and WITHERS 1992; THAMES et al. 1992) while the γ factor for normal tissue complications has been estimated at 4 (THAMES et al. 1992), demonstrating the overall relative flatness of tumor response curves. If treatment-related factors (e.g., increasing the accuracy of dose distribution and eliminating geographical underdosage) were optimized, the change in tumor control probability with dose would be steeper than suggests by the retrospective studies. Under such circumstances the effect of dose escalation on the probability of local control will be maximized.

The application of new methods for accurate radiation treatment planning and delivery, together with improved staging and better assessment of tumor characteristics (e.g., DNA ploidy, proliferative profiles, and radiosensitivity), are expected to improve tumor control probabilities even without the use of dose escalation. Recent comparative studies of CT-assisted two-dimensional treatment planning and the new techniques of three-dimensional (3D) treatment planning, capable of providing complete anatomical and dose information for the entire tumor volume and its surrounding normal tissue (Photon Treatment Planning Collaborative Working Group 1991), have in fact documented significant improvements in target coverage and dose homogeneity with 3D techniques (TEN HAKEN et al. 1989; LEIBEL et al. 1991a). An open question remains as to the need for dose escalation to overcome the inherent radiation resistance of tumor stem cells. Clinical studies currently underway have been designed to test the effect of dose on the probability of local tumor control using the high-precision techniques of 3D conformal photon beam radiation therapy (LEIBEL et al. 1992). These techniques not only are capable of avoiding underdosed regions within the tumor and outright marginal misses, but also enable tumor dose escalation due to meticulous removal of normal tissues from the volume receiving high radiation doses. The feasibility of dose escalation has been demonstrated in several types of human tumors, but its effect on the outcome still needs to be established (LEIBEL et al. 1992). Indeed, there have been concerns that in many human tumors a significant escalation of dose will be necessary before an effect on local control can be detected (THAMES et al. 1992).

10.4 Local Control and Metastatic Dissemination in Experimental Tumors

Several experimental studies in animal models have demonstrated that failure to control the primary tumor leads to increased rates of distant metastases (Table 10.1). Early experiments by KAPLAN and MURPHY (1949) and by VON ESSEN and KAPLAN (1952) demonstrated that subcurative irradiation of a transplanted mammary carcinoma in C57BL mice

Table 10.1. Impact of local control on the incidence of distant metastates in experimental animal studies

Investigators	Mice	Tumor	Treatment	% Lung metastases	
				LC	LF
SHELDON et al. 1974	C_3H/He	Mammary	Radiation	8.0	35
TODOROKI and SUIT 1985	C_3Hf/Sed	FSaII	None	–	35
			Surgery	6.5	26
			Radiation	8.5	56
			Surgery + radiation	7.2	45
RAMSAY et al. 1988	C_3Hf/Sed	SCVII	Radiation	6.9	43
		FSaII	Radiation	3.1	12.5

LC, local control; LF, local failure

resulted not only in local recurrences but also in an increased incidence of pulmonary metastases when compared to unirradiated controls. Subsequently, SHELDON et al. (1974) showed that the incidence of distant metastases after locally curative irradiation was reduced compared to animals in which a local cure was not achieved. Using first-generation transplants of a spontaneous mammary carcinoma in C3H/He mice, they found that the incidence of lung metastases increased from 8% when mice were locally cured by high-dose radiation therapy to 35% in animals with local failure after irradiation. While the rate of metastasis was found to be identical after local cure with either surgery or irradiation, the ultimate incidence of distant metastases was dependent on the size of the tumor at the time of definitive therapy (SHELDON et al. 1974; TODOROKI and SUIT 1985; RAMSAY et al. 1988).

RAMSAY et al. (1988) reported data which demonstrated an association between local relapse and an increase in distant metastases. C3Hf/Sed mice were transplanted with early-generation transplantable tumors into their limbs. When the transplanted tumor reached a diameter of 6 mm, the tumor-bearing limb was either amputated or treated with a TCD_{50} dose of radiation. Animals that suffered local recurrence after irradiation underwent a salvage amputation when the recurrent tumor regained the size of 6 mm. Table 10.1 shows that mice transplanted with SCVII squamous cell carcinoma exhibited a six fold increase in the incidence of metastases (43%) when local relapse occurred, as compared to animals with successful initial local treatment (6.9%). A four fold increase is distant metastases was also observed in a transplanted FSaII spontaneous fibrosarcoma in the same experimental system. A similar phenomenon was observed in experiments published by PETERS (1975), who irradiated transplanted squamous cell carcinoma in WHT/Ht mice with doses of approximately the TCD_{50}. Both the incidence and the probability of death from lung metastases were found to significantly correlate with the probability of local control at the primary site. Furthermore, the slope of the survival curves published in this study for mice which had a local relapse was significantly steeper than that observed when permanent local control was achieved, suggesting that local failure was associated in this system not only with an increased incidence, but also with accelerated dissemination of metastatic clonogens.

10.5 Local Control and Metastatic Dissemination in Human Tumors

Until recently there have been few reports which specifically focused on the impact of local control on the incidence of distant metastases in human tumors. However, retrospective studies of patterns of failure in patients undergoing curative local-regional therapy indicate that human tumors conform in general with the patterns of relapse observed in animal models, exhibiting increased metastatic dissemination after failure to control the primary tumor (Table 10.2).

To analyze the effect of local control on metastatic dissemination, human cancers can be divided into three categories. The first, exemplified by carcinomas of the prostate and breast, includes tumors in which survival is determined by the development of metastatic disease, whereas local tumor progression only rarely impacts on the outcome. The second group includes tumors arising in sites such as the head and neck, in which local failure is frequently the direct cause of the patient's death, while metastatic disease becomes a factor that impacts on the outcome mostly in locally controlled patients. Finally, there are those tumors, including non-small cell lung carcinoma, in which both local failure and distant metastases affect the survival outcomes.

The first category is the most relevant model for examining the impact of local control on the metastatic outcome, as locally failing patients survive long enough to permit evaluation of a possible association with metastatic disease. An analysis of 679 patients with surgically staged B-CN0 prostatic carcinoma treated at the Memorial Sloan-Kettering Cancer Center with interstitial iodine-125 (^{125}I) source implants showed that the actuarial 15-year distant metastasis-free survival rate in 351 locally controlled patients was 77%, compared to 24% in 328 patients who relapsed locally ($P < 0.00001$) (Fig. 10.1) (FUKS et al. 1991b). Thus, in addition to metastases arising from micrometastatic spread before initial treatment (observed in locally controlled patients), there was a two fold increment in metastatic disease which was associated with the failure to control the primary tumor within the prostate. To test the biological significance of this association, a Cox proportional regression analysis of factors affecting the probability of distant metastasis-free survival was performed. Local control was found to be the most significant factor affecting the metastatic outcome. The relative risk of meta-

Table 10.2. Impact of local control on the incidence of distant metastates in human tumors

Investigators	Site	Stage	No. of Patients	% Distant metastases	
				LC	LF
CHAUVET et al. 1990	Breast	pT1/pN0	202	9	20
PEREZ et al. 1987	Lung	T1-3/N0-2	365	46	58
CHUNG et al. 1982	Lung	T1-2/N0-2	118	45	50
		N0	51	24	90
		N1-2	67	52	59
MALISSARD et al. 1991	Lung	T1-3/N0-2	186	42	42
		N0	57	17	67
		N1-2	129	54	47
MERINO et al. 1977	Head and neck	I-IV	5019	8	17
LEIBEL et al. 1991c	Head and neck	I-IV	2860	17	40
LEE et al. 1989	Nasopharynx	I	196	3	20
FUKS et al. 1991b	Prostate	B-C/N0	679	24	77
PEREZ et al. 1986b	Prostate	B-C	317	22	58
KUBAN et al. 1989	Prostate	A2-C	414	19	68
ZAGARS et al. 1991	Prostate	A2-C	601	40	70
PAUNIER et al. 1967	Cervix	I-IV	1705	6	30
ANDERSON and DISCHE 1981	Cervix	IIB-IV	122	30	90
PEREZ et al. 1988b	Cervix	I-IV	1054	18	66
STOKES et al. 1986	Endometrium	I	304	4	50
PEREZ et al. 1988a	Vagina	I-IV	149	20	54
SCHILD et al. 1989	Rectum	B2-C3	139	28	90
VIGLIOTTI et al. 1987	Rectosigmoid	B1-C3	103	32	93
MARKHEDE et al. 1982	Soft tissue sarcoma	All	97	41	71
SUIT et al. 1988	Soft tissue sarcoma	All	204	25	61
GUSTAFSON et al. 1991	Soft tissue sarcoma	All	375	25	56

LC, local control; LF, local failure

static disease subsequent to local relapse was four times greater than the risk without evidence of local failure. Since local control is a potentially transient state, it was necessary to use a period analysis to determine accurately the annual and cumulative risks of distant metastases. The difference in metastatic disease was highly significant, with an $11\% \pm 0.8\%$ annual mean incidence during the 3- to 10-year interval for locally relapsing patients as compared to $1.7\% \pm 0.3\%$ per year for those in local control. The relationship between local failure and the development of metastatic disease was uniformly observed across the spectrum of biological variants, from the less aggressive B1N0–grade 1 lesions to the highly malignant stage B3-C and grade 3 tumors. The median local relapse-free survival for patients with local recurrences who did not receive hormonal therapy before distant metastases were detected was 51 months, compared to a median of 71 months for distant metastasis-free survival in the same patients

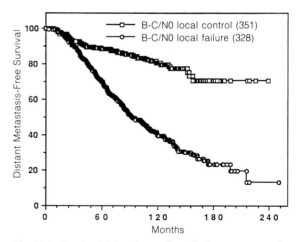

Fig. 10.1. Kaplan-Meier time adjusted distant metastasis-free survival by the local tumor status in 619 patients with stage B-CN0 carcinoma of the prostate treated with ^{125}I implantation. The actuarial distant metastasis-free survival for locally controlled patients was significantly improved compared to those who developed a local recurrence ($P < 0.00001$)

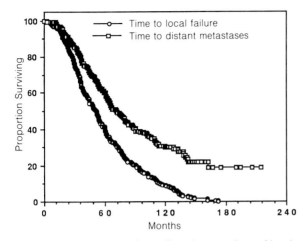

Fig. 10.2. Kaplan-Meier time-adjusted comparison of local relapse-free survival and distant metastasis-free survival in 268 patients with state B-CN0 carcinoma of the prostate who developed local failures after ^{125}I implantation. Because hormonal therapy may delay the detection of distant metastases, only those patients who did not not receive hormonal therapy before distant metastases were detected are included in this analysis. In this cohort of patients the time to detection of the local prostatic tumor recurrence significantly preceded the time to detection of metastatic disease ($P < 0.001$)

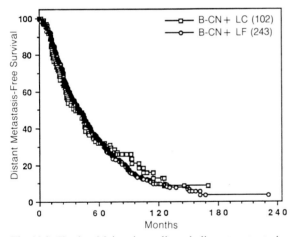

Fig. 10.3. Kaplan-Meier time-adjusted distant metastasis-free survival by the local tumor status in 345 patients with carcinoma of the prostate involving the pelvic lymph nodes treated with ^{125}I implantation. Control of the primary tumor had no impact on the subsequent development of distant metastases in this subgruoup of patients ($P = 0.22$)

($P < 0.001$) (Fig. 10.2), supporting the hypothesis that in patients with local residual tumors metastases are formed and disseminated secondary to regrowth of the occult local residuum (Fuks et al. 1991b).

In contrast to patients without pelvic lymph node metastases, a Cox proportional hazard analysis of 345 patients with pelvic lymph node involvement

showed that control of the primary tumor had no impact on the development of distant metastases (Fig.10.3). The most important covariate affecting distant metastasis-free survival in this group of patients was the number of tumor-containing pelvic lymph nodes, followed by tumor grade and stage, indicating that nodal involvement is an important marker of disseminated disease in prostate carcinoma (LEIBEL et al. 1993).

Increased metastases in patients with locally recurring prostatic carcinoma has also been reported by others, although no other study has separated patients according to pelvic lymph node status. KUBAN et al. (1989) showed that 68% of patients treated with either ^{125}I implantation or external beam irradiation who developed local recurrence ultimately developed distant metastases, whereas only 19% of those who had no evidence of local relapse developed distant metastatic dissemination ($P < 0.001$). When the primary tumor was controlled, the metastatic rate increased with lesser degrees of tumor differentiation and higher stage, suggesting that disease dissemination had preceded therapy in high-grade and advanced-stage tumors. However, when local failure occurred, the incidence of metastases was consistently high across grade and stage categories, suggesting a significant contribution of dissemination from the recurring local tumor. Similarly, ZAGARS et al. (1991) reported a 70% 13-year actuarial incidence of distant metastases in 93 patients with locally recurring stage A2-C prostate carcinoma, compared to 40% in 508 locally controlled patients ($P < 0.001$). Factors that are predictive of metastatic disease were equally distributed between the locally controlled and relapsed patients. The differences in metastatic outcome were most striking in patients with early-stage disease who were less likely to have micro-metastatic dissemination at the time of initial diagnosis. In a series of patients who underwent biopsies after external beam radiotherapy, FREIHA and BAGSHAW (1984) observed that 28 of 39 patients (72%) with positive biopsies subsequently developed metastases compared with 6 of 25 (24%) with negative biopsies.

A similar relationship between metastatic disease and the local outcome was reported in carcinoma of the breast. FISHER et al. (1991) examined the impact of ipsilateral breast tumor recurrences on the development of distant metastatic disease in patients accrued to the National Surgical Adjuvant Breast and Bowel Project (NSABP) trial B-06 (FISHER et al. 1989). This study comprised 1857 women with N0-1M0 breast tumors measuring 4 cm or less in size, randomly assigned to treatment by total mastectomy, lumpectomy and radiation therapy, or lumpectomy alone. Follow-up at 5, 8, and 9 years demonstrated no significant difference in distant disease-free survival or overall survival rates between the three treatment arms. However, by 9 years 43% of women treated by lumpectomy alone and 12% of those treated by lumpectomy and radiation therapy suffered recurrence in the ipsilateral breast. A Cox proportional hazards regression analysis revealed that local recurrence, age, nodal status, nuclear grade, and tumor type were independent covariates that affected the time to distant metastases. However, ipsilateral breast tumor recurrence had the highest regression coefficient, with locally failing patients having a 3.41-fold greater risk of metastatic disease than those who were locally controlled. Ipsilateral breast tumor recurrences impacted on the time to distant disease in both node-negative and nodepositive patients (FISHER et al. 1991). The authors did not present a period analysis of the incidence of distant metastases according to local disease and axillary lymph node status, or other stratifications by covariates that also affect the metastatic outcome. Hence, the conclusion offered by the authors that ipsilateral breast tumor recurrence represents a high-risk marker for metastatic disease rather than a cause of distant spread is not completely substantiated. It is possible that in the ipsilaterally controlled patients, other risk factors such as nodal status and grade outweighed the beneficial impact of local control on the metastatic outcome, leading to an equal rate of metastatic dissemination as observed in the ipsilateral failing patients.

Another recent study on the association of a breast relapse and metastatic disease in axillary lymph node-negative patients was reported by CHAUVET et al. (1990). This study comprised a relatively homogeneous group of 202 patients with pT1pN0 breast carcinoma treated by lumpectomy, axillary dissection and radiation therapy, without adjuvant chemotherapy. Both the overall survival and distant metastasis-free survival rates were significantly increased in locally controlled patients. The 5-year overall survival rates were 87.5% for relapsed and 98.3% for controlled patients ($P < 0.001$), whereas the 5-year distant metastasis-free survival rates were 80.2% for relapsed and 91.3% for controlled patients ($P < 0.001$).

The effect of local relapse on the metastatic outcome was also demonstrated in the categories of patients who frequently succumb to locally recurrent disease. The analysis of this group of patients is, however, complicated due to an attrition by early death from local relapse before metastatic disease has had a chance to become clinically apparent. LEIBEL et al. (1991c) reported the treatment results in 2648 head and neck cancer patients retrieved from the database of the Radiation Therapy Oncology Group (RTOG). A Cox proportional hazards regression analysis showed that local-regional failure had a 3.9- to 15-fold greater effect on increasing the incidence of metastatic disease than tumor site, N-stage, and T-stage, all of which were independent variables affecting the metastatic outcome. Patients who were in local-regional control at 6 months after the beginning of treatment (1874 patients) were compared with surviving patients who relapsed locally by that time point (774 patients). The 5-year time-adjusted distant metastasis-free survival rate was 79% for patients who were in local-regional control at 6 months and 62% for relapsed patients ($P < 0.001$). A period analysis for patients at risk between 6 months and 2.5 years after treatment showed that the incidence of distant metastases was significantly reduced in locally controlled patients ($P < 0.001$). The difference in metastatic risk was highly significant for patients with tumors of the oral cavity, oropharynx, supraglottic larynx, and glottis (19% distant metastases after local-regional failure vs 7% in patients with local-regional control; $P < 0.001$), but was not significant for those with carcinoma of the nasopharynx or hypopharynx (20% distant metastases after local-regional failure vs 23% in patients with local-regional control; $P = 0.455$). As the likelihood of distant metastases in patients with locally controlled nasopharyngeal and hypopharyngeal primaries (23%) was significantly higher than in those with locally controlled primaries at other head and neck sites (7%), it seems that nasopharyngeal and hypopharyngeal carcinomas have a greater propensity for micrometastatic spread at the time of initial diagnosis. Whether local control affects the metastatic outcome in patients with nasopharyngeal and hypopharyngeal tumors who do not develop micrometastatic dissemination before diagnosis remains to be studied. However, LEE et al. (1989), reported that in 196 patients with stage I nasopharyngeal carcinoma, the risk of distant metastasis was 20% in patients with local-regional failure compared to 3% in controlled patients.

Similar difficulties in the analysis of the effects of local failure on the metastatic outcome have been encountered in patients with non-small cell lung carcinoma (NSCLC). PEREZ et al. (1987) found little difference in the overall incidence of distant metastases between locally controlled or locally failing patients (46% vs 58%, respectively). However, at 6 months the incidence of distant metastases in patients with thoracic tumor control was 16.7%, compared to 37.8% in those who relapsed in the thorax. At longer follow-up periods (2 and 3 years), a significant attrition had occurred due to death from local failure or distant metastases or both, and a difference could no longer be demonstrated due to small patient numbers (PEREZ et al. 1986a). CHUNG et al. (1982) reported that in surgically staged T1-2 NSCLC, patients who did not have regional lymph node involvement and who relapsed locally had a significantly greater risk of metastatic disease than those who were locally controlled (90% vs 24%, respectively, $P = 0.001$). Local control did not, however, appear to affect the incidence of distant metastases in patients with N1-2 disease. A similar trend was reported by MALISSARD et al. (1991) in a retrospective study of 186 patients with primary adenocarcinoma of the lung. Local control was not found to have an effect on the risk of distant metastases in node-positive patients, but in node-negative patients, those who were locally controlled had a 17% incidence of distant metastases at 1 year, whereas in those who relapsed locally, the risk was 67%.

Similar associations between local failure and metastatic disease have been reported in carcinoma of the rectum (SCHILD et al. 1989; VIGLIOTTI et al. 1987), uterine cervix (PAUNIER et al. 1967; ANDERSON and DISCHE 1981; PEREZ et al. 1988b; FAGUNDES et al. 1992), endometrium and vagina (STOKES et al. 1986; PEREZ et al. 1988a), and soft tissue sarcoma (MARKHEDE et al. 1982; SUIT et al. 1988; GUSTAFSON et al. 1991) (see Table 10.2). Some of these databases reported only crude overall incidence rates, with no distinction made between node-negative and node-positive patients, and in some cases there was no stratification for biological covariates, such as grade and stage. Nonetheless, these studies provide strong evidence that the association of metastatic disease and local relapse represents a general phenomenon across the spectrum of human tumors, even in tumors with an inherent propensity for early and frequent metastatic dissemination (i.e., carcinomas of the breast, lung, and nasopharynx) or tumors that lead to an early death from local recurrences

(i.e., carcinomas of the head and neck and lung). Furthermore, this generalized association suggests, although it does not prove, a causative rather than an incidental association between the two phenomena.

10.6 Generation and Nature of Metastatic Clonogens in Primary and in Locally Relapsing Tumors

The association between local relapse and metastatic disease can be interpreted as evidence that neoplastic clonogens within locally relapsing tumors are subjected to biological pressures that lead to an accelerated acquisition of a metastatic competence and to an increased potential for metastatic dissemination. The experimental data of RAMSAY et al. (1988) described above are consistent with this hypothesis, as they show that equisize primary and locally relapsing tumors are associated with different rates of lung metastases in two types of transplantable murine tumors. However, this postulate applies only if it is assumed that the ability to metastasize is not a random property equally shared by all tumor cells, but that metastatogenic clonogens are phenotypically and functionally distinct from nonmetastatic tumor cells. The existence of specific tumor phenotypes with metastatic competence was, in fact, introduced by FIDLER in 1973 and has since been confirmed by many investigators (FIDLER 1990). Furthermore, recent investigations on the generation of metastatic phenotypes have indicated that metastatic competence is a product of a mutational process that occurs in tumor clonogens which are primarily nonmetastatic. There is compelling evidence that malignant transformation and tumor progression result from a multistage process of pleiotropic mutagenic events (FEARON and VOGELSTEIN 1990). Alterations in positive and negative regulatory genes seem equally prevalent among human cancers (BISHOP 1991). Genetic instability apparently leads to a series of mutational events, altered transcriptional activations and phenotypic alterations, granting selective advantage to specific neoplastic cells. Metastasis is the ultimate outcome of tumor progression in this selective process (FEARON and VOGELSTEIN 1990; BISHOP 1991; VOGELSTEIN et al. 1989; HOLLSTEIN et al. 1991; KERBEL 1989; SOBEL 1990).

The full details of the mutational processes that lead to maturation of the metastatic phenotype are still unknown. However, existing data, summarized in Table 10.3, indicate that it apparently involves several recessive suppressor genes, dominant regulatory genes, and oncogenes (VOGELSTEIN et al. 1989; HOLLSTEIN et al. 1991; KERBEL 1989; SOBEL 1990; STEEG et al. 1988; LIOTTA et al. 1991), and is also associated with overexpression of suppression of several normal genes (LIOTTA et al. 1991; VLODAVSKY et al. 1988; SLOANE et al. 1981). It appears that it is the accumulation rather than the order of these pleiotropic events that confers in tumor cells that ability to invade and metastasize, thus creating an uncontrollable widespread disease.

The simplest approach to characterizing metastatic phenotypes is by identifying differential gene expressions in primary versus metastatic lesions. In animal models there is evidence that metastasis is associated with alterations in the function of the major histocompatibility complex (MHC) (FELDMAN and EISENBACH 1991). The metastatic competence of mouse 3LL Lewis lung carcinoma cells was found to correlate with suppression of the H-2K^b gene expression (EISENBACH et al. 1984), and this association appeared to be a causal relationship, since transfection of metastatic clones with the H-2K^b genes abrogated their metastatic competence (PLAKSIN et al. 1988). Alterations in MHC gene expression were also demonstrated in human tumors. CORDON-CARDO et al. (1991) recorded the expression of determinants of the HLA class I (HLA A, B, and C) antigens in fresh-frozen tissue specimens obtained from 70 breast, colon bladder, and renal primary tumor lesions, and from either synchronous or metachronous lymph node, lung, or liver metastases available in 44 of the patients. The majority ($>70\%$) of tumor cells in the primary lesions were HLA-positive (observed in 38/70 patients; 54%), especially in patients who did not have clinical evidence of metastatic disease (8/11 patients; 73%). Various degrees of loss of expression were observed in 32 (46%) of the primary lesions, although the neoplastic cells were nearly exclusively HLA non-expressors in only eight (12%) (seven of these were obtained from patients with clinically proven metastatic disease). In contrast, the majority of the metastatic lesions consisted either of predominantly HLA-negative cells (33/44 specimens; 75%) or of mixed populations (10/44 specimens; 23%), and only one metastatic lesion manifested HLA class I antigen expression in more than 70% of its tumor cells ($P = 0.0005$). Of particular interest was the finding that intravascular clusters of tumor cells, representing metastatic tumor

Table 10.3. Genes involved in cancer metastasis

I. Aberrant expressions of dominant and regulatory genes
  a) Suppressed expression of MHC proteins
  b) Ectopic expression of enzymes involved in the metastatic cascade (i.e., plasminogen activator, collagenase type IV, heparanase, cathepsin proteases)
  c) Increased expression of oncogene products (i.e., N-myc, L-myc, EGFr, HER-2/neu)

II. Mutations in recessive suppressor genes
  a) Deletion of nm23 protein
  b) Altered p53 expression
  c) Deletion of the Rb protein

phenotypes enroute to metastatic colonization at remote target organs, consisted predominantly of HLA class I nonexpressors. The pattern of HLA class I suppression in human tumors suggests that it is a characteristic feature of the metastatic phenotype, although occasionally, under undefined paracrine tissue conditions, expression of this gene may be reinduced in metastatic cells.

Other normal genes which exhibit altered functions in metastatic variants are the enzymes involved in the metastatic cascade. These genes are either overexpressed or ectopically expressed in cells with metastatic competence, leading to production and release of the enzymes that participate in the biochemical degradation of extracellular matrix and basement membranes during invasion and metastasis (LIOTTA and STETLER-STEVENSON 1991; VLODAVSKY et al. 1990). This category includes tissue plasminogen activator (VLODAVSKY et al. 1988), collagenase type IV (LIOTTA and STETLER-STEVENSON 1991; LIOTTA et al. 1989), heparanase (VLODAVSKY et al. 1988, 1990; NAKAJIMA et al. 1988), and the cathepsin proteases (SLOANE et al. 1981; TANDON et al. 1990), and their demonstration in tumor cells has been considered as evidence for the presence of metastatic phenotypes.

Another approach to characterize metastasis genes has been by transfection of tested gene constructs into the genome of tumor cells, and testing their effect on the acquisition of metastatic competence. Transfection with one of several oncogenes, including myc, ras, fos, fms, and src, was shown to confer metastatogenicity in various cell systems (MUSCHEL and LIOTA 1988; GREENBERG et al. 1989). The most relevant of these oncogenes to human tumors has been the myc oncogene. Transfection of myc into a neuroblastoma cell line induced metastatic competence (BERNARDS et al. 1989). These data complement clinical studies which have reported amplification of N-myc in advanced metastatic neuroblastoma, as compared to the normal levels observed in early and nonmetastatic stage I and II tumors (SEEGER et al. 1985). Similarly, amplification and overexpression of N-*myc* and L-*myc* have been associated with metastases and small cell lung cancer (GEMMA et al. 1989).

Some genes have been shown to suppress, rather than induce, the metastatic competence upon transfection. For example, transfection with the adenovirus 2 E1a suppressor gene abrogated the metastatic competence of *ras*-transfected rat embryo fibroblasts (POZZATI et al. 1986). Based on these and similar observations, it was postulated that mutagenic deactivation or deletion of recessive suppressor genes may be involved in the metastatogenic transformation. STEEG et al. (1988) reported that mRNA levels of the nm23-H1 suppressor gene were approximately ten-fold higher in two K-1735 murine melanoma lines with low metastatic potential as compared with five highly metastatic K-1735 melanoma cell lines. The human nm23-H1 gene maps to the 17q21 chromosome, and it encodes for a 17-kDa nucleoside diphosphate (NDP) kinase (BIGGS et al. 1990; STAHL et al. 1991). A study by BEVILACQUA et al. (1989) of 27 primary breast tumors showed reductions in cytoplasmic nm23-mRNA levels and in immunoperoxidase detectable 17-kDa nm23 protein in specimens from patients with histological and clinical evidence of highly metastatic tumors. These observations were confirmed by HENNESSY et al. (1991), who reported that patients with high levels of nm23 mRNA in their primary breast tumors exhibited significantly longer disease-free ($P < 0.002$) and overall ($P < 0.003$) survivals than patients with low levels of nm23 mRNA.

In contrast to breast cancer, high rather than low levels of p19/nm23-H1 protein were found in advanced-stage neuroblastoma-associated N-*myc* gene amplification and metastasis (HAILAT et al. 1991). Similarly, HAUT et al. (1991) reported that nm23 mRNA was increased in 13 colonic tumor specimens relative to morphologically normal colon mucosa in the same patients. The latter data are surprising in view of the fact that the same group reported somatic allelic deletions of nm23 in DNA extracts from a variety of human tumors, including carcinoma of the colon (LEONE et al. 1991). Indeed, COHN et al. (1991) found allelic deletions of the nm23-H1 gene in 11 of 21 human colonic tumors and a significant correlation between nm23-H1 allelic deletion in the primary tumors and the eventual development of metastatic spread. The enigma of nm23 and the metastatic competence in

carcinoma of the colon is as yet unresolved. It is possible that the increased levels of nm23 gene products detected in some tumors are produced by a mutated gene which lacks suppressor activity. A similar phenomenon has been described for the p53 suppressor gene in colonic tumors (BAKER et al. 1989).

The p53 gene is another suppressor gene associated with the metastatic potential in several types of tumors (LEVINE et al. 1991). It is located on the chromosome 17p13.1 and encodes a phosphoprotein which localizes to the nucleus and appears to play an essential role in the negative regulation of the G_0–G_1 transition of the cell cycle (LEVINE et al. 1991). The p53 protein does not normally accumulate in the cell, but missense mutations significantly increase its half-life, thereby leading to its accumulation and detectability by immunohistochemical analysis.

Somatic mutations of the p53 gene have been described in patients with tumors of the breast (THOR et al. 1992; ELLEDGE et al. 1992), colon (BAKER et al. 1989; CAMPO et al. 1991), prostate (EFFERT et al. 1992; VISAKORPI et al. 1992), and urinary bladder (PRESTI et al. 1991; DALBAGNI et al. 1993). In a recent study, THOR et al. (1992) reported that patients with mutated p53 in primary breast tumors had a shorter metastasis-free survival ($P = 0.003$) and poorer overall survival ($P = 0.0008$) than patients negative for this protein. VISAKORPI et al. (1992) reported that only 6% of 137 primary prostatic tumors exhibited intense immunostaining for mutated p53, but high levels of mutated p53 accumulation predicted for both a significantly shortened progression-free interval ($P < 0.01$) and poor survival ($P < 0.001$) as compared to patients without evidence of mutated p53 in their tumors. DALBAGNI et al. (1993) reported that p53 mutations and 17p allelic deletions significantly correlated with vascular invasion ($P = 0.021$) and the presence of lymph node metastases ($P = 0.007$) in 60 patients with carcinoma of the bladder.

A third suppressor gene associated with the metastatic potential is the retinoblastoma susceptibility (Rb) gene, located on chromosome 13q14 (FRIEND et al. 1986; LEE et al. 1987). It encodes a 110-kDa nuclear phosphoprotein, believed to function as a cell cycle regulator. Historically, Rb gene deletions were initially described in heritable retinoblastoma (FRIEND et al. 1986). Subsequently, either deletions, rearrangements, or altered expressions of the Rb gene have been described in several types of tumors, including soft tissue and bone sarcomas (FRIEND et al. 1986; REISSMAN et al. 1989; CANCE et al. 1990; WUNDER et al. 1991), bladder (PRESTI et al. 1991; CAIRNS et al. 1991; CORDON-CARDO et al. 1992; ISHIKAWA et al. 1991), renal (ISHIKAWA et al. 1991; ANGLARD et al. 1991), testicular (STROHMEYER et al. 1991), breast (LEE et al. 1988; VARLEY et al. 1989), and small cell lung tumors (HARBOUR et al. 1988; MINNA et al. 1989). CANCE et al. (1990) demonstrated an inverse correlation between the expression of the Rb gene and both metastatic spread and prognosis in patients with soft tissue sarcomas. When the nuclear Rb protein was partially or completely deleted, there was an increased incidence of patients succumbing to metastatic disease, compared to patients in whom the tumor cells exhibited homogeneous and intensive staining of the Rb protein. Examination of 12 metastatic lesions showed a complete or significant deletion of the Rb gene product in all tumor specimens. CORDON-CARDO et al. (1992) evaluated the Rb gene expression in 48 primary bladder tumors from radical cystectomy specimens and reported that survival was significantly decreased in Rb-negative patients compared to those with nomal Rb expression ($P < 0.001$). Since mortality in this group of patients resulted from distant metastases, these data suggest an association between altered Rb protein expression and metastatic disease in bladder tumors.

Taken together, these data strongly suggest that suppressor genes are associated with progression of tumors to the metastatic phase. However, the data also demonstrate that none of these genes is uniformly altered in metastatic phenotypes, disclosing occasionally normal gene expressions in metastatic lesions. This phenomenon indicates that perturbation in the function of any of these genes alone is not sufficient to induce the metastatic phenotype, and it appears that either concurrent or stepwise processes in several suppressor and other metastasis genes are required for the progression of the metastatic conversion.

The realization that a multistep mutational process is associated with the acquisition of the metastatic competence may elucidate the mechanism by which local failure enhances the rate of metastatic disease. It is likely that tumor cell clonogens remaining in residual tumors after failure to eradicate the primary lesion are primed with at least some of the initial genetic events required for completion of the metastatic conversion. The increased mitotic activity and enhanced growth fraction that are typical for the early phases of the regrowth of locally

failing primary residual lesions (TUBIANA 1988; WITHERS et al. 1988) provide an opportunity for an accelerated accumulation of the mutations required for completion of the metastatic transformation. Hence, the incomplete eradication of the primary tumor in patients in whom the multistage metastatic conversion has not been completed before the initial diagnosis leaves behind a small-volume residual tumor that initiates an intensive mitotic activity and thus creates a highly favorable condition for the maturation of premetastatic clonogens and the subsequent development of metastatic disease. This model is consistent with the observations on the temporal development of local relapse and metastatic disease when occurring in the same patients (see Fig. 10.2) described by FUKS et al. (1991b) in carcinoma of the prostate. It is also consistent with the pattern of the temporal appearance of metastatic disease in patients with local control versus those with local relapse described in the same series (FUKS et al. 1991b). This hypothesis also emphasizes the need for complete eradication of the primary tumor during the initial attempt at curative therapy, and serves as a biological basis for the development of studies on the effect of improved local control on the metastatic outcome (FUKS et al. 1991a; LEIBEL et al. 1991b).

10.7 Conclusions

The need to impove local control while minimizing treatment-related toxicities continues to represent a major challenge in the management of localized human cancer. The limited success in controlling localized disease with the currently available modalities and the association of local failure with incurable metastatic disease have stimulated a search for improved methods to accomplish permanent control of the primary tumor at the initial therapeutic attempt. Whereas the maximal potential benefits from modern surgical approaches have probably been realized, recent technological advances in computerized radiation treatment planning and delivery systems have produced opportunities for the application of new high-precision techniques to improve the likelihood of local control (FUKS et al. 1991a; SUIT and URIE 1992; LEIBEL et al. 1992). In addition to brachytherapy, intraoperative radiotherapy, chemical modifiers of the radiation response, and altered fractionation schemes, techniques that improve external beam targeting and the differential dose distribution between tumor and normal tissues exemplify some of the more advanced strategies that are being actively explored. However, such efforts can only be justified if an improvement in local control has a significant impact on the outcome in patients with several different cancers.

Based on the biological considerations discussed in this review, we have proposed the hypothesis that improved local control is likely to decrease the ultimate rates of metastatic disease in several types of tumors (Fuks et al. 1991a; Leibel et al. 1991b). The recently introduced modality of three-dimensional conformal radiation therapy using either protons (Suit and Urie 1992) or photons (Fuks et al. 1991a; Leibel et al. 1992) provides a tool for testing this hypothesis. The studies required to test the hypothesis would be greatly assisted by the availability of predictive indicators to distinguish prospectively between patients who are candidates for cure by local treatment modalities and those who already have micrometastatic dissemination at the time of initial diagnosis, who would also require adjuvant systemic treatments. Based on the demonstration that tumor cells which metastasize are phenotypically distinct from the nonmetastatic variants, the development of such assays may be feasible. Accordingly, at the Memorial Sloan-Kettering Cancer Center we are currently examining primary tumor specimens using a panel of biological and immunological markers to enumerate the frequency of neoplastic cells bearing metastatic phenotype markers and correlate the frequency of such phenotypes with the eventual metastatic outcome. The successful establishment of criteria for predictive indicators of the probability of micrometastatic spread before initial treatment would improve the ability to select the most appropriate therapy for the individual patient and facilitate studies designed to test the impact of local control on the outcome.

Acknowledgements This work was supported in part by grant no. CA 54749 from the National Cancer Institute, Department of Health and Human Services, Bethesda, Md.

References

Alper T (1980) Survival curve models. In: Meyn RE, Withers HR (eds) Radiobiology in cancer-research. Raven, New York, pp 3–18

Anderson P, Dische S (1981) Local tumor control and subsequent incidence of distant metastatic disease. Int J Radiat Oncol Biol Phys 7: 1645–1648

Anglard P, Tory K, Brauch H, et al. (1991) Molecular analysis of genetic changes in the origin and development of renal cell carcinoma. Cancer Res 51: 1071

Baker S, Fearon E, Nigro J, et al. (1989) Chromosome 17 deletions and p53 gene mutations in colorectal carcinoma. Science 244: 217–221

Bentzen SM, Thames HD (1991) Clinical evidence for tumor clonogen regeneration: implications of the data. Radiother Oncol 22: 161–166

Bernards R, Dessain SK, Weinberg RA (1989) N-*myc* amplification causes down-modulation MHC class I antigen expression in neuroblastoma. Cell 47: 667–674

Bevilacqua G, Sobel ME, Liotta LA, Steeg PS (1989) Association of low nm 23 RNA levels in human primary infiltrating breast carcinoma with lymph node involvement and other histopathological indicators of high metastatic potential. Cancer Res 49: 5185–5199

Biggs J, Hersperger E, Steeg PS, et al. (1990) A drosophila gene that is homologous to a mammalian gene associated with tumor metastasis codes a nucleoside disphosphate kinase. Cell 63: 933

Bishop JM (1991) Molecular themes in oncogenesis. Cell 64: 235–249

Brahme A (1984) A. Dosimetric precision requirements in radiation therapy. Acta Radiol Oncol 23: 379–391

Cairns P, Proctor AJ, Knowles MA (1991) Loss of heterozygosity at the RB locus is frequent and correlates with muscle invasion in bladder carcinoma. Oncogene 6: 2305

Campo E, Calle-Martin O, Miquel R, et al. (1991) Loss of heterozygosity of p53 gene and p53 protein in human colorectal carcinoma. Cancer Res 51: 4436–4442

Cance WG, Brennan MF, Dudas ME, Huang C-M, Cordon-Cardo C (1990) Altered expression of the retinoblastoma gene product in human sarcomas. N Engl J Med 323: 1457–1462

Chauvet B, Reynaud-Bougnoux A, Calais G, Panel N, Lansac J, Bougnoux P, Le Floch O (1990) Prognostic significance of breast relapse after conservative treatment in node-negative early breast cancer. Int J Radiat Oncol Biol Phys 19: 1125–1130

Chung CK, Stryker JA, O'Neill M, DeMuth WE (1982) Evaluation of adjuvant postoperative radiotherapy for lung cancer. Int J Radiat Oncol Biol Phys 8: 1877–1880

Cohn KH, Wang F, DeSoto-LaPaix F, et al. (1991) Association of nm23-H1 allelic deletions with distant metastases in colorectal carcinoma. Lancet 338: 722–724

Cordon-Cardo C, Fuks Z, Eisenbach L, Feldman M (1991) Expression of HLA-A, B, C antigens on primary and metastatic tumor cell populations of human carcinomas. Cancer Res 51: 6372–6380

Cordon-Cardo C, Wartinger D, Petrylak D, Dalbagni G, Fair WR, Fuks Z, Reuter VE (1992) Altered expression of the retinoblastoma gene product: prognostic indicator in bladder cancer. J Natl Cancer Inst 84: 1251–1256

Dalbagni G, Presti JC, Reuter VE, et al. (1993) Molecular genetic alterations of chromosome 17 and p53 expression in human bladder cancer. Diag Mol Pathol 2: 4–13

Deacon JM, Peckham MJ, Steel GG (1984) The radioresponsiveness of human tumors and the initial slope of the cell survival curve. Radiother Oncol 2: 317–323

DeVita VT (1983) Progress in cancer management. Cancer 51: 2401–2409

DeVita VT, Lippman M, Hubbard SA, Idhe DC, Rosenberg SA (1986) The effect of combined modality therapy on local control and survival. Int J Radiat Oncol Biol Phys 12: 487–501

Dutreix J, Tubiana M, Dutreix A (1988) An approach to the interpretation of clinical data on tumour control probability-dose relationship. Radiother Oncol 11: 239–258

Effert PJ, Neubauer A, Walter PJ, Liu E (1992) Alterations of the p53 gene are associated with the progression of human prostate carcinoma. J Urol 147: 789–793

Eisenbach L, Hollander N, Greenfeld L, Yakor H, Segal S, Feldman M (1984) The differential expression of H-2K versus H-2D antigens distinguishing low metastatic clones from high metastatic clones is correlated with the immunogenic properties of the tumor cells. Int J Cancer 34: 567–573

Elledge RM, Fukua SAW, Clarck GM, Allerd DC, McGuire WL (1992) Prognostic significance of mutations in the p53 gene in node-negative breast cancer. Proc Am Assoc Cancer Res 33: 253

Fagundes H, Perez CA, Grigsby PW, Lockett MA (1992) Distant metastases after irradiation alone in carcinoma of the uterine cervix. Int J Radiat Oncol Biol Phys 24: 197–204

Fearon ER, Vogelstein B (1990) A genetic model for colorectal tumorigenesis. Cell 61: 759–767

Feldman M, Eisenbach L (1991) MHC class I genes controlling the metastatic phenotype of tumor cells. Semin Cancer Biol 2: 337–346

Fertil B, Malaise EP (1981) Inherent cellular radiosensitivity as a basic concept for human tumor radiotherapy. Int J Radiat Oncol Biol Phys 7: 621–629

Fertil B, Malaise EP (1985) Intrinsic radiosensitivity of human cell lines is correlated with radioresponsiveness of human tumors: analysis of 101 published survival curves. Int J Radiat Oncol Biol Phys 11: 1699–1707

Fidler IJ (1973) Selection of successive tumor lines for metastasis. Nature New Biol 242: 148–149

Fidler IJ (1990) Critical features in the biology of human metastasis: G.H.A. Clowes Memorial Award Lecture. Cancer Res 50: 6130–6138

Fischer JJ, Moulder JE (1975) The steepness of the dose-response curve in radiation therapy. Radiat Biol 117: 179–184

Fisher B, Redmond C, Poisson R et al. (1989) Eight-year results of a randomized clinical trial comparing total mastectomy and lumpectomy with or without irradiation in the treatment of breast cancer. N Engl J Med 320: 822–828

Fisher B, Anderson S, Fisher ER et al. (1991) Significance of ipsilateral breast tumor recurrence after lumpectomy. Lancet 338: 327–331

Fowler JF (1986) Potential for increasing the differential response between tumors and normal tissues: can proliferation rate be used? Int J Radiat Oncol Biol Phys 12: 641–645

Freiha FS, Bagshaw MA (1984) Carcinoma of the prostate: results of post-irradiation biopsy. Prostate 5: 19–25

Friend SH, Bernards R, Rogelj S, Weinberg RA, Rapaport JM, Albert DM, Dryja TP (1986) A human DNA segment with properties of the gene that predisposes to retinoblastoma and osteosarcoma. Nature 323: 643–646

Fuks Z, Leibel SA, Kutcher GE, Mohan R, Ling CC (1991a) Three dimensional conformal treatment: a new frontier in radiation therapy. In: DeVita VT Jr, Hellman S, Rosenberg SA (eds) Important advances in Oncology. J.B. Lippincott, Philadelphia, pp 151–172

Fuks Z, Leibel SA, Wallner KE et al. (1991b) The effect of local control on metastatic dissemination in carcinoma of the prostate: long term results in patients treated with ^{125}I implantation. Int J Radiat Oncol Biol Phys 21: 537–547

Gemma A, Nakajima T, Shiraishi M et al. (1989) *Myc* family gene abnormality in lung cancer and its relation to xenotransplantability. Cancer Res 48: 6025–6028

Greenberg AH, Egan SE, Wright LA (1989) Oncogenes and metastatic progression. Invasion Metastasis 9: 350–378

Gustafson P, Rooser B, Rydholm A (1991) Is local recurrence of minor importance for metastases in soft tissue sarcoma? Cancer 67: 2083–2086

Hailat N, Keim DR, Melhem RF et al. (1991) High levels of p19/nm23 in neuroblastoma are associated with advanced stage disease and with N-*myc* gene amplification. J Clin Invest 88: 341–345

Harbour JW, Lai S-L, Whang-Peng J et al. (1988) Abnormalities in structure and expression of the human retinoblastoma gene in small cell lung cancer. Science 241: 353

Haut M, Steeg PT, Wilson KJV, Markowitz SD (1991) Induction of nm23 expression in human colonic neoplasms and equal expression in colon tumors of high and low metastatic potential. J Natl Cancer Inst 83: 712–716

Hendry JH, Moore JV (1984) Is the steepness of dose-incidence curves for tumour control or complications due to variation before or as a result of irradiation? Br J Radiol 57: 1045–1046

Hennessy C, Henry JA, May FFB, et al. (1991) Expression of the anti-metastatic gene nm23 in human breast cancer: association with good prognosis. J Natl Cancer Inst 83: 281–285

Hollstein M, Sidransky D, Vogelstein B et al. (1991) p53 mutations in human cancers. Science 253: 49–53

Ishikawa J, Xu H-J, Hu S-X et al. (1991) Inactivation of the retinoblastoma gene in human bladder and renal cell carcinomas. Cancer Res 51: 5736–5743

Kaplan HS, Murphy ED (1949) The effect of local roentgen irradiation on the biological behavior of a transplantable mouse carcinoma. I. Increased frequency of pulmonary metastasis. J Natl Cancer Inst 9: 407–414

Kerbel RS (1989) Towards an understanding of the molecular basis of the metastatic phenotype. Invasion Metastasis 9: 329–337

Kuban DA, El-Mahdi AM, Schellhammer PF (1989) Prognosis in patients with local recurrence after definitive irradiation for prostatic cancer. Cancer 63: 2421–2425

Lee AW, Sham JS, Poon YF, Ho JH (1989) Treatment of stage I nasopharyngeal carcinoma: analysis of the patterns of relapse and the results of withholding elective neck irradiation. Int J Radiat Oncol Biol Phys 17: 1183–1190

Lee EYH, To H, Shew J-Y, et al. (1988) Inactivation of the retinoblastoma susceptibility gene in human breast cancers. Science 241: 218

Lee WH, Bookstein R, Hong F, Young LJ, Shew J-Y, Lee EYH (1987) Human retinoblastoma susceptibility gene: cloning, identification and sequence. Science 235: 1394–1399

Leibel SA, Fuks Z, Zelefsky MJ, Whitmore WF Jr (1993) The effects of local and regional treatment on distant metastatic outcome in prostatic carcinoma with pelvic lymph node involvement. Int J Radiat Oncol Biol Phys (to be published)

Leibel SA, Kutcher GJ, Harrison LB et al. (1991a) Improved dose distributions for 3D conformal boost treatments in carcinoma of the nasopharynx. Int J Radiat Oncol Biol Phys 20: 823–833

Leibel SA, Ling CC, Kutcher GJ, Mohan R, Cordon-Cardo C, Fuks Z (1991b) The biological basis of conformal three-dimensional radiation therapy. Int J Radiat Oncol Biol Phys 21: 805–811

Leibel SA, Scott CB, Mohiuddin M, Marcial V, Coia LR, Davis LW, Fuks Z (1991c) The effect of local-regional control on distant metastatic dissemination in carcinoma of the head and neck: results of an analysis from the RTOG head and neck database. Int J Radiat Oncol Biol Phys 21: 549–556

Leibel SA, Kutcher GJ, Mohan R et al. (1992) Three-dimensional conformal radiation therapy at the Memorial Sloan-Kettering Cancer Center. Semin Radiat Oncol 2: 274–289

Leone A, McBride OW, Weston A et al. (1991) Somatic allelic deletion of nm23 in human cancer. Cancer Res 51: 2490–2493

Levine AJ, Momand J, Finalay CA (1991) The p53 tumor suppressor gene. Nature 250: 435–456

Liotta LA, Stetler-Stevenson WG (1991) Tumor invasion and metastasis: an imbalance of positive and negative regulation. Cancer Res 51: 5054s–5059s

Liotta LA, Wewer U, Rao NC et al. (1989) Biochemical mechanisms of tumor invasion and metastases. Adv Exp Med Biol 233: 161–169

Liotta LA, Steeg PS, Stettler-Stevenson WG (1991) Cancer metastasis and angiogenesis: an imbalance of positive and negative regulation. Cell 64: 327–336

Malissard L, Nguyen TD, Jung GM et al. (1991) Localized adenocarcinoma of the lung: a retrospective study of 186 non-metastatic patients from the French Federation of Cancer Institutes—The Radiotherapy Cooperative Group. Int J Radiat Oncol Biol Phys 21: 369–373

Markhede G, Angervall L, Stener B (1982) A multivariate analysis of the prognosis after surgical treatment of soft tissue tumors. Cancer 49: 1721–1733

McMillan TJ (1992) Residual DNA damage: what is left over and how does this determine cell fate? Eur J Cancer 28: 267–269

Menick HR, Garfinkel L, Dodd GD (1991) Preliminary report of the National Cancer Data Base. Ca 41: 7–18

Merino OR, Lindberg RD, Fletcher GH (1977) An analysis of distant metastases from squamous cell carcinoma of the upper respiratory and digestive tracts. Cancer 40: 145–151

Metz CE, Tokars RP, Kronman HB, Griem ML (1982) Maximum likelihood estimation of dose-response parameters for therapeutic operating characteristic (TOC) analysis of carcinoma of the nasopharynx. Int J Radiat Oncol Biol Phys 8: 1185–1192

Minna JD, Schütte, Viallet J et al. (1989) Transcription factors and recessive oncogenes in the pathogenesis of human lung cancer Int J Cancer 4: 32

Munro TR, Gilbert CW (1961) The relation between tumour lethal doses and the radiosensitivity of tumour cells. Br J Radiol 34: 246–250

Muschel R, Liotta RA (1988) Role of oncogenes in metastasis. Carcinogenesis 9: 705–710

Myers MH, Ries LA (1989) Cancer patient survival rates: SEER program results for 10 years of follow-up. CA 39: 21–32

Nakajima M, Irimura T, Nicolson GL (1988) Heparanase and tumor metastasis. J Cell Biochem 36: 157–167

Paunier JP, Delclos L, Fletcher GH (1967) Cause, time of death, and sites of failure in squamous cell carcinoma of the uterine cervix on intact uterus. Radiology 88: 552–562

Perez CA, Brady LW (1992) Overview. In: Perez CA, Brady LW (eds) Principles and practice of radiation oncology, 2nd edn. J.B. Lippincott, Philadelphia, pp 25–26

Perez CA, Bauer M, Edelstein S, Gillespie BW, Birch R (1986a) Impact of tumor control on survival in carcinoma of the lung treated with irradiation. Int J Radiat Oncol Biol Phys 12: 539–547

Perez CA, Pilepich MV, Zivnuska F (1986b) Tumor control in definitive irradiation of localized carcinoma of the prostate. Int J Radiat Oncol Biol Phys 12: 523–531

Perez CA, Pajak TF, Rubin P et al. (1987) Long term observations of the pattern of failure in patients with unresectable non-oat cell carcinoma of the lung treated with definitive radiotherapy. Report by the Radiation Therapy Oncology Group. Cancer 59: 1874–1881

Perez CA, Camel HM, Galakatos AE, Grigsby PW, Kuske R, Buchsbaum G, Hederman MA (1988a) Definitive irradiation in carcinoma of the vagina: long-term evaluation of results. Int J Radiat Oncol Biol Phys 15: 1283–1290

Perez CA, Kuske RR, Camel HM, Galakatos AE, Hederman MA, Kao MS, Walz BJ (1988b) Analysis of pelvic tumor control and impact on survival in carcinoma of the uterine cervix treated with radiation therapy alone. Int J Radiat Oncol Biol Phys 14: 613–621

Peters LJ (1975) A study of the influence of various diagnostic and therapeutic procedures applied to a murine squamous carcinoma and its metastatic behaviour. Br J Cancer 32: 355–365

Peters LJ, Fletcher GH (1983) Causes of failure of radiotherapy in head and neck cancer. Radiother Oncol 1: 53–63

Peters LJ, Withers HR, Thames HD, Fletcher GH (1981) Keynote address—The problem: tumor radioresistance in clinical radiotherapy. Int J Radiat Oncol Biol Phys 8: 101–108

Photon Treatment Planning Collaborative Working Group (1991) State of the art of external photon beam radiation treatment planning. Int J Radiat Oncol Biol Phys 21: 9–23

Plaksin D, Gelber C, Feldman M, Eisenbach L (1988) Reversal of the metastatic phenotype in Lewis lung carcinoma cells after transfection with syngeneic H-2K^b gene. Proc Natl Acad Sci USA 85: 4463–4467

Porter EH (1980) The statistical dose-cure relationships for irradiated tumors. Br J Radiol 53: 336–345

Pozzati R, Muschel RJ, Williams JE, Padmanhabhan R, Howard B, Liotta LA, Khoury G (1986) Primary rat embryo cells transformed by one or two oncogenes show different metastatic potentials. Science 232: 223–227

Presti JC, Reuter VE, Galan T, Fair WR, Cordon-Cardo C (1991) Molecular genetic alterations in superficial and locally advanced human bladder cancer. Cancer Res 51: 5405–5409

Ramsay J, Suit HD, Sedlacek R (1988) Experimental studies on the incidence of metastases after failure of radiation treatment and the effect of salvage surgery. Int J Radiat Oncol Biol Phys 14: 1165–1168

Reissman PT, Simon MA, Lee W-H, Slamon DJ (1989) Studies of the retinoblastoma gene in human sarcomas. Oncogene 4: 839–842

Schild SE, Martenson JA Jr, Gunderson LL, Ilstrup DM, Berg KK, O'Connell MJ, Weiland LH (1989) Postoperative adjuvant therapy of rectal cancer: an analysis of disease control, survival and prognostic factors. Int J Radiat Oncol Biol Phys 17: 55–62

Seeger R, Brodeur G, Sather H et al. (1985) Association of multiple copies of N-myc oncogene with rapid progression of neuroblastoma. N Engl J Med 313: 1111–1116

Sheldon PW, Begg AC, Fowler JF, Lansley IF (1974) The incidence of lung metastases in C3H mice after treatment of implanted tumors with X-rays or surgery. Br J Cancer 30: 342–348

Sloane BF, Dunn TR, Honn KV (1981) Lysosomal cathepsin B: Correlation with metastatic potential. Science 212: 1151–1153

Sobel ME (1990) Metastasis suppressor genes. J Natl Cancer Inst 82: 267–276

Stahl JA, Leone A, Rosengard AM et al. (1991) Identification of a second human nm23 gene, nm23-H2. Cancer Res 51: 445–449

Steeg PS, Bevilacqua G, Kopper L et al. (1988) Evidence for a novel gene associated with low tumor metastatic potential. J Natl Cancer Inst 89: 200–203

Stokes S, Bedwinek J, Kao MS, Camel HM, Perez CA (1986) Treatment of stage I adenocarcinoma of the endometrium by hysterectomy and adjuvant irradiation: a retrospective analysis of 304 patients. Int J Radiat Oncol Biol Phys 12: 339–344

Strohmeyer T, Reissmann P, Cordon-Cardo C et al. (1991) Correlation between retinoblastoma gene expression and differentiation in human testicular tumors. Proc Natl Acad Sci USA 88:6662

Suit HD (1982) Potential for improving survival rates for the cancer patient by increasing the efficacy of treatment of the primary lesion. Cancer 50: 1227–1234

Suit H, Urie M (1992) proton beams in radiation therapy. J Natl Cancer Inst 84: 155–164

Suit HD, Mankin HJ, Wood WC et al. (1988) Treatment of the patient with stage MO soft tissue sarcoma. J Clin Oncol 6: 854–862

Tandon, AK, Clark GM, Chamnes GC, Chirgwin JM, McGuire WI (1990) Cathepsin D and prognosis in breast cancer. N Engl J Med 322: 297–302

Taylor JMC, Wither HR (1992) Dose-time factors in head and neck data. Radiother Oncol 25: 313–315

Ten Haken RK, Perez-Tamayo C, Tesser RJ, McShan DL, Fraass BA, Lichter AS (1989) Boost treatment of the prostate using shaped fixed beams. Int J Radiat Oncol Biol Phys 16: 193–200

Thames HD Jr, Peters LJ, Spanos WS Jr, Fletcher GF (1980) Dose response of squamous cell carcinomas of the upper respiratory and digestive tracts. Br J Cancer 41 [Suppl IV]: 35–38

Thames HD, Schulthheiss TE, Hendy JH, Tucker SL, Dubray BM, Brock WA (1992) Can modest escalations of dose be detected as increased tumor control? Int J Radiat Oncol Biol Phys 22: 241–246

Thomlinson RH, Gray LH (1955) The histological structure of some human lung cancers and the possible implications for radiotherapy. Br J Cancer 9: 539–549

Thor AD, Moore DH, Edgerton SM (1992) Accumulation of p53 tumor supperessor protein: an indipendent marker of prognosis in breast cancer. J Natl Cancer Inst 84: 845–855

Todorki T, Suit HD (1985) Therapeutic advantage in pre-operative single dose radiation combined with concervative and radical surgery in different size murine fibrosarcoma. J Surg Oncol 29: 207–215

Tubiana M (1988) Repopulation in human tumors. Acta Oncol 27: 83–88

U.S. Department of Health and Human Services (1988) Cancer trends: 1950–1985 In: 1987 annual cancer statistics review. NIH Publication NO. 88–2789, Bethesda, Md., pp II.1–II.203

Varley JM, Armour J, Swallow JE et al. (1989) The retinoblastoma gene is frequently altered leading to loss of expression in primary breast tumors. Oncogene 4: 725–729

Vigliotti A, Rich TA, Romsdahl MM, Withers HR, Oswald MJ (1987) Postoperative adjuvant radiotherapy for adeno-carcinoma of the rectum and rectosigmoid. Int J Radiat Oncol Biol Phys 13: 999–1006

Visakorpi T, Kallioniemi OP, Heikkinen A, Koivula T, Isola J (1992) Small group of aggressive, highly proliferative prostatic carcinoma defined by p53 accumulation. J Natl Cancer Inst 84: 883–887

Vlodavsky I, Michaeli RI, Bar-Ner M, Friedman R, Howowitz AT, Fuks Z, Biran S (1988) Involvement of heparanase in tumor metastasis and angiogenesis. Isr J Med Sci 24: 464–470

Vlodavsky I, Korner G, Ishai-Michaeli R, Bashkin P, Bar-Shavit R, Fuks Z (1990) Extracellular matrix-resident growth factors and enzymes: possible involvement in tumor metastasis and angiogenesis. Cancer Metastasis Rev 9: 203–226

Vogelstein B, Fearon ER, Kern SE et al. (1989) Allelotype of colorectal carcinomas. Science 244: 207–211

Von Essen CF, Kaplan HS (1952) Further studies of metastasis of a transplantable mouse mammary carcinoma after roentgen irradiation. J Natl Cancer Inst 12: 883–890

Walsh PC (1987) Adjuvant radiotherapy after radical prostatectomy: is it indicated? J Urol 138: 1427–1428

Weichselbaum RR, Rotmensch J, Swan SA, Beckett MA (1989) Radiobiological characterization of 53 human tumor cell lines. Int J Radiat Biol 56: 553–560

Wither HR, Taylor JMG, Maciejewski B (1988) The hazards of accelerated tumor clonogen repopulation during radio therapy. Acta Oncol 27: 131–146

Wunder JS, Czitrom AA, Kandel R, Andrulis IL (1991) Analysis of alterations in the retinoblastoma gene and tumor grade in bone and soft-tissue sarcomas. J Natl Cancer Inst 83: 194

Zagars GK, Schultheiss TE, Peters LJ (1987) Inter-tumor heterogeneity and radiation dose-control curves. Radiother Oncol 8: 353–362

Zagars GK, von Eschenbach AC, Ayala AG, Schultheiss TE, Sherman NE (1991) The influence of local control on metastatic dissemination of prostate cancer treated by external beam megavoltage radiation therapy. Cancer 68: 2370–2377

11 Cell Loss in Irradiated Tumours

I. Brammer and H. Jung

CONTENTS

11.1 Introduction

The basic objective of radiation therapy of malignant tumours is to obtain local and regional control. This is done by destroying the proliferative capacity of those tumour cells that are responsible for tumour growth. These cells then die, disintegrate and are resorbed, finally leading to tumour shrinkage. Accompanying radical or definitive treatment is the risk of normal tissue damage and physiological alterations. There is a narrow dose range that leads to tolerable acute and chronic side-effects while maximizing the potential for locoregional control. (CALABRESI et al. 1985; PEREZ and BRADY 1987; DEVITA et al. 1989)

Palliative programmes are aimed at reducing the distressing symptoms arising from the primary tumour. Generally radiation is delivered in a relatively short treatment course intended to lead to early regression of the tumour mass. It is therefore of fundamental interest to know more about the principles, mechanisms and kinetics of tumour regression following radiation therapy.

For curative radiotherapy, the rate of tumour regression is of minor importance. The cardinal question is, at the end of treatment, whether the therapy has been sufficient in sterilizing all gross and microscopic disease by killing the very last tumour cell that might be able to repopulate the tumour, thus finally leading to complete and permanent regression (local control). Nevertheless, for clinical praxis there is a need for prognostic factors that might serve as indicators for the efficiency of cell killing achieved during or at least at the end of treatment. Following this line it has frequently been asked whether the probability of final local control (radiocurability) can be derived from the kinetics or the extent of regression (radioresponsiveness).

A reduction in tumour parenchyma mass while preserving the essential supply functions of the stroma is considered a favourable condition for improving the oxygenation state of a tumour. In particular, reducing the number of oxygen-consuming cells and lowering the cell-capillary distances are important factors for improving reoxygenation of hypoxic tumour cells (HORSMAN, Chap. 9, this volume).

In irradiated solid tumours, the loss of radiation-sterilized tumour cells is the main process that leads to depopulation of parenchymal tumour cells from the tumour tissue. This process, in conjunction with atrophy of the tumour stroma, is finally responsible for a radiation-induced tumour regression. Tumour shrinkage is the result of various processes that all are initiated by radiation damage at the time of exposure, finally leading to the loss of cells after hours, days or weeks.

There are typical pathways by which primary lesions develop to become irreversible lethal events. Each mode of cell death is associated with a specific time point of manifestation and is often followed by a typical mode and time sequence of degeneration,

I. BRAMMER, PhD, Institute of Biophysics and Radiobiology, University of Hamburg, University Hospital Eppendorf, Martinistraße 52, 20246 Hamburg, Germany
H. JUNG, PhD, Institute of Biophysics and Radiobiology, University of Hamburg, University Hospital Eppendorf, Martinistraße 52, 20246 Hamburg, Germany

lysis and resorption that specifically influences the kinetics of ultimate cell disappearance.

It must be considered that the overall loss of tumour cells in irradiated tumours is not restricted to cells directly killed by irradiation that subsequently undergo cellular autolysis. In addition, tumour cells may be lost by tissue-related mechanisms, such as histodynamic displacement into necrosis, as well as by the cytotoxic and phagocytic attack of host cells.

In this contribution, the principal modes of cell loss occurring in irradiated tumours are described. Particular emphasis is given to data concerning the kinetics of cell loss, and finally some factors influencing the kinetics of tumour regression are discussed.

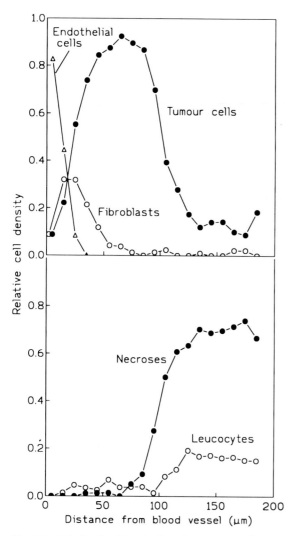

Fig. 11.1. Relative densities of cells and necroses as a function of distance from blood vessel towards coagulative necrosis as determined morphometrically in corded tumour tissue of the rat carcinoma Walker 256. (Data redrawn from BRAMMER et al. 1979)

11.2 Modes of Cell Loss

In irradiated tumours, tumour cells are eliminated by three categories of cell loss mechanisms: (a) by processes that also operate in untreated tumours, (b) by direct cytotoxic action of the radiation insult, and (c) by indirect cytotoxic action of irradiation related to tissue injury and irritation.

11.2.1 Volume Growth-Related Cell Loss

In growing solid tumours there is a continuous loss of cells (COOPER 1973; COOPER et al. 1975; MOORE 1987). Many cells are lost by cell death in situ; some of them die individually from apoptosis or from mitosis-linked cell death, while others die collectively, forming coagulative necrotic areas. Furthermore, cells may be lost by metastasis via vasculature or lymphatics, or by exfoliation if the tumour grows superficially or adjoining a body cavity. When a tumour is irradiated, part of the permanent cell loss, occurring in the tumour just before treatment, will probably continue for some time after treatment.

Cell death in situ is closely related to tumour volume growth. Apoptosis, the so-called programmed cell death, may play a regulatory function in controlling the overall cell population size; it might be considered a residue of normal homeostatic tissue control (KERR and SEARLE 1972, 1980; KERR et al. 1987; SARRAF and BOWEN 1986, 1988; BOWEN and BOWEN 1990; FALKVOLL 1990a). Necrotic regions may accumulate when tumour cell proliferation exceeds stromal growth. Necrotic cell death is regarded as a result of ischaemia, i.e. inadequate supply of essential nutrients and additional insufficient clearance of toxic catabolites (VAUPEL 1979). Studies on tumour tissue cords have illustrated the way in which, in the local absence of newly formed blood vessels, cell death may occur at a critical distance from a nutritive blood vessel (THOMLINSON and GRAY 1955; TANNOCK 1968, 1972; TANNOCK and HOWES 1973; RABES et al. 1978; BRAMMER et al. 1979; HIRST and DENEKAMP 1979; HIRST et al. 1982; JONES and CAMPLEJOHN 1983; MOORE et al. 1983, 1984, 1985).

A typical pattern of the spatial organization of the main cellular elements in tumour tissues is shown in Fig. 11.1. For the rat carcinoma Walker 256, the relative cell densities of various morphologically characterized cell types have been measured as a function of distance from the nearest blood vessel (BRAMMER et al. 1979). Endothelial cells, fibroblasts and tumour parenchyma cells together with diverse leucocytes and some isolated necrotic cells (probably apoptoses) form a viable tissue layer, about 100 μm in thickness (measured in fixed tissue), that extends between blood vessels and necrotic areas. Cell kinetic studies have shown that cells may die because they are pushed across the border into necrosis by proliferation of those cells that are closer to the supplying vessel. In rapidly growing rodent tumours the time for a cell to cross the viable tissue layer is about 36–52 h (MOORE et al. 1985).

After irradiation, tumours may still increase in volume, even if further cell divisions are instantly blocked. The reason is that cells, even if blocked in G_2 phase, keep on growing and increase in size. In addition, inflammatory cells infiltrate the tumour tissue at enhanced rates, leading to histodynamic cell movements and any kind of cell death related to these spatial changes (MOORE et al. 1983; JUNG et al. 1990).

A disproportion between parenchymal tumour cell mass and functional supporting stromal tissue evolves not only from a high proliferation rate of tumour cells exceeding the rate of neovascularization, but also from any treatment-induced reduction in the capacity of the vasculature. After irradiation with higher doses or many fractions, vascular stasis, thrombosis and changes of endothelial cells have been observed and related to a necrotic breakdown of tumour tissue, in particular in the central parts of the tumours (YAMAURA and MATSUZAWA 1979; FALKVOLL 1990b; ZYWIETZ 1990).

11.2.2 Mitotic Death

Mitotic cell death is the most common form of direct cell kill in tumours exposed to intermediate doses (1–20 Gy) of ionizing radiation (DENEKAMP 1986; HENDRY and SCOTT 1987). When tumours are irradiated, the proliferating cells are usually transiently blocked at specific positions of the cell cycle, sometimes at the G_1-S transition or, more frequently, in the G_2 phase (FRINDEL et al. 1970; DEMEESTERE et al. 1980; ZYWIETZ and JUNG 1980; FURUSE and KASUGA 1983). When they are released from the block and enter mitosis (VON SZCZEPANSKI and TROTT 1975; ROCKWELL et al. 1978), they often show chromosome aberrations (HERMENS 1973; KOVACS et al. 1976; ROWLEY et al. 1980). Frequently, acentric chromosome fragments are lost from the cell nucleus; the number of these

so-called micronuclei (FALKVOLL 1990a,b; GEORGE et al. 1988, 1989) often shows a close relationship to subsequent cell death and necrosis. Other types of chromosome aberrations may also contribute to cell death, such as dicentrics, which may result in an anaphase bridge, thus leading to cell death in mitosis.

The time course of mitosis-linked cell death may be illustrated from Fig. 11.2 showing, for comparison, the relative changes in the average DNA content (BRAMMER and VOGLER, unpublished work) and the average nuclear volume of the tumour cells (JUNG et al. 1981) as observed for the rat rhabdomyosarcoma R1H at various times after irradiation with 15 Gy of x-rays.

The average DNA content of the tumour cells was determined by flow cytometry (BECK et al. 1981). The cells were released from the tumour tissue by mechanical and enzymatic dissociation. The single-cell suspension was stained for DNA using a fluorescent dye. The frequency distribution of the cellular DNA content was measured using a flow cytometer. From the resulting DNA histogram, in which the hyperploid tumour cells are clearly separated from the host cells, the average cellular DNA content was calculated.

The average nuclear volume of the tumour cells was determined by microscopic morphometry

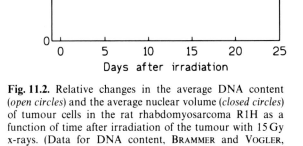

Fig. 11.2. Relative changes in the average DNA content (*open circles*) and the average nuclear volume (*closed circles*) of tumour cells in the rat rhabdomyosarcoma R1H as a function of time after irradiation of the tumour with 15 Gy x-rays. (Data for DNA content, BRAMMER and VOGLER, unpublished work; data for nuclear volume redrawn from JUNG et al. 1981)

(BRAMMER and JUNG 1987). Conventional tumour cross-sections were scanned systematically and the nuclear profiles of the tumour cells were analysed according to stereological methods. From the mean so-called chord length, the mean nuclear diameter was calculated and converted to volume.

The average cellular DNA content increased after irradiation and reached a maximum after 1–2 days, indicating a transient accumulation of cells in G_2 phase. After release from the block by day 2, the DNA content decreased steadily to control level (redistribution). Nuclear volume also increased immediately after irradiation. The initial rise and the first maximum reflects the increase in DNA content resulting from the G_2 block. This is followed by a pronounced enlargement of nuclear volume, which is due to nuclear oedema associated with the onset of necrosis. The decrease in the average volume observed after day 10 does not mean that the cell nuclei return to normal size but more probably reflects that the swollen cells disintegrate (depopulation) and that surviving cells overgrow the population (repopulation).

11.2.3 Interphase Death

In previous years, the term "interphase death" (or "intermitotic death") was widely used to charac-

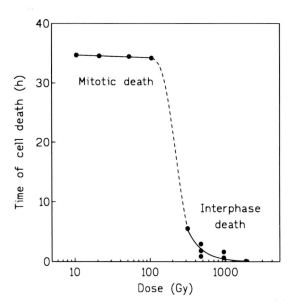

Fig. 11.3. Time of cell death of cultured mammalian cells L5178Y irradiated with single doses of x-rays as a function of dose. On the *ordinate* the time required to reach eosin staining in 50% of the exposed cells is plotted. (Data redrawn from GOLDSTEIN and OKADA 1969; dose transformed by equating 1 Gy to 0.1 kR)

terize any mode of fast radiation-induced cell death, in contrast to the mode of mitosis-linked death (CASARETT 1980; HALL 1988). However, it appears more useful to restrict this term to processes that not only occur soon after irradiation but also require much larger doses than those needed to cause a similar amount of mitotic death. Interphase death is the dominant mode in tissues with fixed post-mitotic cells, such as the long-lived neurones or skeletal muscle cells or the short-lived granulocytes, erythrocytes or superficial epithelial cells, which all are extremely radioresistant when the direct loss of these cells is considered. It does not appear adequate to use the term "interphase death" to characterize, for example, the rapid death of highly sensitive cells, such as small lymphocytes. This mode of death is now attributed to the formation of apoptosis (see Sect. 11.2.4).

Figure 11.3 illustrates the relationship between interphase and mitotic death (GOLDSTEIN and OKADA 1969). Interphase death was observed for cultured cells after radiation doses exceeding 100 Gy and occurred within a few hours. By contrast, mitotic cell death developed after much lower doses and required about 35 h to result in eosin staining in 50% of the exposed cells.

Because of the extremely high doses required, interphase cell death probably does not contribute substantially to the cell loss in tumours irradiated with moderate doses. However, there are some reports on morphologically defined processes of early cell death that occur in irradiated tumours within a few hours or 1 day after treatment (TANNOCK and HOWES 1973; YAMAURA and MATSUZAWA 1979; MOORE 1983; FUJIWARA and WATANABE 1990). This might be interpreted as radiation-induced apoptotic cell death.

11.2.4 Apoptotic Death

Apoptosis is another mode of cell death that may be induced by ionizing radiation (KERR et al. 1987). In addition, there exists indirectly caused apoptosis mediated by radiation-induced inflammation (GOLDSTEIN et al. 1991), the pathways of which are discussed in the Sect. 11.2.5. Some aspects of a possible mechanism by which radiation may generate apoptosis directly in proliferating cells are included in a model published recently (LANE 1992). The model is based on the p53 protein, which is able to monitor the integrity of cellular DNA and to inhibit replication. When DNA is damaged by irradiation, p53 accumulates and switches off new DNA replication. Thus, cycling cells are arrested in G_1 phase, which allows extra time for DNA damage repair. If repair fails, p53 may trigger cell suicide by apoptosis. Correspondingly, cells in which the p53 pathway is inactivated, e.g. by mutation, are not arrested in G_1 and replicate their damaged DNA; if repair in G_2 also fails, they run the risk of dying in mitosis or developing mutants or aneuploidy. If this model holds true, then the frequency of radiation-induced apoptosis in a cell population might be related to the state of endogenous p53 protein (KASTAN et al. 1991). Since the p53 gene, sometimes termed a tumour-suppressor gene, is the most frequently mutated gene thus far identified in human cancers, it is not known at present to what extent apoptoses contribute to cell death in irradiated tumours (HARRIS and LOWENTHAL 1982).

It is well documented that some normal cell types, such as lymphocytes (HEDGES and HORNSEY 1978; GERACI et al. 1974; PROMWICHIT et al. 1982; EIDUS et al. 1990; KRUMAN et al. 1991) or intestinal epithelial cells (HENDRY and POTTEN 1982; HENDRY et al. 1982; IJIRI and POTTEN 1984), die by apoptosis after relatively low radiation doses. Since the onset of morphological changes usually occurred within a few hours after irradiation and before the first post-treatment mitoses were observed, apoptosis was previously described as another type of interphase cell death. This time course of the appearance of apoptoses and mitoses after a single dose of radiation is illustrated by Fig. 11.4 (IJIRI and POTTEN 1984).

The number of apoptotic cells and mitoses was determined by microscopic morphometry. Histological preparations of crypts were sectioned longitudinally. Sections were scanned completely and the apoptoses and mitoses were scored.

The number of apoptotic cells in the crypt epithelium of the small intestine of mice increased within a few hours after exposure, remained high for 1 day and declined thereafter. By contrast, mitoses decreased immediately after irradiation and did not recover significantly before day 2. This was followed by an overshoot due to partial synchrony.

Tumours show a certain rate of apoptoses during undisturbed growth (see Sect. 11.2.1). Apoptoses induced by irradiation were observed in melanomas irradiated with single doses of x-rays (FALKVOLL 1990a). The number of cells expressing morphological attributes of apoptosis increased with time after exposure and reached a maximum value which was higher for higher doses; thereafter, the numbers

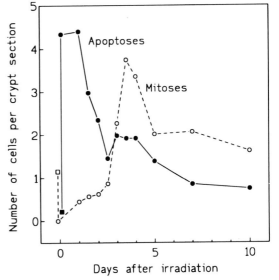

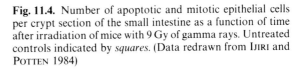

Fig. 11.4. Number of apoptotic and mitotic epithelial cells per crypt section of the small intestine as a function of time after irradiation of mice with 9 Gy of gamma rays. Untreated controls indicated by *squares*. (Data redrawn from IJIRI and POTTEN 1984)

declined to control levels, thus showing somewhat similar kinetics to normal tissue (Fig. 11.4). In tumours, the highest number of apoptotic cells was observed after resumption of mitotic divisions, whereas in normal tissue this maximum occurred earlier. The time course might be explained by the above-mentioned model: Immediately after exposure only those cells that are either in G_1 at the time of treatment or triggered from G_0 to G_1 may be affected by a block at the G_1–S transition and thus run the risk of apoptosis. The other cells exposed in S and G_2 must first proceed to the next mitosis. Only those cells that have not died during the following mitosis may be blocked at G_1–S and die via apoptosis (KASTAN et al. 1991; KRUMAN et al. 1991; MARTINEZ et al. 1991). If this model holds true, then apoptosis must no longer be termed "interphase death".

11.2.5 Inflammation-Related Cell Loss

The acute inflammatory response, which generally takes place in tissue damaged by irradiation, is able to modify the extent and the time sequence of the overall cell loss occurring after treatment in at least two different ways. One process is the phagocytic action of inflammatory cells, i.e. granulocytes and mononuclear phagocytes, which resorb the major portion of the directly killed cells. The other process is the cytotoxic potential of activated inflammatory cells and associated humoral mediators, which might lead to additional cell killing.

Various biochemical events have been discussed with respect to their potential for initiating the early inflammatory response observed after irradiation (MICHALOWSKI 1989; WALDEN and FARZANEH 1990). One of the fastest events, which occurs within a few hours after exposure, is the production of eicosanoids, i.e. prostaglandins, prostacyclin, thromboxanes and leukotrienes. These substances are produced following radiochemical modification of membrane phospholipids by the metabolism of arachidonic acid (STEEL et al. 1988; VICKER et al. 1991). They are known to act as important mediators in the

genesis of inflammation (LEWIS 1986; GILMAN et al. 1990). The early biological events include a dose-dependent increase in permeability of the endothelium of the fine vasculature (POTCHEN et al. 1972; FUJIWARA and WATANABE 1990), subsequent extravasation and oedema, as well as diapedesis of blood cells into extravascular interstitial spaces (CASARETT 1980; ALTMAN and GERBER 1983).

An accumulation of host cells following irradiation has been observed in a number of different tumours (STEPHENS et al. 1978; NUESSE et al. 1985; TENFORDE et al. 1990). Figure 11.5 shows the density of host cells as observed in the R1H tumour at various times after single-dose irradiation (JUNG et al. 1981, 1990; BRAMMER et al. 1992).

The numerical density of host cells, i.e. the number of cells per gram of tissue, was determined in two different ways. In one study (JUNG et al. 1990; comparing 7.5, 15 and 30 Gy x-rays), cell density was calculated from three measured parameters: the total amount of cellular DNA per gram (measured biochemically), the DNA content per cell of host and tumour cells and the numerical ratio of host to tumour cells (both values were derived from DNA histograms measured by flow cytometry). In the other studies [comparing 15 Gy x-rays (JUNG et al. 1981) and 5 Gy neutrons (BRAMMER et al. 1992)], the density of host cells was calculated from two measured parameters: the numerical density of tumour cells (determined by microscopic morphometry) and the numerical ratio of host to tumour cells (measured by flow cytometry).

Following x-irradiation, the host cell density increased after all doses applied. This increase is mainly attributed to an enhanced infiltration of irradiated tumours by blood-borne inflammatory cells, rather than to a rapid proliferation of those host cells present in the tumour stroma. Host cells accumulating in x-irradiated R1H tumours have recently been shown to consist mainly of mononuclear phagocytes (Fig. 11.6) and granulocytes (TARNOK 1988). In tumours irradiated with 7.5, 15 or 30 Gy x-rays, inflammatory cells accumulated earlier and to a higher maximum concentration after higher doses, suggesting that the intensity of the stimulus for inflammation increased with radiation dose. After 5 Gy neutrons (which is isoeffective to 15 Gy x-rays with respect to cell kill) the maximum host cell concentration was reached about 12 days after treatment, whereas for 15 Gy x-rays an equal density was found already after 7 days, indicating that neutrons might be less effective for evoking early inflammation than for cell killing.

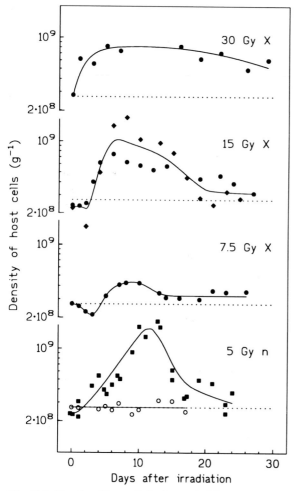

Fig. 11.5. Density of host cells in the rat rhabdomyosarcoma R1H as a function of time after irradiation of the tumour with single doses of 200-kVp x-rays (*X*) or 14-MeV neutrons (*n*). [Data redrawn from JUNG et al. 1981 (*rhombi*); JUNG et al. 1990 (*open and closed circles*); BRAMMER et al. 1992 (*squares*)]

Inflammatory cells, once in the tissue, mature or are activated; they secrete additional inflammatory mediators and enzymes (KAMPSCHMIDT and WELLS 1968) as well as reactive oxygen metabolites from respiratory burst reactions (VICKER et al. 1991). The time course of some events associated with radiation-induced acute inflammation are shown in Fig. 11.6. The data plotted were obtained from enzyme-histochemical studies on the changes occurring in the population of mononuclear phagocytes of the R1H tumour after irradiation with a single dose of 15 Gy x-rays (TARNOK and BRAMMER 1990).

At various times after irradiation R1H tumours transplanted on syngeneic WAG/Rij rats were excised. For each tumour frozen sections were stained using four different enzyme-histochemical methods: the total population of mononuclear phagocytes was determined from cells stained by α-naphthylacetate esterase and by chloroacetate esterase, the subpopulation of macrophages was stained by tartrate-resistant acid phosphatase, and the fraction of activated or exudate macrophages was intensely stained by both tartrate-resistant acid phosphatase and cytochrome c oxidase. For each cell type the volume density in the tumour was determined microscopically by the point counting method. The reciprocal value of the nuclear-cytoplasmic ratio was taken as a measure for cytoplasmic volume changes as related to nuclear size.

After irradiation of the R1H tumour with 15 Gy x-rays, the density of all mononuclear phagocytes was doubled during the first day and remained elevated for 2 weeks. The first rise was paralleled by that of macrophage density. This might be due to immigration of blood-borne macrophages and maturation of monocytes present in the tissue at the time of exposure. At later times a second increase in macrophage density was observed. Two waves of high cellularity, around day 1 and day 8, were also found for the activated or exudate macrophages. This might point to two distinct phases of enhanced inflammatory activity. The first might be associated with early membrane changes and possibly apoptosis (Fig. 11.4), while the second might be due to delayed and protracted mitotic cell death (Fig. 11.2). The volume ratio of cytoplasm/nucleus of mononuclear phagocytes increased significantly within 6 h, followed by a second slight increase near day 8. Since macrophages contain more cytoplasm than monocytes, the two peaks at days 1 and 8 might reflect the time course observed for the macrophage density, whereas the fast increase within the first few hours might be due to enlarge-

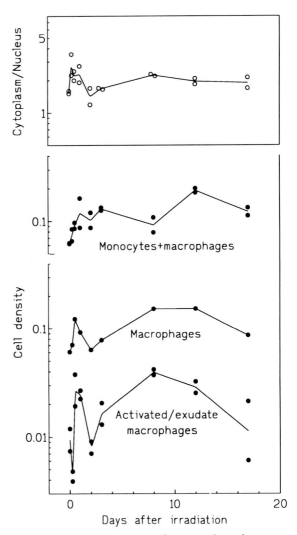

Fig. 11.6. Population changes of mononuclear phagocytes in the rat rhabdomyosarcoma R1H with time after irradiation of the tumour with 15 Gy x-rays. *Lower chart*: Relative cell density of total population (monocytes and macrophages), of all macrophages, and of activated or exudate macrophages. *Upper chart*: Volume ratio of cytoplasm/nucleus of total population. (Data redrawn from TARNOK and BRAMMER 1990)

ment of the stained perinuclear area caused by an immediate radiation-induced extracellular release of the investigated enzymes (WATKINS 1975).

Macrophages and granulocytes are mainly responsible for the resorption of dying cells. In addition, these cells might be cytotoxic. Activated macrophages are possibly capable of killing tumour cells in a non-specific manner (VAN DER BOSCH et al. 1991; HIGUCHI et al. 1990; SCHWAMBERGER et al. 1991). Potential mediators of macrophage-mediated cytotoxicity are enzymes, tumour necrosis factor (TNF; cytokines) or activated oxygen. TNF kills tumour cells by initiating apoptosis (BOWEN and BOWEN 1990). Activated granulocytes also produce activated oxygen and might therefore contribute to the cytotoxic potential of the inflammatory process (KLEBANOFF 1982; NATHAN et al. 1989). In addition immunological reactions mediated by lymphocytes, either non-specifically (NK cells) or specifically (T cells), might occur when tumour cell antigens are altered by radiochemical reactions (TENFORDE et al. 1990).

11.3 Kinetics of Cell Loss

At least three fundamentally different approaches have been proposed to determine the overall loss of tumour cells in irradiated solid tumours.

According to the first model, the rate of total cell loss is derived indirectly from the difference between the rate of cell production and the rate of actual growth of the whole cell population (IVERSEN 1967; REFSUM and BERDAL 1967; STEEL 1967, 1968, 1977; ROTI ROTI et al. 1978). In untreated tumours, the cell production rate of the tumour cell population may be determined by using ^{3}H-thymidine labelling techniques and autoradiography (STEEL 1977; AHERNE et al. 1977; DENEKAMP 1982). The actual growth rate of the tumour cell population is estimated from the growth rate of the tumour volume corrected for necrotic volume fractions (TANNOCK 1969; LALA 1972). However, in irradiated tumours, cell production rate as well as population growth rate may hardly be measured by this method, since severe disturbances of cell cycle progression and rapid changes of cell composition of the tumour tissue invalidate the assumptions underlying this model (HERMENS 1973; JUNG et al. 1981).

In the second approach, the rate of overall cell loss was calculated from the loss of radioactivity measured in situ for tumours that had been labelled by incorporating ^{125}I- or ^{131}I-iododeoxyuridine into nuclear DNA. This method is based on the assumption that the disintegration of a dead cell in situ (or any other kind of cell loss) results in loss of the incorporated radioactivity from the tumour (PORSCHEN and FEINENDEGEN 1969; BEGG 1977; DETHLEFSEN et al. 1977; PORSCHEN et al. 1978; KELLEY et al. 1981; HOFER 1987). The applicability of this technique to irradiated tumours appears to be very limited, since labelled host cells infiltrate the tumour tissue (FRANKO and KALLMAN 1980; FRANKO et al. 1980) and some of the radioactivity is either retained in necrotic regions (PORSCHEN

et al. 1983) or reutilized after release from dying cells (FRANKO et al. 1980).

The third method is a relatively direct approach. Here, the rate of cell loss is determined from the rate at which the number of non-clonogenic tumour cells per tumour decreased with time after treatment (JUNG et al. 1981, 1990; BRAMMER et al. 1992). For this approach, the number of tumour cells per tumour must be determined at different time intervals after treatment, e.g. by microscopic morphometry (BRAMMER and JUNG 1987) or by combined biochemical and flow cytometric DNA measurements (BECK et al. 1981; JUNG et al. 1990). Furthermore, the colony-forming ability of the tumour cells has to be assessed by a conventional in vitro colony assay. From the colony-forming fraction of irradiated tumour cells, normalized to the plating efficiency of untreated cells, the clonogenic fraction is obtained. The remaining fraction represents the fraction of radiation-induced non-clonogenic tumour cells from which, by multiplication with the number of all tumour cells, the number of non-clonogens is derived.

The kinetics of depopulation, i.e. the time course of the decrease in radiation-induced non-clonogenic tumour cells with time, has been quantified for the rat rhabdomyosarcoma R1H following single doses of x-rays (JUNG et al. 1981, 1990) or neutrons (BRAMMER et al. 1992).

The number of non-clonogenic tumour cells per tumour was calculated from three measured parameters: (a) the tumour mass taken from in situ volume, (b) the non-clonogenic fraction of the tumour cells as derived from in vitro colony assay and (c) the numerical density of tumour cells, i.e. the number per gram of tumour tissue. The latter parameter was determined in two different ways, as described for Fig. 11.5.

Figure 11.7 shows that depopulation after single-dose irradiation occurred in two phases: After an initial lag period, the number of non-clonogenic tumour cells decreased with exponential kinetics. In tumours exposed to x-rays, the duration of the lag period decreased (from 3.8 ± 1.4 to 1.5 ± 1.0 and 0 ± 0.7 days) with increasing radiation dose (from 7.5 to 15 and 30 Gy). For 5 Gy neutrons, the lag period (1.3 ± 1.9 days) was comparable to that observed for 15 Gy x-rays (these doses lead to the same survival level). Following the lag period, depopulation occurred with exponential kinetics. The steepness of the slope of the corresponding curves increased with increasing radiation dose.

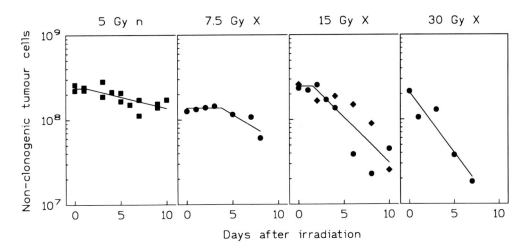

Fig. 11.7. Depopulation kinetics in irradiated tumours. The number of non-clonogenic tumour cells per tumour recorded for the rat rhabdomyosarcoma R1H is plotted as a function of time after irradiation of the tumour with single doses of 200-kVp x-rays (*X*) or 14-MeV neutrons (*n*). [Data redrawn from JUNG et al. 1981 (*rhombi*); JUNG et al. 1990 (*circles*); BRAMMER et al. 1992 (*squares*)]

Figure 11.8 shows the rate of depopulation as calculated from the slope of the exponential curves (Fig. 11.7) by linear regression analysis. In tumours irradiated with 5 Gy neutrons, depopulation occurred significantly more slowly than was observed for 15 Gy x-rays. Since both doses are isoeffective for cell killing, this result clearly indicates that the rate of depopulation is not directly related to the amount of cell killing induced. From the smoothed curve shown in Fig. 11.8 it appears that the energy deposited is the primary determinant of the rate of depopulation, rather than the degree of cell killing induced by irradiation.

11.3.1 Proliferation of Doomed Cells

In the following, the question of whether proliferation of doomed cells influences the rate of depopulation following irradiation is discussed. In principle, like in any other cell population, the population of non-clonogenic tumour cells may change in size (cell number) at a rate which is given by the difference between the cell production rate and the cell loss rate (STEEL 1977). Production of non-clonogens may arise, if at all, from proliferation of so-called doomed-to-die cells and/or from abortive divisions of clonogenic cells giving rise to non-clonogenic descendants. For higher radiation doses the latter process is without any relevance, since survival is about 5% or below 0.1% following 15 or 30 Gy, respectively. If proliferation of doomed cells does not occur, the rate of decline in the number of

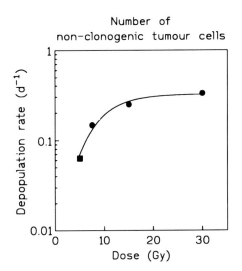

Fig. 11.8. Rate of depopulation in the rat rhabdomyosarcoma R1H after irradiation with single doses of 200-kVp x-rays (*circles*) or 14-MeV neutrons (*squares*). The data plotted as a function of radiation dose were calculated from the number of non-clonogenic tumour cells (Fig. 11.7) by linear regression analysis

non-clonogenic tumour cells (Fig. 11.7), termed the depopulation rate, reflects directly the loss rate of radiation-killed tumour cells.

For 7.5 Gy x-rays, the data for the lag period are also compatible with a modest increase during the initial period of 4 days, but certainly not with an increase by a factor of 2 or more, as would be anticipated if division of doomed cells occurred in vivo at a rate comparable to that observed in vitro (ELKIND et al. 1963; TROTT 1974; JUNG 1982).

Proliferation of doomed cells is frequently discussed as an explanation for the further increase in volume of irradiated tumours (CURTIS et al. 1973; STREFFER and VAN BEUNINGEN 1991), as is generally observed for several days following treatment even when high doses have been applied. However, it appears questionable whether this conclusion from the in vitro to the in vivo situation is justified by the experimental data available at present.

11.3.2 Modes of Cell Loss in Irradiated Tumours

When judged exclusively from the radiation doses applied, mitotic death followed by necrosis (Fig. 11.2) should be the dominant mode of cell degeneration leading to the observed depopulation. However, the results in Fig. 11.7 imply that mitotic death cannot be the only way in which the tumour cells are lost after higher doses. In principle, irradiated proliferating cells may only die from mitotic death after having entered mitosis, and this means that they must have been released from the G_2 block. Since mitoses are delayed by G_2 arrest for about one cell cycle duration per 15 Gy (DENEKAMP 1982), a lag period of 0.5, 1 or 2 days should be expected for 7.5, 15 or 30 Gy, respectively. If most of the tumour cells in an irradiated tumour were to respond in this manner, depopulation should start later the higher the dose. This is just the opposite of what was observed for the R1H tumour. Therefore, at least in the tumours irradiated with 30 Gy, which show an approximately immediate loss of nonclonogens, a significant proportion of cells must be lost via another mode which is not linked to mitosis, but occurs before the cells have left the G_2 block.

Instantaneous cell loss might be related to histodynamic movements in the transition region between capillaries and necrosis (Fig. 11.1). Even if cell division is completely blocked following high radiation doses, the cells continue to increase in volume until they have reached G_2 phase, where they are arrested. In addition, an enhanced infiltration of inflammatory cells as well as oedematous alterations may lead to a further increase in volume. By these processes, nonclonogenic tumour cells might be pushed into necrotic regions where they are lysed and disintegrate.

Rapid cell death by apoptosis (Fig. 11.4) might possibly be involved in an early cell loss of irradiated tumours, as a result of either direct cell damage or attack by cytotoxic host cells. There are some reports on morphologically defined processes of early cell death in irradiated tumour tissue adjacent to capillaries that occur within a few hours to 1 day after exposure (TANNOCK and HOWES 1973; YAMAURA and MATSUZAWA 1979; MOORE 1983; FUJIWARA and WATANABE 1990).

Unfortunately, the experimental data available at present do not allow estimation of the extent to which these processes contribute to the overall cell loss occurring in irradiated tumours.

11.3.3 Depopulation and Host Cells

As shown in Fig. 11.7 following x-irradiation, there was a lag period prior to depopulation, the length of which decreased with increasing x-ray dose. Similar lag periods were observed prior to immigration of host cells (Fig. 11.5). Furthermore, the steepness of the initial rise in the concentration of host cells, the maximum concentration reached and the persistence of the elevated level of host cells increased with increasing radiation dose (Fig. 11.5). Thus, it is tempting to look for a relationship between the rate of depopulation and the concentration of host cells.

In Fig. 11.9 the ratio of the number of host cells to the number of non-clonogenic tumour cells is plotted as a function of time after irradiation. For all conditions studied, this ratio showed an increase, since the number of host cells increased and that of non-clonogenic tumour cells decreased in the time interval considered. Except for 7.5 Gy x-rays, immediately after irradiation this ratio was close to 1. This means that the tumours contained about equal numbers of host and tumour cells, and most ($>95\%$) of the tumour cells were non-clonogenic. In the tumours exposed to 7.5 Gy x-rays, the number of tumour cells was also equal to that of host cells. However, since only 56% of the tumour cells were non-clonogenic, each non-clonogenic tumour cell on average was faced by about two host cells. Later, after the onset of depopulation and host cell accumulation, the ratio increased with time, as was also found for the other conditions.

Figure 11.10 shows the rate of increase in the ratio of host cells to non-clonogenic tumour cells as calculated from the slope of the curves shown in Fig. 11.9 by linear regression analysis. The calculated values increased in a dose-dependent manner.

An elevated density of host cells implies that the tumours contain a higher concentration of inflammatory cells (Fig. 11.6), which could account for the quicker removal of non-clonogenic tumour cells

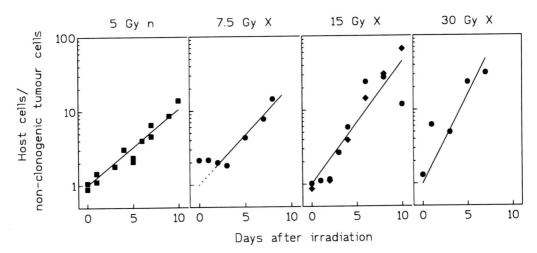

Fig. 11.9. Numerical ratio of host cells to non-clonogenic tumour cells in the rat rhabdomyosarcoma R1H as a function of time after irradiation of the tumour with single doses of 200-kVp x-rays (*X*) or 14-MeV neutrons (*n*), calculated from the number of host cells per tumour [derived from host cell density (Fig. 11.5) and tumour volume (data not shown)] and the number of non-clonogenic tumour cells per tumour (Fig. 11.7)

observed for higher doses. This conclusion is supported by the neutron data. After irradiation with 5 Gy neutrons, the accumulation of host cells occurred more slowly (Fig. 11.5) and the rate of depopulation was significantly lower (Fig. 11.8) than observed for 15 Gy x-rays. Consequently, the neutron-sterilized tumour cells, the number of which was about the same as for 15 Gy x-rays (Fig. 11.7, day 0), were exposed to a considerably smaller number of host cells (Fig. 11.10), which might account for the slower removal of non-clonogenic tumour cells observed for neutrons as compared to x-rays.

This hypothesis is further supported by two recent experiments performed on a subline of the R-1 rhabdomyosarcoma (TENFORDE et al. 1990; AFZAL et al. 1991). It was shown that infiltrating host cells removed clonogenic tumour cells from irradiated tumours, but were not cytotoxic to unirradiated tumour cells; thus, radiochemical damage and modification of the outer cell membrane of irradiated tumour cells was discussed to explain their enhanced immunogenicity (TENFORDE et al. 1990). For 7 Gy of neon ions, which caused the same amount of cell killing as was found for 20 Gy x-rays, the loss of clonogens with time after treatment was lower by a factor of 2 as compared to x-rays (AFZAL et al. 1991). This indicates that the stimulus for inflammation is not directly correlated to the amount of cell killing but rather to the energy dose deposited by irradiation. Therefore, fewer host cells were attracted and activated in neon-irradiated

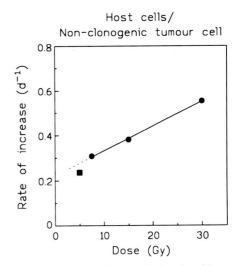

Fig. 11.10. Rate of increase in the numerical ratio of host cells to non-clonogenic tumour cells in the rat rhabdomyosarcoma R1H irradiated with single doses of 200-kVp x-rays (*circles*) or 14-MeV neutrons (*square*) as a function of dose. The data plotted were calculated from the numerical ratio of host cells to non-clonogenic tumour cells (Fig. 11.9) by linear regression analysis

tumours. This is in qualitative agreement with the neutron data discussed above.

11.4 Kinetics of Tumour Regression

Tumours usually respond to radiotherapy by volume regression. The period of regression either ends with the onset of recurrent growth when the dose has been insufficient (partial response) or proceeds to complete and permanent regression as found for curative doses (complete response).

Tumour volume curves representing typical regression patterns after different radiation treatments are shown in Figs. 11.11 and 11.12.

Transplanted tumours of the rat rhabdomyosarcoma R-1 were exposed to single doses of x-rays (Fig. 11.11; BARENDSEN 1968; BARENDSEN and BROERSE 1969). Tumours of the rat rhabdomyo-

sarcoma R1H were treated with a total dose of 75 Gy x-rays given in 30 fractions of 2.5 Gy within an overall treatment time of either 19 days (ten fractions per week) or 67 days (three fractions per week) (Fig. 11.12; VOGLER 1986). Tumour volume was determined in situ by caliper measurements. The maximum rate of regression achieved by a certain treatment was read off from the steepest tangent aligned to the corresponding volume curve. The data for regression rate shown in Fig. 11.13 were derived graphically from volume curves recorded for the rat rhabdomyosarcomas R-1 (BARENDSEN and BROERSE 1970) or R1H (VOGLER 1986; ZYWIETZ, unpublished work) after irradiation with x-rays or neutrons applied in various fractionation schedules with different but constant doses per fractions. The dose per day was calculated by dividing the total dose by the overall treatment time (in days), thus yielding the average dose applied per day.

Following irradiation with high single doses (Fig. 11.11), tumour volume increased slightly for a few days. Then tumour shrinkage was observed for doses exceeding 10 Gy. The rate of regression increased with dose (data not shown) and appeared to approach a maximum value of 0.2 (20%) per day, which is approximately the rate measured for the highest dose applied (50 Gy). Similar tendencies may be deduced from various volume curves published for animal tumours exposed to high single doses (THOMLINSON 1960; ABDELAAL and NIAS 1979; ABDELAAL et al. 1980; TROTT and KUMMERMEHR 1982).

During fractionated irradiation (Fig. 11.12), tumour volume continued to increase for some time

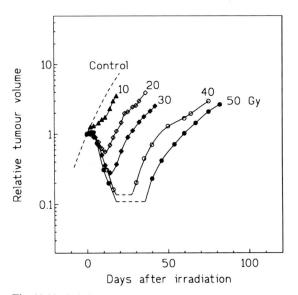

Fig. 11.11. Relative tumour volume of the rat rhabdomyosarcoma R-1 as a function of time after irradiation of the tumour with single doses of x-rays. [Data redrawn from BARENDSEN 1968 (50 Gy); BARENDSEN and BROERSE 1969]

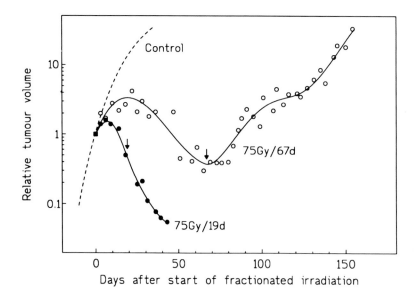

Fig. 11.12. Relative tumour volume of the rat rhabdomyosarcoma R1H as a function of time after start of fractionated irradiation of the tumour with a total dose of 75 Gy x-rays given within different overall treatment times. *Arrows* indicate end of treatment. (Data redrawn from VOGLER 1986)

after the start of treatment, although at a lower rate than in untreated controls. About one-third of the total dose or one-third of the overall treatment time was required to achieve growth arrest. Thereafter, the tumours started shrinking.

In Fig. 11.13 the maximum rate of regression obtained for fractionated irradiation is plotted as a function of the average dose per day. For x-rays, the rate of regression was lower, the lower the average dose per day. For doses exceeding 3 Gy per day, the observed regression rate approached a level that was comparable to the highest rate found after high single-dose irradiation. A similar dose dependence could be shown to exist for the Lewis lung carcinoma of the mouse (BECK-BORNHOLDT et al. 1985).

11.4.1 Depopulation

The maximum rate of volume shrinkage for high doses was 20% per day (Fig. 11.13). The highest rate of depopulation of non-clonogenic tumour cells observed for 30 Gy was 30% per day (Fig. 11.8). From this it is evident that tumour shrinkage occurs at a rate considerably lower than the rate at which the tumour is depleted from radiation-sterilized tumour cells. Considering the massive infiltration of irradiated tumours by host cells (Fig. 11.5), this difference may easily be explained. These processes lead to a (transient) reduction in the density of tumour cells, as has been observed for various animal tumours (BARENDSEN and BROERSE 1969; TANAKA et al. 1979; ROWLEY et al. 1980; JUNG et al. 1981, 1990).

Further evidence that tumour regression is not simply correlated to depopulation comes from the neutron data. Fractionated irradiation with 15-MeV neutrons at about 1.1 Gy per day resulted in a regression rate that was comparable to the rate caused by x-rays at about 2.5 Gy per day (Fig. 11.13; BARENDSEN and BROERSE 1970). This corresponds to an RBE for volume regression of 2.3, which is at variance with the RBE value of about 1 observed for cellular depopulation (Fig. 11.8). The lower value was attributed to the very early inflammatory reaction occurring within a few hours after (first) exposure at an intensity which was related to physical dose rather than to the degree of cell killing. In fractionated treatments, except for the first fraction, the tumour is already inflamed. Thus, the second wave of inflammation mediated by cell death (Fig. 11.6) may predominate and consequently

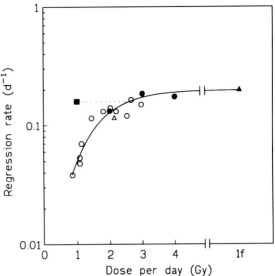

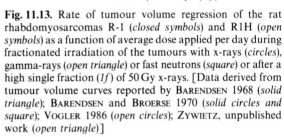

Fig. 11.13. Rate of tumour volume regression of the rat rhabdomyosarcomas R-1 (*closed symbols*) and R1H (*open symbols*) as a function of average dose applied per day during fractionated irradiation of the tumours with x-rays (*circles*), gamma-rays (*open triangle*) or fast neutrons (*square*) or after a high single fraction (*1f*) of 50 Gy x-rays. [Data derived from tumour volume curves reported by BARENDSEN 1968 (*solid triangle*); BARENDSEN and BROERSE 1970 (*solid circles and square*); VOGLER 1986 (*open circles*); ZYWIETZ, unpublished work (*open triangle*)]

determine the rate of resorption for the whole period of fractionated treatment. So the RBE of neutrons for depopulation during and after fractionated irradiation might be different from that observed after single doses; it might be similar to the RBE for cell killing, but this is rather speculative at present.

11.4.2 Stroma

Removal of dead tumour cells is the main prerequisite for tumour shrinkage, but by no means the only factor responsible for volume reduction. Besides the parenchymal tumour cells, normal cells (termed host cells in tumour transplants) represent an essential compartment of tumour structure. There are fixed stromal cells, mainly endothelium cells and fibroblasts forming blood vessels and connective tissue, and infiltrating leucocytes, mainly inflammatory cells (Fig. 11.1; TANNOCK 1970; DVORAK 1986; KAISER 1989). Furthermore, the volume of a solid tumour is not completely filled by cells but also contains extracellular spaces. Vascular volume may change with time after irradiation (RUBIN and

CASARETT 1966; THOMLINSON 1973), and interstitial spaces vary greatly in volume and composition of filling due to exudation, oedema, necrosis or fibrosis (CASARETT 1980; ALTMAN and GERBER 1983).

From these remarks it is evident that any change with time in the overall volume of a tumour depends in a highly complex fashion on the response of all of its components (JUNG 1983). Correspondingly, a wide spectrum of volume responses may be observed during or after radiation treatment. If the dose has been sufficiently high, most tumours do shrink, some rapidly, others more slowly (DENEKAMP 1972; KOVACS et al. 1977). But there are also examples where tumour volume does not respond significantly to irradiation—where, upon completion of depopulation, the tissue has been found to consist of a fibrotic matrix almost free of tumour cells (KUMMERMEHR 1985; CHOI et al. 1979).

11.5 Concluding Remarks

The aim of this chapter has been to give a rough account of the extreme complexity of cellular reactions that occur in transplantable animal tumours following irradiation. In particular, it has been shown that the processes associated with cell death and removal of radiation-sterilized cells from tumour tissue are far from being understood in great detail. At least in part, this is because the experimental methods applicable for studying cell loss from irradiated tissue are not highly developed. Thus, there is a great need for further research in this area of tumour radiobiology, not only with the aim of obtaining further and possibly more relevant data on cell loss processes, but also with respect to improving and extending the arsenal of experimental methods that might be applied for studying these phenomena.

References

Abdelaal AS, Nias AHW (1979) Regression, recurrence and cure in an irradiated mouse tumour. JR Soc Med 72; 100–105

Abdelaal AS, Wheldon TE, Clarke BM (1980) Perturbation of the growth kinetics of C3H mouse mammary carcinoma by irradiation of tumour and host and by attempted pre-immunization of host. Br J Cancer 41: 567–576

Afzal SMJ, Tenforde TS, Kavanau KS, Curtis SB (1991) Repopulation kinetics of rat rhabdomyosarcoma tumors following single and fractionated doses of low-LET and high-LET radiation. Radiat Res 127: 230–233

Aherne WA, Camplejohn RS, Wright NA (1977) An introduction to cell population kinetics. Arnold, London

Altman KI, Gerber GB (1983) The effect of ionizing radiations on connective tissue. Adv Radiat Biol 10: 237–304

Barendsen GW (1968) Responses of cultured cells, tumours and normal tissues to radiations of different linear energy transfer. In: Ebert M, Howard A (eds) Current topics in radiation research, vol IV. North-Holland, Amsterdam, pp 295–356

Barendsen GW, Broerse JJ (1969) Experimental radiotherapy of a rat rhabdomyosarcoma with 15 MeV neutrons and 300 kV x-rays. I. Effects of single exposures. Eur J Cancer 5: 373–391

Barendsen GW, Broerse JJ (1970) Experimental radiotherapy of a rat rhabdomyosarcoma with 15 MeV neutrons and 300 kV x-rays. II. Effects of fractionated treatments, applied five times a week for several weeks. Eur J Cancer 6: 89–109

Beck HP, Brammer I, Zywietz F, Jung H (1981) The application of flow cytometry for the quantification of the response of experimental tumours to irradiation. Cytometry 2: 44–46

Beck-Bornholdt HP, Peacock JH, Stephens TC (1985) Kinetics of cellular inactivation by fractionated and hyperfractionated irradiation in Lewis lung carcinoma. Int J Radiat Oncol Biol Phys 11: 1171–1177

Begg AC (1977) Cell loss from several types of solid murine tumour: comparison of ^{125}I-iododeoxyuridine and tritiated thymidine methods. Cell Tissue Kinet 10: 409–427

Bowen ID, Bowen SM (1990) Programmed cell death in tumours and tissues. Chapman and Hall, London

Brammer I, Jung H (1987) Morphometry of irradiated tumors. In: Kallman RF (ed) Rodent tumor models in experimental cancer therapy. Pergamon, New York, pp 97–100

Brammer I, Zywietz F, Jung H (1979) Changes of histological and proliferative indices in the Walker carcinoma with tumour size and distance from blood vessel. Eur J Cancer 15: 1329–1336

Brammer I, Zywietz F, Beck-Bornholdt HP, Jung H (1992) Kinetics of depopulation, repopulation and host cell infiltration in the rhabdomyosarcoma R1H after 14 MeV neutron irradiation. Int J Radiat Biol 61: 703–711

Calabresi P, Schein PS, Rosenberg SA (1985) Medical oncology: basic principles and clinical management of cancer. Macmillan, New York

Casarett GW (1980) Radiation histopathology. CRC Press, Boca Raton

Choi CH, Sedlacek RS, Suit HD (1979) Radiation-induced osteogenic sarcoma of C3H mouse: effects of Corynebacterium parvum and WBI on its natural history and response to irradiation. Eur J Cancer 15: 433–442

Cooper EH (1973) The biology of cell death in tumours. Cell Tissue Kinet 6: 87–95

Cooper EH, Bedford AJ, Kenny TE (1975) Cell death in normal and malignant tissues. In: Klein G, Weinhouse S (eds) Advances in cancer research, vol 21. Academic, New York, pp 59–120

Curtis SB, Barendsen GW, Hermens AF (1973) Cell kinetic model of tumour growth and regression for a rhabdomyosarcoma in the rat: undisturbed growth and radiation response to large single doses. Eur J Cancer 9: 81–87

Demeestere M, Rockwell S, Valleron AJ, Frindel E, Tubiana M (1980) Cell proliferation in EMT6 tumours treated with single doses of x-rays or hydroxyurea. II. Computer simulations. Cell Tissue Kinet 13: 309–317

Denekamp J (1972) The relationship between the 'cell loss factor' and the immediate response to radiation in animal tumours. Eur J Cancer 8: 335–340

Denekamp J (1982) Cell kinetics and cancer therapy. Charles C. Thomas, Springfield, Ill

Denekamp J (1986) Cell kinetics and radiation biology. Int J Radiat Biol 49: 357–380

Dethlefsen LA, Sorensen J, Snively J (1977) Cell loss from three established lines of the C3H mouse mammary tumor: a comparison of the ^{125}I-UdR and the ^{3}H-TdR-autoradiographic methods. Cell Tissue Kinet 10: 447–459

DeVita VT, Hellman S, Rosenberg SA (1989) Cancer: principles and practice of oncology. J.B. Lippincott, Philadelphia

Dvorak HF (1986) Tumors: wounds that do not heal. N Engl J Med 315: 1650–1659

Eidus LK, Korystov YN, Dobrovinskaja OR, Shaposhnikova VV (1990) The mechanism of radiation-induced interphase death of lymphoid cells: a new hypothesis. Radiat Res 123: 17–21

Elkind MM, Han A, Volz KW (1963) Radiation response of mammalian cells grown in culture. IV. Dose dependence of division delay and postirradiation growth of surviving and nonsurviving Chinese hamster cells. J Natl Cancer Inst 30: 705–721

Falkvoll KH (1990a) The occurrence of apoptosis, abnormal mitoses, cells dying in mitosis and micronuclei in a human melanoma xenograft exposed to single dose irradiation. Strahlenther Onkol 166: 487–492

Falkvoll KH (1990b) Histological study of the regrowth of a human melanoma xenograft exposed to single dose irradiation. APMIS 98: 758–764

Franko AJ, Kallman RF (1980) Cell loss and influx of labeled host cells in three transplantable mouse tumors using [^{125}I]UdR release. Cell Tissue Kinet 13: 381–393

Franko AJ, Kallman RF, Rapacchietta D, Kelley SD (1980) ^{125}IUdR loss as a measure of tumour cell loss: influence of reutilization and influx of labelled host cells. Br J Cancer 41 [Suppl IV]: 69–73

Frindel E, Vassort F, Tubiana M (1970) Effects of irradiation on the cell cycle of an experimental ascites tumour of the mouse. Int J Radiat Biol 17: 329–337

Fujiwara K, Watanabe T (1990) Effects of hyperthermia, radiotherapy and thermoradiotherapy on tumor microvascular permeability. Acta Pathol Jpn 40: 79–84

Furuse T, Kasuga T (1983) Difference in ^{3}H-thymidine incorporation after irradiation between murine B16 melanoma and squamous cell carcinoma in vivo. Gann 74: 232–239

George KC, van Beuningen D, Streffer C (1988) Growth, cell proliferation and morphological alterations of a mouse mammary carcinoma after exposure to x-rays and hyperthermia. Recent Results Cancer Res 107: 113–117

George KC, Streffer C, Pelzer T (1989) Combined effects of x-rays, Ro 03–8799, and hyperthermia on growth, necrosis, and cell proliferation in a mouse tumor. Int J Radiat Oncol Biol Phys 16: 1119–1122

Geraci JP, Thrower PD, Jackson KL, Christensen GM, Fox MS (1974) The r.b.e. of cyclotron fast neutrons for interphase death in rat thymocytes in vitro. Int J Radiat Biol 25: 403–405

Gilman AG, Rall TW, Nies AS, Taylor P (1990) Goodman and Gilman's the pharmacological basis of therapeutics. Pergamon, New York

Goldstein R, Okada S (1969) Interphase death of cultured mammalian cells (L5178Y). Radiat Res 39: 361–373

Goldstein P, Ojcius DM, Young JDE (1991) Cell death mechanisms and the immune system. Immunol Rev 121: 29–65

Hall EJ (1988) Radiobiology for the radiologist. J.B. Lippincott, Philadelphia

Harris AW, Lowenthal JW (1982) Cells of some cultured lymphoma lines are killed rapidly by x-rays and by bleomycin. Int J Radiat Biol 42: 111–116

Hedges MJ, Hornsey S (1978) The effects of x-rays and neutrons on lymphocyte death and transformation. Int J Radiat Biol 33: 291–300

Hendry JH, Potten CS (1982) Intestinal cell radiosensitivity: a comparison for cell death assayed by apoptosis or by a loss of clonogenicity. Int J Radiat Biol 42: 621–628

Hendry JH, Scott D (1987) Loss of reproductive integrity of irradiated cells, and its importance in tissues. In: Potten CS (ed) Perspectives on mammalian cell death. Oxford University Press, Oxford, pp 160–183

Hendry JH, Potten CS, Chadwick C, Bianchi M (1982) Cell death (apoptosis) in the mouse small intestine after low doses: effects of dose-rate, 14.7 MeV neutrons, and 600 MeV (maximum energy) neutrons. Int J Radiat Biol 42: 611–620

Hermens AF (1973) Variations in the cell kinetics and the growth rate in an experimental tumour during natural growth and after irradiation. PhD Thesis. Radiobiol Inst TNO, Rijswijk

Higuchi M, Higashi N, Taki H, Osawa T (1990) Cytolytic mechanisms of activated macrophages: tumor necrosis factor and L-arginine-dependent mechanisms act synergistically as the major cytolytic mechanisms of activated macrophages. J Immunol 144: 1425–1431

Hirst DG, Denekamp J (1979) Tumour cell proliferation in relation to the vasculature. Cell Tissue Kinet 12: 31–42

Hirst DG, Denekamp J, Hobson B (1982) Proliferation kinetics of endothelial and tumour cells in three mouse mammary carcinomas. Cell Tissue Kinet 15: 251–261

Hofer KG (1987) Heat potentiation of radiation damage versus radiation potentiation of heat damage. Radiat Res 110: 450–457

Ijiri K, Potten CS (1984) The re-establishment of hypersensitive cells in the crypts of irradiated mouse intestine. Int J Radiat Biol 46: 609–623

Iversen OH (1967) Kinetics of cellular proliferation and cell loss in human carcinomas. Eur J Cancer 3: 389–394

Jones B, Camplejohn RS (1983) Stathmokinetic measurement of tumour cell proliferation in relation to vascular proximity. Cell Tissue Kinet 16: 351–355

Jung H (1982) Postirradiation growth kinetics of viable and nonviable CHO cells. Radiat Res 89: 88–98

Jung H (1983) Radiation effects on tumours. In: Broerse JJ, Barendsen GW, Kal HB, van der Kogel AJ (eds) Radiation research. Nijhoff, Amsterdam, pp 427–434

Jung H, Beck HP, Brammer I, Zywietz F (1981) Depopulation and repopulation of the R1H rhabdomyosarcoma of the rat after x-irradiation. Eur J Cancer 17: 375–386

Jung H, Krueger HJ, Brammer I, Zywietz F, Beck-Bornholdt HP (1990) Cell population kinetics of the rhabdomyosarcoma R1H of the rat after single doses of x-rays. Int J Radiat Biol 57: 567–589

Kaiser HE (1989) Stroma, generally a non-neoplastic structure of the tumor. In: Liotta LA (ed) Influence of tumor development on the host. Kluwer Academic, Dordrecht, pp 1–8

Kampschmidt RF, Wells D (1968) Acid hydrolase activity during the growth, necrosis, and regression of the Jensen sarcoma, Cancer Res 28: 1938–1943

Kastan MB, Onyekwere O, Sidransky D, Vogelstein B, Craig RW (1991) Participation of p53 protein in the cellular response to DNA damage. Cancer Res 51: 6304–6311

Kelley SD, Kallman RF, Rapacchietta D, Franko AJ (1981) The effect of x-irradiation on cell loss in five solid murine tumours, as determined by the ^{125}IUdR method. Cell Tissue Kinet 14: 611–624

Kerr JFR, Searle J (1972) A suggested explanation for the paradoxically slow growth rate of basal-cell carcinomas that contain numerous mitotic figures. J Pathol 107: 41–44

Kerr JFR, Searle J (1980) Apoptosis: its nature and kinetic role. In: Meyn RE, Withers HR (eds) Radiation biology in cancer research. Raven, New York, pp 367–384

Kerr JFR, Searle J, Harmon BV, Bishop CJ (1987) Apoptosis. In: Potten CS (ed) Perspectives on mammalian cell death. Oxford University Press, Oxford, pp 93–128

Klebanoff SJ (1982) Oxygen-dependent cytotoxic mechanisms of phagocytes. In: Gallin JI, Fauci AS (eds) Advances in host defense mechanisms, vol I. Raven, New York, pp 111–162

Kovacs CJ, Hopkins HA, Evans MJ, Looney WB (1976) Changes in cellularity induced by radiation in a solid tumour. Int J Radiat Biol 30: 101–113

Kovacs CJ, Evans MJ, Wakefield JA, Looney WB (1977) A comparative study of the response to radiation by experimental tumors with markedly different growth characteristics. Radiat Res 72: 455–468

Kruman II, Matylevich NP, Beletsky IP, Afanasyev VN, Umansky SR (1991) Apoptosis of murine BW 5147 thymoma cells induced by dexamethasone and γ-irradiation. J Cell Physiol 148: 267–273

Kummermehr J (1985) Measurement of tumour clonogens in situ. In: Hendry JH, Potten CS (eds) Cell clones. Livingstone, Edinburgh, pp 215–222

Lala PK (1972) Age-specific changes in the proliferation of Ehrlich ascites tumor cells grown as solid tumors. Cancer Res 32: 628–636

Lane DP (1992) p53, guardian of the genome. Nature 358: 15–16

Lewis GP (1986) Mediators of inflammation. Wright, Bristol

Martinez J, Georgoff I, Martinez J, Levine AJ (1991) Cellular localization and cell cycle regulation by a temperature-sensitive p53 protein. Genes Dev 5: 151–159

Michalowski AS (1989) A case for humoral radiopathology. Br J Radiol 62: 1114–1114

Moore JV (1983) Cytotoxic injury to cell populations of solid tumours. In: Potten CS, Hendry JH (eds) Cytotoxic insult to tissue. Churhill Livingstone, Edinburgh, pp 368–404

Moore JV (1987) Death of cells and necrosis of tumours. In: Potten CS (ed) Perspectives on mammalian cell death. Oxford University Press, Oxford, pp 295–325

Moore JV, Hopkins HA, Looney WB (1983) Response of cell populations in tumor cords to a single dose of cyclophosphamide or radiation. Eur J Cancer Clin Oncol 19: 73–79

Moore JV, Hopkins HA, Looney WB (1984) Tumour-cord parameters in two rat hepatomas that differ in their radiobiological oxygenation status. Radiat Environ Biophys 23: 213–222

Moore JV, Hasleton PS, Buckley CH (1985) Tumour cords in 52 human bronchial and cervical squamous cell carcinomas: inferences for their cellular kinetics and radiobiology. Br J Cancer 51: 407–413

Nathan C, Srimal S, Farber C et al. (1989) Cytokine-induced respiratory burst of human neutrophils: dependence on extracellular matrix proteins and CD11/CD18 integrins. J Cell Biol 109: 1341–1349

Nuesse M, Afzal SMJ, Carr B, Kavanau K (1985) Cell cycle kinetic measurements in an irradiated rat rhabdomyosarcoma using a monoclonal antibody to bromodeoxyuridine. Cytometry 6: 611–619

Perez CA, Brady LW (1987) Principles and practice of radiation oncology. J.B. Lippincott, Philadelphia

Porschen W, Feinendegen L (1969) In-vivo-Bestimmung der Zellverlustrate bei Experimentaltumoren mit markiertem Joddeoxyuridin. Strahlentherapie 137: 718–723

Porschen W, Gartzen J, Gewehr K, Muehlensiepen H, Weber HJ, Feinendegen LE (1978) In vivo assay of the radiation sensitivity of hypoxic tumour cells; influence of γ-rays, cyclotron neutrons, misonidazole, hyperthermia and mixed modalities. Br J Cancer 37 [Suppl III]: 194–197

Porschen R, Porschen W, Muehlensiepen H, Feinendegen LE (1983) Cell loss from viable and necrotic tumour regions measured by ^{125}I-UdR. Cell Tissue Kinet 16: 549–556

Potchen EJ, Kinzie J, Curtis C, Siegel BA, Studer RK (1972) Effect of irradiation on tumor microvascular permeability to macromolecules. Cancer 30: 639–642

Promwichit P, Sturrock MG, Chapman IV (1982) Depressed DNaseI inhibitor activity and delayed DNA damage in x-irradiated thymocytes. Int J Radiat Biol 42: 565–571

Rabes HM, Carl P, Rattenhuber U (1978) Determination of proliferative compartments in human tumors. Experientia 34: 1510–1511

Refsum SB, Berdal P (1967) Cell loss in malignant tumours in man. Eur J Cancer 3: 235–236

Rockwell S, Frindel E, Valleron AJ, Tubiana M (1978) Cell proliferation in EMT6 tumors treated with single doses of x-rays or hydroxyurea. I. Experimental results. Cell Tissue Kinet 11: 279–289

Roti Roti JL, Bohling V, Dethlefsen LA (1978) Kinetic models of C3H mouse mammary tumor growth: implications regarding tumor cell loss. Cell Tissue Kinet 11: 1–21

Rowley R, Hopkins HA, Betsill WL, Ritenour ER, Looney WB (1980) Response and recovery kinetics of a solid tumour after irradiation. Br J Cancer 42: 586–595

Rubin P, Casarett G (1966) Microcirculation of tumors. Part II: The supervascularized state of irradiated regressing tumors. Clin Radiol 17: 346–355

Sarraf CE, Bowen ID (1986) Kinetic studies on a murine sarcoma and an analysis of apoptosis. Br J Cancer 54: 989–998

Sarraf CE, Bowen ID (1988) Proportions of mitotic and apoptotic cells in a range of untreated experimental tumours. Cell Tissue Kinet 21: 45–49

Schwamberger G, Flesch I, Ferber E (1991) Tumoricidal effector molecules of murine macrophages. Pathobiology 59: 248–253

Steel GG (1967) Cell loss as a factor in the growth rate of human tumours. Eur J Cancer 3: 381–387

Steel GG (1968) Cell loss from experimental tumours. Cell Tissue Kinet 1: 193–207

Steel GG (1977) Growth kinetics of tumours. Clarendon, Oxford

Steel LK, Hughes HN, Walden TL (1988) Quantitative, functional and biochemical alterations in the peritoneal cells of mice exposed to whole-body gamma-irradiation. I. Changes in cellular protein, adherence properties and enzymatic activities associated with platelet-activating factor formation and inactivation, and arachidonate metabolism. Int J Radiat Biol 53: 943–964

Stephens TC, Currie GA, Peacock JH (1978) Repopulation of γ-irradiated Lewis lung carcinoma by malignant cells and host macrophage progenitors. Br J Cancer 38: 573–582

Streffer C, van Beuningen D (1991) Cellular radiobiology. In: Scherer E, Streffer C, Trott K R (eds) Radiopathology of organs and tissues. Springer, Berlin, pp 1–31

Tanaka N, Tanabe C, Okumura Y, Murakami K (1979) Post-irradiation kinetics of the C3H/He mouse mammary carcinoma as regards tumor volume regrowth time and cell loss. Strahlentherapie 155: 58–62

Tannock IF (1968) The relation between cell proliferation and the vascular system in a transplanted mouse mammary tumour. Br J Cancer 22: 258–273

Tannock IF (1969) A comparison of cell proliferation parameters in solid and ascites Ehrlich tumours. Cancer Res 29: 1527–1534

Tannock IF (1970) Population kinetics of carcinoma cells, capillary endothelial cells, and fibroblasts in a transplanted mouse mammary tumor. Cancer Res 30: 2470–2476

Tannock IF (1972) Oxygen diffusion and the distribution of cellular radiosensitivity in tumours. Br J Radiol 45: 515–524

Tannock IF, Howes A (1973) The response of viable tumor cords to a single dose of radiation. Radiat Res 55: 477–486

Tarnok A (1988) Histochemischer Nachweis und Quantifizierung der Leukozyten im unbehandelten und bestrahlten Rhabdomyosarkom R1H der Ratte. PhD Thesis, University of Hamburg

Tarnok A, Brammer I (1990) Population kinetics and nuclear/ cytoplasmic ratio of mononuclear phagocytes in the x-irradiated rhabdomyosarcoma R1H. In: Burger G, Oberholzer M, Vooijs GP (eds) Advances in analytical cellular pathology. Excerpta Medica, Amsterdam, pp 281–282

Tenforde TS, Kavanau KS, Afzal SMJ, Curtis SB (1990) Host cell cytotoxicity, cellular repopulation dynamics, and phase-specific cell survival in x-irradiated rat rhabdomyosarcoma tumors. Radiat Res 123: 32–43

Thomlinson RH (1960) An experimental method for comparing treatments of intact malignant tumours in animals and its application to the use of oxygen in radiotherapy. Br J Cancer 14: 555–576

Thomlinson RH (1973) Radiation and the vascularity of tumours. Br Med Bull 29: 29–32

Thomlinson RH, Gray LH (1955) The histological structure of some human lung cancers and the possible implications for radiotherapy. Br J Cancer 9: 539–549

Trott K R (1974) Relation between division delay and damage expressed in later generations. In: Ebert M, Howard A (eds) Current topics in radiation research, vol II. North-Holland, Amsterdam, pp 336–337

Trott K R, Kummermehr J (1982) Split dose recovery of a mouse tumour and its stroma during fractionated irradiation. Br J Radiol 55: 841–846

van der Bosch J, Rueller S, Horn D, Schlaak M (1991) Monocyte-mediated growth control and the induction of tumor cell death. Pathobiology 59: 243–247

Vaupel P (1979) Oxygen supply to malignant tumors. In: Peterson HI (ed) Tumor blood circulation: angiogenesis, vascular morphology and blood flow of experimental and human tumors. CRC Press, Boca Raton, pp 143–168

Vicker MG, Bultmann H, Glade U, Haefker T (1991) Ionizing radiation at low doses induces inflammatory reactions in human blood. Radiat Res 128: 251–257

Vogler H (1986) Zelluläre Inaktivierungskinetik beim Rhabdomyosarkom R1H der Ratte während fraktionierter Röntgenbestrahlung. PhD Thesis, University of Hamburg

von Szczepanski L, Trott K R (1975) Post-irradiation proliferation kinetics of a serially transplanted murine adenocarcinoma. Br J Radiol 48: 200–208

Walden TL, Farzaneh NK (1990) Biochemistry of ionizing radiation. Raven, New York

Watkins DK (1975) Lysosomes and radiation injury. In: Dingle JT, Dean RT (eds) Lysosomes in biology and pathology, vol 4. North-Holland, Amsterdam (Frontiers of Biology, vol 43) pp 147–166

Yamaura H, Matsuzawa T (1979) Tumour regrowth after irradiation: an experimental approach. Int J Radiat Biol 35: 201–219

Zywietz F (1990) Vascular and cellular damage in a murine tumour during fractionated treatment with radiation and hyperthermia. Strahlenther Onkol 166: 493–501

Zywietz F, Jung H (1980) Partial synchronization of three solid animal tumours by x-rays. Eur J Cancer 16: 1381–1388

Subject Index

List of Contributors

K. KIAN ANG, M.D.
Professor of Radiotherapy
Department of Radiotherapy
The University of Texas
M.D. Anderson Cancer Center
1515 Holcombe Blvd.
Houston, TX 77030-4095
USA

M. BAUMANN, M.D.
Department of Radiation Therapy
University of Hamburg
University Hospital Eppendorf
Martinistraße 52
20246 Hamburg
Germany

SOREN M. BENTZEN, Ph.D.
Danish Cancer Society
Department of Experimental Clinical Oncology
Nørrebrogade 44
DK-8000 Aarhus C
Denmark

INGO BRAMMER, Ph.D.
Institute for Biophysics and Radiobiology
University of Hamburg
Martinistraße 52
20246 Hamburg
Germany

W. BUDACH, M.D.
Department of Radiation Therapy
University of Essen
Hufelandstraße 55
45147 Essen
Germany

EKKEHARD DIKOMEY, Ph.D.
Institute for Biophysics and Radiobiology
University of Hamburg
Martinistraße 52
20246 Hamburg
Germany

ZVI FUKS, M.D.
Department of Radiation Oncology
Memorial Sloan-Kettering Cancer Center
New York, NY 10021
USA

MICHAEL R. HORSMAN, Ph.D.
Danish Cancer Society
Department of Experimental Clinical Oncology
Nørrebrogade 44
DK-8000 Aarhus C
Denmark

H. JOHNS, BSc.
CRC Gray Laboratory
P. O. Box 100, Mount Vernon Hospital
Northwood, Middlesex HA6 2JR
England

MIKE C. JOINER, Ph.D.
CRC Gray Laboratory
P. O. Box 100, Mount Vernon Hospital
Northwood, Middlesex HA6 2JR
England

HORST JUNG, Ph.D.
Institute for Biophysics and Radiobiology
University of Hamburg
Martinistraße 52
20246 Hamburg
Germany

STEVEN A. LEIBEL, M.D.
Department of Radiation Oncology
Memorial Sloan-Kettering Cancer Center
New York, NY 10021
USA

B. MARPLES, Ph.D.
B.C. Cancer Research Centre
601 West 10 Ave.
Vancouver, B.C. V5Z 1L3
Canada

LESTER J. PETERS, M.D.
Professor of Radiotherapy
Head, Division of Radiotherapy
John G. and Marie Stella Kenedy Chair
The University of Texas
M.D. Anderson Cancer Center
1515 Holcombe Blvd.
Houston, TX 77030–4095
USA

A. TAGHIAN, M.D.
Department of Radiation Oncology
Massachusetts General Hospital
Harvard Medical School
Fruit Street
Boston, MA 02114
USA

H.D. THAMES, Ph.D.
Helen Buchanan and Stanley Joseph Seeger
Research Professor
Department of Biomathematics
The University of Texas
M.D. Anderson Cancer Center
1515 Holcombe Blvd.
Houston, TX 77030-4095
USA

K.R. TROTT, M.D.
Professor, Radiation Biology Department
St. Bartholomew's Medical College
Charterhouse Square
London EC1M 6BQ
England

GEORGE D. WILSON, M.D.
CRC Gray Laboratory
Mount Vernon Hospital
P. O. Box 100
Northwood, Middlesex HA6 2JR
England

H. RODNEY WITHERS, M.D. DSc.
Professor, Department of Radiation Oncology
UCLA Medical Center
Los Angeles, CA 90024-1714
USA

Springer-Verlag
and the Environment

We at Springer-Verlag firmly believe that an international science publisher has a special obligation to the environment, and our corporate policies consistently reflect this conviction.

We also expect our business partners – paper mills, printers, packaging manufacturers, etc. – to commit themselves to using environmentally friendly materials and production processes.

The paper in this book is made from low- or no-chlorine pulp and is acid free, in conformance with international standards for paper permanency.